A Concise Clinical Text

Neurology: A Concise Clinical Text

Michael Swash, MD (London) FRCP MRCPath
Consultant Neurologist
The London Hospital, St Mark's Hospital and
Newham General Hospital

and

Martin S. Schwartz MD (Baltimore)
Consultant Clinical Neurophysiologist
Atkinson Morley's Hospital
and St George's Hospital

Baillière Tindall
London · Philadelphia · Toronto · Sydney · Tokyo

31.95

Baillière Tindall   24–28 Oval Road
  WB Saunders   London NW1 7DX, England

        The Curtis Center
        Independence Square West, Philadelphia, PA 19106-3399, USA

        1 Goldthorne Avenue
        Toronto, Ontario M8Z 5T9, Canada

        Harcourt Brace Jovanovich Group (Australia) Pty Limited
        32–52 Smidmore Street, Marrickville, NSW 2204, Australia

        Harcourt Brace Jovanovich (Japan) Inc.
        Ichibancho Central Building, 22–1 Ichibancho
        Chiyoda-ku, Tokyo 102, Japan

British Library Cataloguing in Publication Data
Swash, Michael, *1939–*
  Neurology.
  1. Medicine. Neurology
  I. Title   II. Schwartz, Martin S. (Martin Samuel)
  616.8

  ISBN 0-7020-1382-X   **60638**

Typeset by Dobbie Typesetting Limited
Printed in Great Britain by Cambridge University Press

iv

Contents

Preface

All textbooks are products of their times. There are many difficulties in achieving a balanced and relevant account of diseases of the nervous system, and it is almost inevitable that the personal interests and preoccupations of the authors will intrude. On the other hand, there is much to be gained from the clarity of view of an account of the practice of neurology seen as a whole, rather than from the uncritically detailed accounts found in multi-author texts. Neurology has a very wide remit, being concerned not only with those diseases that are exclusive to the nervous system, but with the effects of other diseases on the nervous system, including trauma, vascular disease and the infections. In recent years the introduction of increasingly powerful and non-invasive methods of imaging the structure of the nervous system, and of lesions within it, has profoundly altered the everyday practice of neurology. It is now possible to assess the effects of treatment in diseases that could previously be evaluated only by clinical examination. In addition the accuracy of diagnosis and the localization of surgically-accessible lesions has been improved immeasurably. As a result, much of the dogma and mystique surrounding neurological diagnosis has disappeared, and the emphasis in neurological and neurosurgical practice has moved towards the exploration of effective treatments. The illustrations in this book are intended to demonstrate the scope and importance of these investigational methods. Relatively few illustrations of patients have been included, since we feel that this experience can more effectively be obtained at the bedside. Indeed, the fundamentals of clinical method as applied to neurology will be found in *Hutchison's Clinical Methods*; this book is concerned more with neurological symptoms and syndromes, and with their investigation and treatment.

It is an old aphorism that all disorders other than that suffered by the patient are of secondary importance; because of the relatively large number of familial and rare metabolic diseases that may afflict the nervous system this is, perhaps, more true of neurology than of other specialties. Clearly, the student and physician must have some basic knowledge of these disorders, as well as a detailed understanding of the common conditions that affect the nervous system, even if only to direct investigation in the appropriate direction, and to refer the patient to the appropriate expert for further advice on management. This book should provide enough background information to achieve this level of clinical expertise.

It has become fashionable to teach medicine in relation to clinical problems, rather than diseases. In the sense that this approach is concerned with the relief of symptoms rather than the treatment of diseases this is relevant when the physician is confronted by a patient suffering from the effects of several different disorders all affecting the nervous system, or when, as in the case of headache, the symptom has no clear organic cause. However, when the primary disorder is clearly defined, as in stroke, or infection of the nervous system, it is more practicable to achieve resolution of symptoms by cure of the underlying disease, as far as this is possible. The layout of chapters in this book reflects the practicalities of combining these problem-oriented and disease-oriented approaches into clinical practice.

We hope that this book will prove useful not only as a source of information to students and young physicians, but in stimulating them with something of our own excitement for neurology in this era of increasing scientific understanding and of more effective treatments. For these reasons we have chosen to begin with an historical introduction and to end with a brief list of relevant recommendations for further reading, arranged according to chapter order. Happy reading!

Michael Swash
Martin S. Schwartz

Acknowledgements

As in any major task, the writing of a textbook inevitably involves co-operation and help from family, friends and colleagues. We thank Caroline and Lee for their forbearance while we have enjoyed ourselves writing this book. Dr Paul Butler, Consultant Neuroradiologist at The London Hospital, kindly provided many of the radiological illustrations. We thank Professor Victor Dubowitz and Dr John Heckmatt, of Hammersmith Hospital, for Figure 14.1. Figure 8.1 and Figure 8.2 are reproduced from "Epidemiology of Head Injuries in England and Wales" by J. H. Field, published by HMSO in 1976, and Figures 9.5 and 9.6 are reproduced from "Multiple Sclerosis" by E. O'Brien, published by the Office of Health Economics in 1987. Figure 9.5 is originally derived from work by Kurtzke and Figure 9.6 from work by Swingler and Compston. Mrs Adrienne Raine faultlessly typed the manuscript.

Historical Introduction

The word 'neurology' was introduced by Thomas Willis (1621–1675) to describe the study of the nervous system. In its modern context this term is used to describe the study of the diseases of the nervous system rather than aspects of clinical or non-clinical neuroscience. Before Willis the schools of natural philosophy of ancient Greece and of the Roman Empire devised functional concepts of mind, movement and sensation that led to appraisals of neuron activity that have echoes even in modern times. Aristotle (382–322 B.C.) and Galen (129–199 A.D.) combined philosophical and observational ideas, including anatomical dissections of the brain, but this work, itself, must be considered in relation to the earlier contributions made in ancient Egypt. The Galenic doctrines derived from this synthesis of anatomy, clinical observation and philosophy became rigidly codified, stultifying further exploration so that the work of Islamic physicians between 900 and 1400 A.D. (Fig. 1) was largely ignored in the western world during medieval and early Renaissance times. The Renaissance in Italy provided a stimulus for new observation and Vesalius (1514–1564), in his anatomical work *De Humani Corporis Fabrica* (1543) laid the foundation for most subsequent studies in his emphasis on observation of natural phenomena (Fig. 2), rather than study of codified Galenic doctrine. These anatomical studies provided a framework for new ideas on brain function and particularly for Descartes' concept of the unity of brain and mind as formulated in his book *De Homine* (1662). Descartes' formulation of the mind/brain identity problem was susceptible to experimental analysis and led directly, or indirectly, to the theory of reflex action, to the neuron theory, to the concept of afferent and efferent systems (Fig. 3), and to understanding of the indirect relationships of psychological, physiological, and anatomical constructs of the brain and its functions that characterize modern ideas of the nervous system.

Modern neurology is concerned with the understanding, investigation, management and treatment of diseases of the central and peripheral nervous systems. This includes a wide variety of primary diseases of the nervous system, and disorders of other bodily

1

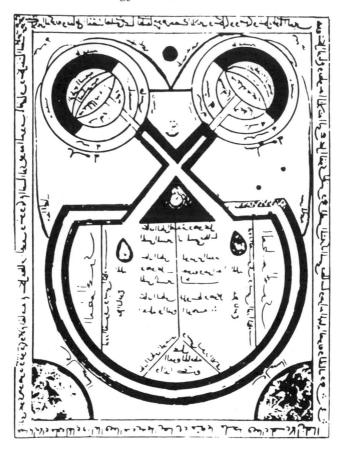

Fig. 1 Schematic diagram of the eye, optic nerves and brain; an Islamic drawing, probably 11th century (reproduced from Clarke and Dewhurst, *An Illustrated History of Brain Function*, Sandford Publications, Oxford, 1972).

systems that involve the nervous system itself. In the past, neurology has been much concerned with the categorization of symptoms, and with the attribution of certain symptom complexes to lesions of particular structures in the nervous system. There is also a long-standing tradition in neurology for studies of psychological disorders, including dementia, psychotic disorders and hysteria. These differing approaches to the clinical practice of neurology diverged in the early part of the 20th century, but have recently come closer together with the development of new approaches to investigation and treatment of disorders of the nervous system, for example, neuropharmacology, molecular genetics and new imaging techniques. Thus, the psychoses, such as schizophrenia

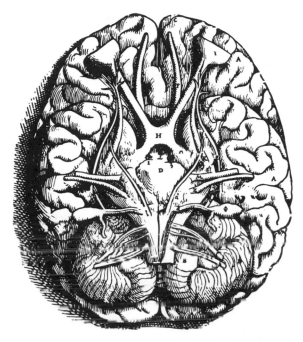

Fig. 2 The base of the brain, showing the frontal and temporal lobes, cerebellum, optic chiasm and cranial nerves; from Vesalius, *De Humani Corporis Fabrica*, 1543.

and bipolar depression, are now again seen as diseases of the brain.

Development of concepts in neurology

It is difficult now to read medieval accounts of disease and relate them to modern diagnostic patterns. This difficulty arises because, in former times, clinical disorders were described in general terms, without established clinical method, and without any underlying concept of the significance of clinical observations considered in relation to the underlying physiological and morphological abnormalities. Thomas Willis, in his books and lectures, strove to order this chaos of uncharacterized description. In doing so, he overturned the Galenical doctrines, and supplanted them with the beginnings of the method of clinical science. Willis described the major arterial anastomoses of the base of the brain and provided succinct descriptions of stroke, involuntary movement disorders, epilepsy, headache, CSF rhinorrhoea and myasthenia gravis. He wrote on sensation and the concepts of voluntary and

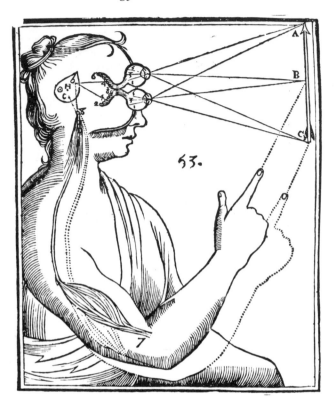

Fig. 3 Descartes' drawing, from De Homine (1662), illustrating his concept of the afferent and efferent systems of nervous action, and showing the optic chiasm.

involuntary movement, and recognized that the cerebral hemispheres rather than the ventricles, were the seat of nervous action. His studies of anatomy included injections of ink into the carotid arteries of the neck in order to investigate the perfusion of the brain and anterior pituitary gland, and he knew that carotid occlusion was a cause of stroke. These 17th-century observations provided the framework for the rationalist investigators of the 18th and early 19th centuries. Sir Thomas Bell (1774–1882) demonstrated the motor function of the anterior roots, and the sensory function of the posterior roots, an observation that provided the foundation for the demonstration of reflex action by Marshall Hall (1790–1857). The latter notion led to the development of the concept of reflex action that lay at the heart of the work of Sherrington (1857–1952) and his followers, based on experimental anatomical and physiological observations on spinal and cerebral activity, and on motor control.

This school of physiology was particularly important because it led to the application of physiological techniques in the study of disabilities resulting from lesions in the human nervous system, exemplified especially by the work of Denny Brown (1901–1981) and his colleagues.

Cortical function was considered in its psychological and behavioural aspects by Hughlings Jackson, especially in relation to temporal lobe epilepsy and aphasia, but the principle of anatomical localization in cortical function was exemplified by Gall (1757–1828) and Spurzheim (1776–1832), who recognized the significance of the difference between grey and white matter in the brain. Gall later used this concept in developing phrenology, an influential if erroneous concept of the localization of brain function. Localization of a psychological function within the brain was first clearly delineated by Broca (1824–1880) who observed that aphasia occurred with a lesion in the third left frontal convolution of the brain. Fritsch (1838–1927) and Hitzig (1838–1907) showed that stimulation of the exposed cortex resulted in contraction of the opposite side of the body, a concept refined by Ferrier (1843–1928) to establish the existence of the motor cortex in man. Ferrier was an important intellectual link in British neurology between the clinical observations and theories of Hughlings Jackson and the experimental studies of Sherrington. Henschen (1847–1930) showed that the calcarine cortex was concerned with vision.

Clinical diagnosis of neurological disease

Advances in neurology developed increasingly broadly from this anatomical and physiological foundation. Recognition of diseases by their clinical features became a fundamentally important part of medical education and practice, especially in neurology. Some disorders, for example Parkinson's disease (Parkinson 1755–1824), were known by their clinical features long before any description of their pathology was available. In other instances, for example Huntington's chorea, the genetic background of the clinical disorder formed part of the definition of the syndrome, allowing its separation from other clinically similar involuntary movement disorders. Multiple sclerosis, on the other hand, is a disorder with a wide range of clinical features. Recognition of this disease was achieved by clinicopathological correlation, an important method in the subsequent development of clinical neurology. Charcot (1825–1893) defined certain clinical syndromes, particularly a triad of intention tremor, nystagmus, and scanning speech (all now recognized as cerebellar signs) and linked these observations with the pathology of the disorder (1868). The characteristic plaque-like lesions of demyelination and hardening of the brain (*sclerose en plaque*) were first described by Cruveilhier (1791–1874) working in Paris in 1835. These observations led gradually to the establishment of diagnostic criteria, and to the recognition of the clinical limits of the disorder. Since then much has been learned about the pathophysiology of the disease particularly about immunological abnormalities in the CSF and genetically-determined susceptibility, although the cause of the disease remains unknown. Diagnosis has been improved by application of these clinical findings and by new techniques, for example evoked potential studies and, especially, by detecting the plaques in the brain in life by magnetic resonance imaging.

Many neurological diseases, especially the degenerative diseases, do not occur in other species. However, infections of the nervous system, some genetic diseases, epilepsy, tumours and the effects of toxic substances on the peripheral and central nervous system have been extensively investigated in animal models. These experiments have led to detailed understanding of the pathophysiological mechanisms of these disorders, of the capacity for repair, and of the effects of treatment. However, the lack of an animal model for the neurodegenerative disorders remains a limiting factor in achieving understanding of these conditions.

Medical treatment of neurological disease

Neurology was, until recently, limited in its capacity for treatment. Epilepsy is an example of the change in emphasis towards therapy that has occurred. Bromides were introduced for their anticonvulsant properties in 1857 by Locock (1799–1875), a physician in the York dispensary. The introduction of phenobarbitone in 1912 by Hauptmann marked the beginning of the era of effective therapy. Phenytoin was synthesized as a result of a series of experiments designed to elucidate the structural aspects of phenobarbitone that conferred its anticonvulsant effect, without the other unwanted effects, particularly drowsiness and depression, and this drug was introduced into clinical practice following formal clinical trials by Merritt and Putnam (1938) in Boston, USA. Additional effective anticonvulsant drugs have been introduced since 1950.

Modern neurology evolved from an earlier era in which the emphasis was on the location of lesions in the nervous system and the establishment of concepts of disordered function. Hughlings Jackson (1835–1911) introduced ideas that were particularly formative. Jackson used the method of clinical observation to delineate positive and negative effects of lesions, meaning the release of lower-level functions, and the loss of function consequent on the lesion.

Jackson used this notion to construct a hierarchical theory of brain function that incorporated evolutionary concepts, the higher levels being functionally super-imposed on the lower. Weir Mitchell (1829–1914), working in Philadelphia, used a similar approach in evaluating peripheral nerve lesions studied in the American Civil War. These concepts of the functional and structural organization of the nervous system were a key factor in the development of neurophysiological and anatomical investigation in later years.

Much was learned in these early studies from clinical findings, especially by study of epilepsy, but subsequent advances have been determined more by the application of technical approaches to the underlying physiological, pathological and immunological abnormalities.

Surgical treatment of neurological disorders

Surgical treatment of disease in the nervous system was probably known not only in the ancient world, but in neolithic Europe, since trophine holes have been recognized in skulls from these civilizations. Whether these were always placed therapeutically or for other, perhaps religious reasons, is unknown but trephination for cranial trauma was recommended in the Hippocratic writings, and clinical observations on head injuries were described in the Edwin Smith papyrus from ancient Egypt. Although attempts were made to drain temporomastoid abscesses in the 18th century the first successful surgical drainage of cerebral abscess was achieved by MacEwen (1848–1934) in 1881. Macewen successfully removed a parietal meningioma in 1879, and Bennett and Godlee operated on a cerebral glioma at The National Hospital, Queen Square, in 1884. Horsley (1857–1916) removed a spinal meningioma, diagnosed and localized by Gowers (1845–1915) in 1887, with subsequent recovery of spastic paraplegia. This is generally regarded as marking the first successful neurosurgical procedure. Major advances in aseptic surgery, in anaesthesia, and in surgical technique were necessary before neurosurgery could be applied more widely to diseases of the nervous system. These improvements were largely introduced by the work of Harvey Cushing (1856–1939) and his pupils, especially Dandy (1886–1946).

Investigation of neurological disease

One of the foremost requirements of the modern era of medical and surgical treatment of neurological disease is accurate diagnosis, both in relation to pathology and localization. Apart from systemic investigations, for example tests for syphilis and other infections, or metabolic disorders, a number of investigative methods have evolved specific to the nervous system. The first of these was lumbar puncture introduced by Quincke (1842–1922) in 1891 for the relief of hydrocephalus. Quincke later used this technique to diagnose tuberculous and purulent meningitis, and haemorrhages in the nervous system. Clinical neurophysiology developed from the concept that brain activity depended in some way on electricity. Caton (1842–1926), working in Liverpool, discovered waxing and waning electrical potentials in the brain of a rabbit in 1875. These potentials, representing the electroencephalogram (EEG) were recorded through the intact skull by Berger (1873–1941) in 1929. The EEG was used initially for localization of epileptic foci but was adapted by Grey Walter in 1936 for the localization of tumours, based upon the characteristic slow wave activity associated with neoplasms. The electrical activity of nerves was studied by Helmholtz (1821–1894) who measured the motor conduction velocity

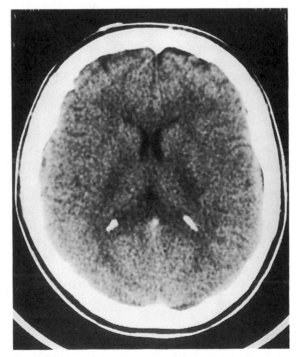

Fig. 4 Normal computerized tomographic X-ray scan (CT scan) of the brain, showing the lateral ventricles, the deep central white matter, and the calcified choroid plexuses in the two occipital horns of the lateral ventricles. The centrally-located pineal gland is also calcified. The sulcal markings of the brain are just visible near the skull margin.

using a string galvanometer in 1850. Recordings of electrical activity from muscle were achieved by Piper in 1909, but were introduced into clinical practice only after the invention of the co-axial needle electrode by Adrian and Bronk in 1929. Evoked potentials in the brain can be recorded from visual, auditory and somatosensory stimulation, using a digital amplifier to remove irrelevant background activity. This technology was pioneered by Dawson (1912–1983) in 1950, using a photographic subtraction method.

Imaging of the nervous system is a fundamental requirement for localization. Prior to Roentgen's discovery of X-rays in 1895 only the first cranial nerve could be visualized, using the ophthalmoscope, invented by Helmholz in 1851. Radiology of the skull was systematically investigated by Schiller (1874–1957), working in Vienna. Walter Dandy used air to delineate the ventricular system by ventricular puncture (1918) and then by lumbar puncture (air encephalography) in 1919. Myelography, a technique to visualize the spinal roots and spinal cord within the spinal canal, was introduced by Sicard (1872–1929) in 1921, an advance that depended on the use of a radio-opaque iodized oil, lipiodol. This contrast medium has been superseded by water-soluble substances, still based on iodine as a radio-opaque substance. Cerebral angiography

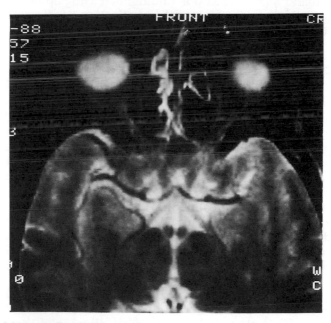

Fig. 5 Magnetic Resonance Imaging (MRI) scan of the same region of the brain in a normal subject, showing the eyes, optic nerves, optic chiasm and optic tracts.

was developed by Moniz (1874–1955) in 1927 but has been refined by improvements in contrast media, by selective catheterization techniques, and by digital subtraction technology, which allows the image to be processed in the computer before hard copy is produced on film.

Neuroradiology was revolutionized by Hounsfield in 1971. Hounsfield, working in the laboratories of EMI, used computing methods to derive transverse images of the brain, using Piezo-electric detectors rather than X-ray film, and rotating the X-ray beam around the patient's head, in the method now known as computerized axial tomography (CAT or CT scanning) (Fig. 4). CT scanning derives images based on the absorbence of X-rays in the brain, but the derivation of the image in the computer allows very fine details to be seen. Magnetic resonance imaging utilizes activation of protons by a radio-frequency current in a uniform high strength magnetic field to derive an image, using a similar computerized method to produce axial cross-sectional images of the brain. Magnetic resonance imaging (MRI) (Fig. 5) enables visualization of lesions in the brain and spinal cord based on their water or fat content, rather than on their X-ray absorbence, and therefore offers a direct biological assessment of the brain in relation to this aspect of function and anatomy. MRI is finding increasing application both in localization and in biological investigation of diseases of the nervous system.

Future trends

The availability of modern methods of imaging the nervous system, and of physiological and immunological assessment of diseases of the brain and peripheral nervous system has greatly enhanced diagnostic specificity both in relation to localization, function, and pathogenesis. Furthermore, these methods enable treatment by physical methods to be applied more accurately to the diseased part of the nervous system, thus decreasing morbidity and mortality from these forms of treatment. With greater understanding of the immunological and pharmacological abnormalities associated with diseases of the nervous system it is likely that medical treatment will become increasingly effective. Thus, some of the disorders described in the following pages of this book, that remain, for the moment, untreatable may shortly yield.

It is an old adage in neurology that although a disorder may be rare, for the patient suffering from the condition it is the only disorder in the whole spectrum of diseases of the nervous system, or of other systems, that has any significance. This is the essential conundrum of the clinical practice of medicine.

Governments come and go, fashions change, the prevalence of different disorders varies from generation to generation, but there are always people with diseases and disabilities, common or rare, who require help in understanding and alleviating their problem. Only the informed physician or surgeon can offer help.

1

Symptoms and Signs

Effective management of the patient with a neurological disorder requires recognition that the nervous system is involved. Thus, understanding of the pathological process and definition of the disability are necessary before an appropriate treatment plan can be determined. Management involves not only specific medical or surgical treatment, but also non-specific therapies, such as physiotherapy. In addition, it is often useful to define methods for assessing progress, such as clinical assessment of particular abnormalities, e.g. extent of sensory loss or severity of weakness, or more objective investigations, such as nerve conduction velocity, CT scanning or biochemical indices of change in a disease process. From the patient's point of view, recovery from the illness consists not so much of cure of the disease, but of relief from symptoms; this distinction should always be kept in mind. Indeed, symptoms can frequently be alleviated, even in incurable conditions.

The nervous system is complex, and the range and scope of clinical abnormality, consisting of the symptoms and signs elicited by the examiner, are enormous. Thus a disorder such as stroke may present with one or more of many different symptoms; indeed different physicians may be impressed by slightly different aspects of the syndrome in the same patient. Thus, the pattern of symptoms and signs is a consequence of the interaction between patient and doctor, rather than an absolute and immutable state of affairs. The direction of the clinical assessment, and the investigations planned will be determined by the doctor's impression of the clinical syndrome. This should always be tempered by the patient's own wishes in relation to the objectives of the consultation.

Approach to neurological disorders

Neurological disorders are sometimes difficult for the patient to describe. When the brain itself is diseased there may be impairment of judgement, thinking or memory, leading to difficulties in conceptualizing the nature of disability, or language itself may be abnormal (aphasia) so that the basic tools of communication are disturbed. Even when the intellect and sensorium are unaffected, as in patients with spinal cord or peripheral nerve disorders, the features of neurological disease are so much outside ordinary experience that many patients cannot adequately describe them without help. The physician must learn to guide the patient through the symptoms in relation to his or her own concept of the nature of neurological disease. Thus the patient may complain of blackouts, a word that has almost no neurological meaning. The patient will initially deny any more specific feature to the symptom but with a little encouragement, most easily established by enquiring about the circumstances, frequency, duration and earliest component of the altered consciousness, it is readily established that the episodes are likely to be due to epilepsy, syncope or other cause, e.g. hypoglycaemia or transient ischaemic attack.

Patients are often so astonished by their symptoms that they are initially reluctant to describe them in detail, and only when the doctor shows understanding does the whole story come out. Patients with complex partial seizures are understandably unwilling to tell a doctor of whom they know very little that they are troubled by repetitive hallucinations or sensory experiences that have a peculiarly compelling sense of other-worldliness.

The patient's view of the problem is compounded by his or her own experience of disease. Thus the patient with headache may be concerned by the possibility of cerebral tumour, experienced in a relative, and may present a description of the headache stressing those particular features that caused concern, and neglecting those that are more relevant such as the social factors that have led to the symptom as a consequence of stress.

Disturbed sensation is a particularly difficult problem. There is impairment of sensation resulting from damage to a peripheral nerve, or central sensory pathway; this may involve all sensory function or be relatively selective, affecting certain types of sensation and sparing others. Thus, in spinal lesions, pain and temperature sensation may be impaired while position sense, vibration and tactile discrimination (light touch) are normal (dissociated sensory loss). This reflects relatively selective damage to the phylogenetically older, small fibre, nociceptive afferent system represented in the human by the spinothalamic tracts. Damage to sensory pathways may also result in spontaneous unpleasant or painful sensations, resulting from disturbance of afferent input, or loss of inhibitory neuronal activity in dorsal horn, thalamus or other central structures.

Similarly, abnormalities of movement and posture can result from loss of function in motor pathways at peripheral or central level in the nervous system. Rather different clinical syndromes develop when there is damage to higher motor centres or pathways, since there is then a more complex disturbance of function, with loss of higher control mechanisms, and release of hierarchically lower control systems.

Consequences of lesions in the nervous system

Lesions in the nervous system cause clinical consequences as a result of the localization of the lesion itself, and the time course of the development of the lesion. These two factors are considered later in this chapter. Acute lesions exemplify four processes by which symptoms and signs may result. These are not all present at any given moment in the course of the disease but they are relevant to understanding disabilities resulting from damage to the nervous system, and the compensatory processes that result. *Firstly*, acute lesions cause temporary disturbance of function. This disturbance of function initially involves parts of the brain not directly involved in the lesion, in addition to the dysfunction caused by the lesion itself. The clinical deficit at this stage may be severe, but recovery is likely in the few hours or days after the onset, leaving a deficit of function related directly to the lesion. Thus in ischaemic stroke the initial functional deficit is much greater than the final clinical outcome, reflecting the effects of a penumbra of ischaemic tissue in the neighbourhood of the infarcted tissue which may recover function in the course of the illness, and the physiological ('cerebral shock') disruption of function resulting from sudden impairment of function in nearby nervous tissue. *Secondly*, irreversible deficit occurs as a consequence of destruction of tissue by the acute lesion. This is ascertained by the final clinical outcome. This deficit of function consists of those functions that are impaired or no longer possible, and thus represents a negative consequence of the lesion. *Thirdly*, released phenomena may interfere with function. After a stroke, there is spasticity, increased reflexes, released flexor reflexes including the extensor plantar response, and sometimes dystonia and involuntary movements also occur. Hughlings Jackson regarded these released phenomena as representing function in phylogenetically primitive parts of the brain released by the lesion from hierarchical levels of higher control but they are now seen as disturbances of function of parts of the command system involved in motor control. This system consists of a distributed system of interrelated points of contact in a complex chain of neuronal pathways leading to a final common path. The latter consists of task-groups of motor neurons innervating motor units in muscles. A similar concept can be applied to the somatosensory and other afferent systems. *Fourthly*, excessive neuronal discharge in or near a cortical lesion may result in focal or generalized epilepsy. The risk of this complication increases, in most circumstances, with time following the lesion, possibly because of maturational factors in recovering cells and pathways related to the lesion.

Temporal factors and symptomatology

The time factor in the development of a lesion is important in determining the resulting symptoms and signs. In general, acute lesions produce severe dysfunction and slowly developing lesions cause much less marked clinical abnormality. Indeed, very slowly progressive lesions, such as meningiomas, may be entirely symptomless until complications such as epilepsy, increased intracranial pressure or stroke-like episodes occur at a stage when the tumour is large and has caused extensive compression and displacement of the brain. Sudden spinal cord compression due to trauma causes immediate flaccid paraplegia, with the later development of spasticity; gradually progressive cord compression causes a slowly progressive spastic paraplegia. In the former spinal shock causes a 'negative' clinical syndrome, and in the latter there is a combination of negative and positive features.

Other factors

As in disease of other systems, the potential for recovery is greater in children and young people than in the elderly. In addition, disease affecting the developing or maturing nervous system produces clinical features that are modified subsequently by the process of maturation of undamaged pathways normally in close functional relation with the damaged structures. Thus children younger than 2 years can tolerate lesions in the dominant hemisphere, and yet develop adequate language capability by transference of language to the presumed non-dominant hemisphere. Beyond the age of 5 years this potential for functional adaptation of the homologous non-dominant hemisphere is lost.

Recovery from a single lesion in the brain, e.g. a stroke, is often excellent, but the potential for recovery after a second lesion is not so great. Further, the second lesion may produce clinical defects apparently greater than would be expected if this were the only brain lesion. Von Monakow used the term diaschisis to describe this phenomenon, and suggested that it was due to functional interference with neuronal systems and pathways at a distance from the second lesion, occurring because of metabolic or physiological abnormalities in these systems that made them vulnerable. He also used this term to explain cerebral or spinal shock; no adequate understanding of these clinically important phenomena is yet available.

Patterns of functional disturbance
in disease of the nervous system

The neurologist, in assessing a patient with suspected neurological disease, looks for patterns of functional disturbance related to disease of particular parts of the nervous system, or characteristic of certain diseases or syndromes. Thus, Parkinson's disease is usually immediately recognizable, although its clinical manifestations, especially resting tremor, akinesia and rigidity, are themselves complex phenomena that are difficult to understand in physiological terms. On the other hand, hemiplegia, consisting of weakness of one side of the body with spasticity, can occur with lesions at different levels in the central nervous system (CNS) and as a consequence of many different underlying disease processes. Frequently, precise recognition of the location of the lesion in the nervous system is of little importance. However, the aetiology of the lesion determines the outcome, and the possibility of treatment, and much modern investigative effort is directed more towards aetiology than to location of lesions. The anatomical location and limits of lesions in the nervous system are particularly important in planning surgical treatment, and are also useful in the clinical diagnosis of patients with more than one lesion in the nervous system, especially in multiple sclerosis and stroke. However, modern imaging methods, especially X-ray CT scanning and magnetic resonance imaging (MRI) have transformed this concept by introducing accurate methodologies for localization that have led to new concepts in understanding of the effects of lesions in different parts of the CNS.

Recognition of the common clinical syndromes resulting from neurological disease is useful both in making a diagnosis and in planning management. Diagnosis implies understanding of pathogenesis as well as location of the lesion or lesions causing disability; this requires temporal information on the course of the disorder that can only be obtained from the history. Although a knowledge of neuroanatomy and neurophysiology in relation to commonly occurring clinical syndromes is interesting, in most clinical circumstances it is not necessary for formulating diagnosis. Localization is especially helpful in diseases in which multiple lesions occur, e.g. stroke and multiple sclerosis, and when this information is required as part of the investigation prior to surgical treatment. The commonly occurring clinical syndromes are listed in Table 1.1.

Many of these clinical syndromes can be immediately associated with disease of certain parts of the brain. In many such disorders

Table 1.1 *Common neurological syndromes.*

A. Motor disorders
    Upper motor neuron syndrome
      hemiplegia
      paraplegia
      quadriplegia
      pseudobulbar palsy
    Lower motor neuron syndrome
      peripheral neuropathy
      root lesions
      anterior horn cells
      bulbar palsy
    Cerebellar syndromes
      truncal ataxia
      limb ataxia
      oculomotor syndromes
    Extrapyramidal syndromes
      Parkinson's disease
      involuntary movements
      dystonia
    Combinations of motor syndromes

B. Sensory disorders
    Peripheral nerve and root syndromes
    Spinal cord
      sensory levels
      dissociated sensory loss
    Higher pathways sensory syndromes

C. Disorders of vision
    Optic nerve and chiasm (and retina)
    Optic radiation
    Occipital cortex (cortical blindness)
    Higher visual pathways (visual agnosias and other
      perceptual disorders)
    Diplopia

D. Disorders of higher mental function
    Language disorders
    Memory disorders
    Visuo-spatial disorders (right parietal lobe syndrome)
    Agnosia and apraxia
    Frontal lobe disorder
    Dementia and delirium
    Psychological disturbances
      hysteria, depression, psychotic disorders

E. Autonomic and sphincter disturbances
    Incontinence/retention of urine or faeces
    Disturbances of cardiovascular reflexes
    Disturbed sexual function
    Disturbances of the enteric nervous system

F. Seizures (see Chapter 2)

certain associations of symptoms or signs suggest particular diagnoses, for example the association of optic atrophy with impaired visual acuity, cerebellar ataxia and diplopia suggests multiple sclerosis. The pattern of sensory loss and the type of sensory disorder may give clues to the underlying cause of a peripheral neuropathy, for example diabetic neuropathy (Chapter 13). This process of pattern recognition is reliable in diagnosis and is more practical than attempts to learn long lists, for example of the causes of cerebellar ataxia. Clinical experience of the common clinical syndromes is invaluable in the process of diagnosis, and in the recognition of unusual disorders.

Motor disorders

Disorders of the motor system represent some of the commonest presentations of serious neurological disease.

Upper motor neuron syndromes

The upper motor neuron consists of the corticospinal tract, arising from motor cells in the motor cortex and synapsing with motor neurons in the brain stem motor nuclei and in the grey matter of the anterior horn of the spinal cord. Lesions in this system cause *weakness, spasticity, increased tendon reflexes* and *extensor plantar responses*. The weakness is typically most marked in fine, co-ordinated movements of the fingers and hands, and also particularly involves shoulder abduction, hip flexion and dorsiflexion of the feet. Even with major corticospinal lesions the patient can learn to walk, since hip extensors and plantar flexion of the foot are strong. This 'pyramidal' or 'corticospinal' distribution of weakness involves movements rather than individual muscles, so that individual muscles may be recruited for some tasks but not for others, e.g. wrist dorsiflexion is weak but these muscles contract strongly during clenching of the fist.

Spasticity develops during the hours or days after an acute corticospinal lesion; the tendon reflexes may be depressed initially but soon become increased as the phase of cerebral or spinal shock passes. In patients with minor corticospinal lesions the fully developed syndrome is not present. The most sensitive indices of minor corticospinal tract disease are increased reflexes and an extensor plantar response. Spasticity is often difficult to detect. In longstanding upper motor neuron syndromes some wasting of muscles may develop. The extensor plantar response (Babinski's sign) is the most important physical sign in clinical neurology. It consists of dorsiflexion (extension) of the large toe, fanning of the other toes and flexor withdrawal of the leg in response to scratching the lateral aspect of the sole of the foot. This motor response consists of contraction of the muscles that are weak to voluntary effort in the upper motor neuron syndrome, illustrating the impairment of excitation and inhibition resulting from the corticospinal lesion.

The level of the lesion in the upper motor neuron determines the distribution of the clinical abnormality. For example, upper motor neuron facial weakness, consisting of marked weakness of the lower face with relative sparing of the upper face is a feature of corticospinal disease rostral to the seventh nerve nucleus. In cervical cord disease there is often lower motor neuron involvement in the arm and upper motor neuron involvement in the ipsilateral leg or, more commonly, in both legs (Chapter 15). When there is disease in the deep white matter of a cerebral hemisphere, e.g. a cerebral infarct, there are frequently associated abnormal postures and rigidity representing spastic dystonia, resulting in a characteristic flexed upper limb and extended lower limb, most marked in the erect posture.

Hemiplegia, consisting of upper motor neuron syndrome affecting one side of the body, is usually due to a lesion in the contralateral cerebral hemisphere or brain stem above the level of the decussation of the pyramids in the medulla. *Spastic paraplegia* consists of spastic weakness of both legs with bilateral extensor plantar responses. It is usually due to spinal cord disease but it can also occur with bilateral cerebral infarction, with parasagittal tumours involving the leg areas of motor cortex or, sometimes, with hydrocephalus which causes damage to the corticospinal fibres subserving the legs as they are stretched around the dilated lateral ventricles. *Spastic quadriplegia* consists of upper motor neuron syndrome causing paralysis in all four limbs. It is due to disease in the cervical spinal cord but may rarely result from extensive bilateral white matter degeneration in the brain or brain stem. In the latter instances there is invariably an associated pseudobulbar palsy. *Pseudobulbar palsy* consists of spastic weakness of the bulbar musculature with dysarthria, dysphagia and released involuntary crying and laughter, due to damage to the cortico-bulbar descending motor pathways, e.g. with multiple sclerosis or multiple cerebral infarcts.

Lower motor neuron syndromes

The lower motor neuron consists of the components of the motor unit, i.e. the motor neuron cell, axon and peripheral nerve, motor end plates and the muscle fibres innervated by this motor neuron. Lesions of the lower motor neuron cause weakness, atrophy, loss of tendon reflexes and, sometimes, fasciculation in affected muscles. Fibrillation potentials can be detected in denervated muscles by electromyography. The plantar response is flexor, but may be absent when weakness is severe.

In *peripheral neuropathy* there is symmetrical lower motor neuron weakness and wasting in the distal parts of the extremities. If the neuropathy is due to damage to the peripheral nerve myelin, weakness may also be present proximally, since the whole nerve is then involved, but axonopathies (Chapter 13) cause strikingly distal involvement. There is usually associated sensory impairment. Lesions of isolated peripheral nerves, e.g. median or radial nerves, cause lower motor neuron involvement in these distributions. *Root and plexus lesions* cause segmentally-distributed lower motor neuron syndromes which, as in mononeuropathies, are usually associated with sensory involvement. *Anterior horn cell diseases* cause lower motor neuron wasting and weakness, which is proximal, distal or generalized, but not necessarily symmetrical, without sensory disturbance, and with decreased reflexes. Fasciculation at rest is a characteristic feature of motor neuron disease, but it also occurs with root lesions. Motor neuron disease, however, is usually associated with a combination of lower and upper motor neuron involvement (Chapter 12). *Bulbar palsy* consists of degeneration of motor cells in the cranial nerve nuclei causing lower motor neuron signs in this distribution, including facial and mandibular weakness and wasting, wasting of the tongue, and dysarthria and dysphagia. Nasal regurgitation of fluids is a common problem in bulbar palsy, and the voice may also be affected from vocal cord weakness.

Cerebellar syndromes

Disease of the cerebellum typically causes cerebellar ataxia, a motor disorder in which there is inco-ordination and inaccuracy in performance of movement tasks in relation to amplitude and velocity of the planned movement so that the target is missed, by undershooting or overshooting. Multiple corrective movements are inserted into the planned movement. Speech may similarly be involved, causing a break-up of sentences into separate syllables (scanning speech). *Ataxia* may involve limbs, when it is often unilateral, and ipsilateral to a lateral cerebellar lesion, or the trunk, when it is due to midline cerebellar lesions, especially affecting the vermis, as in alcoholic cerebellar degeneration. *Nystagmus* consists of a jerking rhythmic conjugate movement of the eyes, with a fast and slow phase; it may be lateral, vertical or rotary depending on the location of the lesion. In most patients nystagmus is due to brain stem or labyrinthine disease, rather than cerebellar disease, and limb ataxia may also result from lesions in the cerebellar connections in the cerebellar peduncles or brain stem. Other disturbances of ocular movement may result from disease in brain stem connections

Table 1.2 *Gait disorders.*

Upper motor neuron syndromes

Hemiplegia:	circumduction of leg with inability to flex hip and dorsiflex against gravity. Triple flexion of upper limb.
Paraplegia:	scissoring, stiff-legged gait with tilting of pelvis to compensate for inability to lift legs against gravity; flexed posture.

Lower motor neuron syndromes

Foot drop:	common peroneal nerve palsy or L5/S1 root lesion causes weakness of dorsiflexion and eversion of foot: the leg is raised excessively to compensate.
Quadriceps weakness:	knee extension weak, leading to sudden falls and difficulty rising from a chair or descending stairs.
Proximal weakness:	difficulty climbing stairs, rising from the floor, a rolling gait. Arms cannot be lifted above shoulder height. Axial weakness may be present.
Peripheral neuropathy:	usually a combination of weakness and sensory loss, causing unsteadiness.

Cerebellar syndromes
Ataxia (unsteadiness) and inability to walk on a narrow base. Often worse on turning suddenly.

Extrapyramidal syndromes
Shuffling gait in Parkinson's disease, with forward flexion and loss of righting responses. Gait may be festinant. Tremor of upper limbs and face Dystonic involuntary movements in other extrapyramidal syndromes.

Sensory ataxia
Impaired posterior column sensation causes cerebellar-like ataxia, markedly worsened with eyes closed. Romberg positive.

Apraxia of gait
Loss of concept of walking, may be associated with tiny short rapid steps (*marche à Petitpas*) resembling ballet steps.

Hysteria
Bizarre, exaggerated, non-physiological gait disorder in which the patient miraculously does not fall; worse when deliberately observed.

involving cerebellar pathways and these, e.g. ocular flutter, may superficially resemble nystagmus.

Extrapyramidal syndromes

The basal ganglia are concerned with postural reflexes in walking, reaching, and changing posture. Disorders of this system cause characteristic syndromes such as Parkinson's disease (Chapter 11), in which there is a combination of akinesia, rigidity and resting tremor, and other syndromes, consisting of involuntary movements, e.g. chorea (Chapter 11), or a tendency to develop fixed postures, e.g. dystonia and choreoathetosis (Chapter 11). There are associated upper motor neuron signs only if the corticospinal tracts are involved. These disorders may be non-progressive, e.g. in cerebral palsy, or progressive as in degenerative conditions such as Parkinson's disease or Huntington's chorea.

Combinations of motor syndromes

In some disorders, e.g. multiple sclerosis, cerebellar and upper motor neuron involvement occur simultaneously and it may be difficult to ascribe individual components of the clinical deficit to these two processes. In motor neuron disease upper and lower motor neuron involvement co-exist so that a wasted, fasciculating muscle exhibits an increased tendon jerk. A similar combination of upper and lower motor neuron involvement is common in biceps or triceps muscles in patients with cervical myelopathy due to cervical spondylosis. In stroke, when there is infarction in the deep cerebral white matter, dystonia often accompanies spastic weakness, and choreo-athetosis. Dystonia and upper motor neuron signs are common manifestations of the cerebral palsy syndrome (Chapter 18).

Gait disorders

Much can be learned from watching the patient walk, especially if the patient is not aware of the observation. Thus, observing the gait as the patient enters a consulting room, before beginning the consultation, is especially valuable (see Table 1.2).

Sensory disorders

Lesions of afferent pathways may result in decreased sensory threshold and discriminative capacity (Jacksonian negative features) and, sometimes, in abnormal sensory experiences (positive features). The latter may be unpleasant or even painful, and their physiology is, as yet, incompletely understood.

In clinical neurology *lesions of the posterior columns* are associated with impairment of fine discriminative sensation, including light touch, two-point discrimination, recognition of texture, position sense and vibration. Lesions of this pathway in the spinal cord or brain stem also lead to a profound disorder of the ability to manipulate small objects in the fingers, and to sensory ataxia and chorea-like movements of the fingers of the outstretched hands that are worsened with the eyes closed. Lesions of the *lateral spinothalamic tracts* are associated with impairment of pain and temperature sensation, and sometimes with spontaneous pain in the affected zones or with a sensation of pain in response to light contact (allodynia). When the spinothalamic tracts are selectively damaged, and the posterior columns are spared, as in syringomyelia, intrinsic cord neoplasms or anterior spinal artery distribution infarction, there is impairment of pain and temperature sensation with sparing of other modalities of sensation (dissociated sensory loss).

Lesions of the *peripheral sensory pathway*, for example in mononeuropathies or peripheral neuropathies, lead to sensory disturbance in an appropriate distribution. In symmetrical peripheral neuropathy this is typically of stocking and glove type, with an upper level of normality that varies somewhat according to the type and intensity of the test stimulus. Allodynia, neuralgia, or even spontaneous pain, as in causalgia, may also occur with lesions in the peripheral sensory pathway, but especially after trauma or compression, in which the myelin covering of the sensory axons is disturbed leading to 'crosstalk' (ephaptic transmission) between neighbouring axons, and a disturbance of the pattern of afferent traffic in the nerve.

In *spinal cord disease*, there may be a sensory level, below which sensation is abnormal or absent. In progressive disorders, such as cord compression from an extrinsic tumour, e.g. meningioma, the sensory level gradually ascends from the feet to reach the segmental level of the lesion. This reflects compression of the laminated pathways in the posterior columns and spinothalamic tracts. Hemicompression of the cord rarely results in the *Brown-Séquard syndrome*, consisting of ipsilateral disturbances of posterior column sensation and corticospinal tract function, with contralateral loss of lateral spinothalamic tract function. The sacral segments tend to be spared. In *high cervical cord lesions* there may be impaired pain and temperature sensation on the face because of involvement of the spinal tract of the trigeminal nerve. In *cauda equina lesions* the sacral segments, in the perianal region, buttocks and posterior thighs are selectively affected, and in *conus medullaris lesions* this is associated with extensor plantar responses. In *cervical myelopathy* due to cervical spondylosis, root pain in the arms may be prominent but radicular sensory impairment is slight in the cervical segments, despite severe spastic paraplegia, with a sensory level.

Thalamic and parietal lesions may cause severe, intractable burning and contact-sensitive pain in addition to contralateral hemisensory loss. This syndrome is frequently also associated with mislocalization of sensory stimuli in the affected area and with a foreshortening of the body image so that the affected limbs are perceived as smaller than those of the normal side. In rare instances, the limbs may be denied as belonging to the patient (anosagnosia).

Disorders of vision. Visual disturbances are important not only because they can result in severe disability, but because they are highly reliable in localizing lesions in the central nervous system. The whole visual pathway, from retina to occipital and association cortex, is contained within the cerebral hemispheres, in the supratentorial compartment of the brain. Patients with visual disturbances must therefore have dysfunction in this part of the neuraxis.

The visual pathway consists of retinae, optic nerves, optic chiasm and optic tracts, terminating in the lateral geniculate bodies.

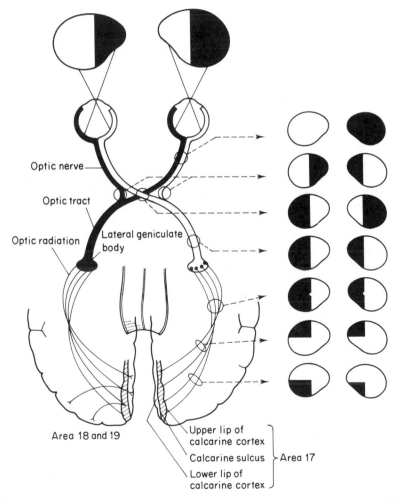

Fig. 1.1 Diagrammatic representation of the optic chiasm and visual pathways, and the visual field disorders associated with lesions in the different parts of these pathways.

The optic radiations project through the deep white matter of the cerebral hemispheres to terminate in the calcarine cortex, in the occipital lobes of the two hemispheres (Fig. 1.1). Visual information is fed forward from the primary visual cortex into the association cortex in the posterior parietal regions, and downwards into the upper brain stem in relation to orienting reflexes. Connections to the frontal lobes are important in initiating ocular movements (frontal eye fields).

Visual disturbances consist of alterations in visual acuity, which reflect abnormalities in central, macular vision; and of alterations in visual fields. In addition, patients with cerebral lesions, especially temporal and parietal lesions, rarely experience more complex aberrations of vision, for example, visual hallucinations, disorders of colour perception and disturbances of higher perceptual function leading to selective problems with visual orientation and visual recognition (visual agnosia). Retinal disease itself can cause colour blindness, impaired acuity, scotomas (shadows or zones of lost vision), or hallucinations of flashes of light (teichopsias or photopsias).

Visual acuity

This is an objective measurement, but in assessing patients with neurological disorders it is important to check the acuity with correction of any defect in the eye itself, especially refractive errors, or to recognize the presence of corneal disease or other disturbance of light transmission through the eye. Visual acuity can be tested with reading cards, or with test types at 6 metres (or 20 feet in the USA). Colour vision can be tested with suitable colour charts, e.g. Ishihara plates.

Visual fields

The fields of vision in each eye must be tested separately, and then conjugately in order to assess the presence of hemianopia or homonymous hemianopia or other field defect. This can be assessed by sitting in front of the patient and testing the limits of vision to finger movement, or to a red pinhead, by confrontation, or by formal perimetry using special equipment. The fields can be tested in the perimeter to static stimuli or to moving stimuli (static and kinetic perimetry). Simple clinical confrontation testing is sensitive and accurate, because the examiner is comparing the patient's field with his own. The central fields are as important as the peripheral fields, since they may be selectively involved in optic nerve and optic chiasm disorders, especially multiple sclerosis and pituitary tumours.

The various field disturbances resulting from lesions at different sites in the visual pathways are shown in Fig. 1.1. Lesions in the optic nerve cause unilateral loss of vision, or central scotomas. In multiple sclerosis decreased acuity, with central scotoma and loss of colour discrimination are characteristically associated with demyelination in the optic nerve. Some patients experience photopsias, localized flashes of light, on moving the eyes. Pituitary tumours or other lesions in the anterior part of the chiasm cause *bitemporal hemianopia*, due to compression of the crossing fibres from the nasal parts of the retinae which subserve the temporal fields of vision. This is often incomplete and sometimes associated with impaired central (macular) vision. *Homonymous hemianopia* can be due to lesions in one optic tract, in the optic radiation, or in the occipital cortex, usually due to infarction, haemorrhage or tumour. In patients with lesions in the *temporal lobe* there is a tendency for the hemianopia to be denser or even restricted to the homonymous upper quadrants, since the temporal loop of the optic radiation subserves vision above the horizontal meridian. Conversely, *parietal lesions* may cause inferior quadrantanopsia.

In lesions of the *posterior visual pathway*, posterior to the geniculate bodies, impaired vision even if total, as in cortical blindness from occipital infarction, is associated with normal pupillary light reactions, since the afferent limb of the light reaction leaves the optic tract just anterior to the lateral geniculate bodies. Thus in total anterior lesions of the visual pathway the pupillary light reaction is absent. In patients with *parieto-occipital lesions*, in whom there is predominant involvement of visual association cortex, the sydrome of visual agnosia develops. This consists of imperception and denial of the reality of blindness, an extreme form of visual agnosia. Other, related defects may occur, especially difficulty recognizing faces (prosopagnosia), visual impersistence and abnormal persistence of objects (palinopsia) and visual disorientation. These visuospatial disorders are particularly associated with disorders of the right parietal lobe.

Diplopia

Double vision is a common neurological syndrome. It may be due to disease in the external ocular muscles or orbits, e.g. myasthenia gravis, orbital tumours or fractures, or more commonly to decompensated minor squint of a congenital type. It may also be due to weakness of an external ocular muscle, or group of muscles, due to disease of the third, fourth or sixth cranial nerves, or to brain stem disease causing disparity in movement of the two eyes due to interference with the conjugate control mechanisms.

In *infranuclear lesions* there is involvement of the third, sixth and fourth cranial nerves, or a combination of these. Thus a sixth nerve lesion causes weakness of lateral movement of the eye, a fourth nerve lesion causes impairment of downward movement of the eye, and a third nerve lesion causes weakness of all movements except lateral and downward deviation. The pupil is usually fixed and dilated, but may be normal if the pupillomotor fibres in the nerve are spared, as is almost invariable in diabetic oculomotor nerve infarction. In myasthenia gravis there are variable signs with diplopia and gaze palsy, and this responds to treatment with cholinergic drugs (Chapter 14).

In *supranuclear lesions* there is impairment of movement of *both* eyes in one direction of gaze (conjugate gaze palsy). Weakness of *lateral conjugate gaze* results from pontine or hemispheric disease; weakness of *conjugate upward gaze* follows lesions of the central mid brain or thalamic region. In *internuclear ophthalmoplegia*, due to a lesion of the ipsilateral medial longitudinal fasciculus in mid brain or upper pons, there is weakness of adduction on the affected side, together with rhythmic nystagmus of the abducting eye. In multiple sclerosis, the commonest cause of this syndrome, the lesion is often bilateral. Slow following, or *pursuit* movements are separately controlled in the brain from rapid, preprogrammed *saccadic* ocular movements. In Huntington's chorea and in Parkinson's disease pursuit movements are slowed and interrupted; in parieto-occipital lesions saccadic movements may be impaired toward the midline in the affected field.

Nystagmus consists of an involuntary, usually conjugate rhythmic oscillation of the eyes with a slow corrective phase, and a fast phase in the direction of the lesion. It results from disturbance of labyrinthine, eighth nerve, vestibular, brain stem or cerebellar pathways, and commonly occurs also from the effect of drugs such as phenobarbitone, phenytoin and diazepam. *Optokinetic nystagmus* is a normal phenomenon in which a rapidly moving object is followed with a slow pursuit, and a saccade is used in the reverse direction to fixate a following object, as in 'railway train nystagmus'. Abnormalities in this response occur in parietal and brain stem lesions.

Pupillary responses

Examination of the pupils is a classical and important part of the neurological examination. *Horner's syndrome* is probably the commonest pupillary abnormality (Fig. 1.2). It results from a lesion in the cervical sympathetic chain or its central connections in the spinal cord and brain stem. The pupil is small, with ptosis, enophthalmos and lack of sweating on the ipsilateral forehead. The *Argyll Robertson pupil* consists of a small, irregular pupil that fails to react to light directly or consensually, but which reacts briskly to accommodation; this abnormality is characteristic of neurosyphilis,

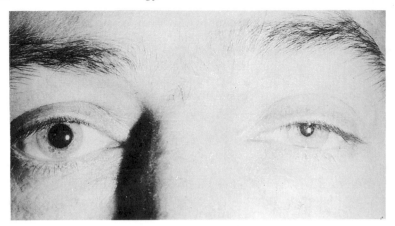

Fig. 1.2 Horner's syndrome. There is ptosis, enophthalmos and a small, normally-reactive pupil.

but may also occur in diabetes mellitus. It is usually bilateral. The *Adie pupil* (*tonic pupil*), part of the Holmes–Adie syndrome, consists of a pupil that is tonically dilated, but which may be small when first seen; the pupil dilates slowly in the dark and constricts slowly with light or accommodation and is usually a unilateral abnormality. In the full syndrome there is ipsilateral or bilateral absence of tendon reflexes. It is due to loss of parasympathetic innervation to the pupillary muscle. In *optic neuritis* there is relative reduction of the direct light reaction on the affected side, so that the consensual reaction to light on the opposite side is more powerful than the direct light stimulus. This is a feature of an afferent pupillary defect, usually due to demyelination but also found in other lesions of the optic nerve (Gunn pupil).

Disorders of higher cerebral function

Much of the fundamental knowledge of cortical function is based on clinical studies of patients with localized cerebral lesions, in the context of missile injuries sustained in the First and Second World Wars, and other lesions, especially infarcts and neoplasms. Thus the main clinical syndromes of cerebral disorders, especially language disturbances, memory disorders, visuo-spatial disorders, personality disturbances and dementia, have been associated with lesions in relatively well-circumscribed parts of the brain. However, the severity of the clinical syndrome does not necessarily coincide with the size of the lesion. Acute lesions produce abrupt and more severe clinical deficit than chronic or slowly progressing lesions, perhaps because of diaschisis, the concept introduced by von Monakow in 1911 (see above).

Temporal lobe lesions

The temporal lobes are concerned with olfactory and auditory perception. The visual radiation projects deeply through temporal lobe white matter and may be involved in temporal lesions. The left temporal lobe is involved in language function, and both temporal lobes have important roles in visual memory and in the recognition of complex images such as faces. Both temporal lobes, especially the hippocampus and amygdala, are important in short-term memory.

Seizures are a common manifestation of temporal lobe disease, especially tumours and abscesses deep in the anterior part of the temporal lobe. The seizures are typically psychomotor (partial epilepsy) in type with olfactory, visual and auditory hallucinations, reiterated fragments from memory and, sometimes, focal motor components affecting face and hand.

Parietal lobe lesions

The parietal lobes function as associational cortex for intercalated functions involving integration of frontal, temporal and occipital cortex. The *right parietal lobe* is concerned especially with visuo-spatial function including visual and geographical orientation, synthesis of the internalized body image from somatosensory, and visual and motor information. The anterior part of parietal cortex consists of the primary sensory cortex. The *left parietal lobe* is involved with language function, particularly with writing, reading, calculation and speech perception involving the integration of auditory and visual components.

Lesions of either parietal sensory cortex will cause contralateral disturbance of tactile discrimination, including astereognosis and vibration and position sense loss, but relatively less involvement of pain and temperature sensation. *Right parietal lesions* cause contralateral neglect of visual, tactile and auditory space, or even denial of the opposite limb. There is sometimes impaired memory for spatial location (geographic memory) with route-finding difficulties. Dressing apraxia, consisting of inability to conceptualize the shape and orientation of clothing, and constructional apraxia, as shown by copying complex figures or constructing shapes with small building blocks, are characteristic right parietal deficits. Prosopagnosia, difficulty recognizing faces, also occurs with right parietal lesions. *Left parietal lesions* cause receptive or sensory dysphagia, often with jargon utterances and inappropriate responses to the auditory environment. Contralateral spatial neglect is less common with left than with right sided parietal lesions. Gerstmann's syndrome, consisting of agraphia, acalculia, finger agnosia and right/left disorientation, is classically associated with left parietal disease; however, it is rare for all four components to occur together in the same patient.

Hemianopia in right parietal disease is sometimes described as 'complex', meaning that it is associated with visual neglect, impairment of perception of the midline of visual space and with other phenomena, including disorientation in the homonymous field deficit, and illusions or hallucinations in this field. These phenomena are serious disabilities since they interfere with rehabilitation.

Frontal lesions

The frontal lobes are involved with personality, initiation of activity and emotional drive, planning and judgement, speech expression and social graces, and with motor function. They contain the primary motor cortex and the associational motor cortex. The left frontal lobe is specialized for language.

Lesions of the *left inferior frontal lobe* cause aphasia. There is impairment of verbal fluency and perseveration of previously uttered phrases may affect spontaneous and conversational verbal communication. *Right frontal lesions* are relatively silent and most recognized clinical syndromes associated with frontal lobe disease occur in patients with bilateral frontal lobe disease. *Frontal lobe lesions* cause impairment of abstract thinking, loss of drive and spontaneity in thought and behaviour. This leads to an apathetic state, with inability to plan, impairment of problem-solving abilities, impairment of learning of abstract information, rigidity and inflexibility in thought and behaviour and focal disturbances, including contra-lateral hemiparesis and impaired conjugate gaze to the opposite side. Incontinence is common with frontal lobe disease, consisting of inappropriate micturition, with urge incontinence. The gait may be disturbed with small steps (Brun's frontal ataxia) and there may be motor and ideational apraxia. *Motor apraxia* consists of an inability to formulate a complex motor task in the absence of other causative clinical deficit, e.g. upper or lower motor neuron lesion. Primitive reflexes are often released, especially a plastic rigidity in opposition to passive movements in any plane (gegenhalten: literally 'go-stop'), palmar and plantar grasp and traction reflexes, and inappropriately maintained postures, sometimes resembling catatonia. Focal motor seizures, and status epilepticus are typical features of frontal lobe tumours or infections involving frontal lobe.

Occipital lesions

Field defects, cortical blindness and visual agnosia occur with occipital lesions, since this part of the cortex is particularly concerned with visual perception. Specific disturbances of visual persistence, colour and face perception and of three-dimensional perception also occur. The macular part of the visual field is represented at the tip of each occipital lobe, and the peripheral fields deeply within the calcarine cortex. Superficial injuries to the occipital lobes, as in blunt trauma, may therefore involve central fields, and penetrating wounds, as in gunshot injuries, particularly affect the peripheral fields.

Speech disorders

Disorders of *language* (*aphasia*) are associated with disease in the left frontal, temporal and parietal lobes. Disorders of *articulation* (dysarthria) are usually due to disease of the larynx, mouth, tongue, brain stem or basal ganglia, but can arise also with frontal lobe disease. Cerebellar, pseudobulbar and extrapyramidal dysarthrias can be recognized clinically, usually associated with other features of disease in these systems. Cultural speech idioms must be considered in assessing speech cadence and character.

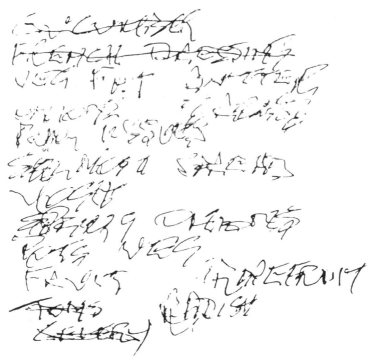

Fig. 1.3 Agraphia in an aphasic patient. There are errors in spacing, letter formation, and spelling.

Aphasia consists of disturbances of articulation, fluency, naming, repetition, comprehension, reading, writing and the use of other symbols, e.g. mathematical or musical symbols (Fig. 1.3). It is almost always due to left hemisphere disease. Left frontal lesions particularly affect articulation and fluency; left temporal lesions disturb fluency, verbal comprehension, repetition and writing, with paraphasias. Parietal lesions disturb associative functions, especially writing and repetition (conduction aphasia). Descriptions of aphasia are confusing because of the use of psychological or anatomical classifications. A simple approach is to classify aphasia as *anterior* or *posterior*. In the former, fluency is impaired and there are hesitations and problems with word recall, but comprehension is normal. In posterior lesions, words are produced relatively readily, but incorrectly and comprehension is severely impaired. The patient does not perceive or monitor errors accurately.

Handedness and cerebral dominance

The concept of *cerebral dominance* arose from the observation of Broca, in the 19th century, that language was usually localized in the left cerebral hemisphere. Since much of the higher cortical activity associated with human behaviour is verbal, or verbally-encoded, the language-based hemisphere was termed dominant and the contralateral, usually the right, hemisphere non-dominant. Hand preference is commonly associated with language, so that most people are right-handed. In more than 90% of right-handed people speech is located in the left hemisphere. The situation in left-handed people is more complex; 50% have right-sided speech localization, 40% left-sided and 10% bilateral language representation. These figures imply that some left-handed people have suffered damage to the left hemisphere in early life, and that a few right-handed people will develop dysphasia with right hemisphere lesions. Language localization is accompanied by asymmetry of the two sides of the brain. The area of the operculum, i.e. the superior surface of the temporal lobe, in the Sylvian fissure is greater on the dominant side.

Development dyslexia, a disorder in which there is an inborn difficulty with reading, spelling and writing, with mirror writing, is associated with left-handedness, suggesting an abnormality of cerebral dominance. Stuttering is also associated with left-handedness. Cerebral dominance is established during infancy, but it is possible for a child to reacquire language after a left-hemisphere injury up to the age of 3 or 4 years, presumably by using the undamaged right hemisphere.

The right hemisphere is itself specialized, especially for attention, emotional responses and visuo-spatial function; it is therefore not necessarily intrinsically subservient to the left hemisphere.

Memory disorders

Memory is impaired with lesions of the temporal lobes, hippocampus, mammillary bodies, fornices and medial thalamic nuclei. Memory is a complex function, and separate syndromes of impaired immediate and short-term memory, and long-term memory are recognized. In addition, alterations of spatial, visual, tactile and other modality-specific aspects of memory can sometimes be discerned, particularly in patients with diffuse or generalized degenerative brain disease. *Short-term memory* is impaired in Wernicke-Korsakoff syndrome, transient global amnesia, post-traumatic encephalopathy, post-encephalitic syndromes, and especially in Alzheimer's dementia and other degenerative dementias.

Short-term memory is assessed by analysis of the history and by testing recall of a simple sentence, a sequence of words or of seven digits forwards and backwards. Performance in immediate recall and short-term recall, after a delay of a few minutes with or without a period of intervening distraction, is tested. Recall of recent daily activities, e.g. meals, visits, conversations, etc., are also reliable data.

Longer term memory is tested by assessing knowledge of public and personal events; various standardized protocols are used for this purpose.

Dementia

The syndrome of dementia implies global impairment of mental function (see Chapter 10). However, memory is the most readily assessable aspect of mental function at the bedside, and it is

Table 1.3 *Mental status questionnaire (MSQ).*

	Score
Where are we now?	1
Where is this place?	1
What is today's *date, month, year*?	3
How old are you?	1
When is your birthday?	1
What year were you born?	1
Who is the Prime Minister?	1
Who was the previous Prime Minister?	1

Table 1.4 *The mini mental state examination.*

Orientation—1 point for each correct answer
  What is the:
    time
    date
    day
    month
    year   5 points
  What is the name of this:
    ward
    hospital
    district
    town
    country   5 points

Registration
  Name three objects
  Score 1,2,3 points according to how many are repeated
  Re-submit list until patient word perfect in order to use this
    for a later test of recall
  Score only first attempt   3 points

Attention and calculation
  Have the patient subtract 7 from 100 and then from the
    result a total of five times. Score 1 point for each correct
    subtraction   5 points

Recall
  Ask for the three objects used in the registration test, one
    point being awarded for each correct answer   3 points

Language
  1 point each for two objects correctly named (pencil and
    watch)   2 points
  1 point for correct repetition of 'No ifs, ands and buts'   1 point
  3 points if three-stage commands correctly obeyed 'Take this
    piece of paper in your right hand, fold it in half, and place
    it on the floor'   3 points
  1 point for correct response to a written command such as
    'close your eyes'   1 point
  Have the patient write a sentence. Award 1 point if the sentence
    is meaningful, has a verb and a subject   1 point
  Test the patient's ability to copy a complex diagram of two
    intersected pentagons   1 point
Total score 30

characteristically affected early in the course of most dementias, especially in Alzheimer's disease. The mental state must be examined in a formal, systematic and semi-quantitative way. Several bedside protocols are available (Table 1.3).

A score of 9–10 in the MSQ is normal; scores of 6–8 represent slight mental confusion, 3–5 moderate confusion and 0–2 severe confusion. The other test in common clinical use is the Mini Mental State Examination (Table 1.4). A total score of 30 is possible. This test differs from the mental status questionnaire in that the score achieved is, to some extent, dependent on educational level. Scores between 21 and 30 are normal, but scores lower than 21 are associated with cognitive impairment. These two tests are not capable of differentiating focal and diffuse cerebral disease. More complex tests, such as the Wechsler Adult Intelligence Score (WAIS) and specific tests of other cortical functions are used by cognitive psychologists in diagnosis and assessment of patients.

Psychological disturbances and neurological disease

This term is used to describe abnormalities of thought, behaviour, personality and mood not directly due to brain lesions. The limits of this concept are indefinable, since some functional disorders, such as schizophrenia and manic-depressive psychosis, are classified as non-organic psychoses although it is recognized that they are due, at least in part, to biochemically determined brain dysfunction.

The syndromes listed in Table 1.5 may present to the neurologist as a neurological symptom, such as headache, dizziness or memory disturbance, or to the psychiatrist with changes in mood or affect. Other symptoms affecting other bodily systems are well-known in other specialties, e.g. chest pain, diarrhoea and abdominal pain. In some patients the psychological disturbance leads to medical consultation, revealing an underlying disorder, such as mild Parkinson's disease, or Huntington's chorea. In others, the psychological disturbance is a complication of severe brain disease, e.g. in frontal tumours, Alzheimer's dementia or severe multiple sclerosis.

Table 1.5 *Psychological disturbances, related to neurological disease.*

Anxiety states
Depression
Conversion hysteria
Post-traumatic syndrome
Dementia and delirium
(see Chapter 10)

Anxiety states

Anxious patients are common, but anxiety of sufficient degree to be a disabling problem is less frequent, forming part of a personality disorder in which the patient is unable to cope with the ordinary events and stresses of life. In the latter patients the main response to external events is emotionally determined and rational explanations are not heeded. There may be a variety of symptoms suggestive of autonomic dysfunction, especially tachycardia, palpitations, dry mouth, blurred vision, breathlessness, weakness and fatiguability, frequency of micturition, diarrhoea and constipation, and abdominal discomfort. Panic attacks, consisting of overwhelming anxiety and fear for which there may be no subsequent memory, occur in some patients. These may be mistaken for epilepsy or other serious organic disorders.

Anxiety may be induced by external life events, such as the death of a relative, psychosexual problems, redundancy and divorce, and in these cases the prognosis is dependent on resolution of the causative problem. Anxiety related to real or imagined disease is more difficult to manage since even extensive negative investigation may not reassure the patient. Psychotherapy can be effective and sedative or tranquillizer medication is useful. The latter should be used only in short courses unless all else has failed because of the risk of habituation to benzodiazepines. Uncontrolled anxiety can lead to phobias concerning specific external objects or situations, and these carry a poor prognosis.

Depression

The cardinal features of depression are feelings of sadness and inadequacy, slowness of thought and movement, poor concentration, loss of initiative, poor grooming, insomnia with early waking and impotence. The overall sadness of affect is recognized by friends and relatives. When appropriate to external events, such as bereavement, this is a normal response but when continued inappropriately or occurring in response to a minor problem it is termed *reactive depression*. *Endogeneous depression* arises spontaneously as part of a major psychiatric illness often associated with swings into relative elation (manic-depressive illness or bipolar depression).

Reactive depression is common in neurological clinics, where it may present with difficulty with memory and concentration, headache, dizziness and anxiety. For example, fear of neurological illness such as brain tumour may lead to anxiety, tension, headache and depression. Investigation will exclude the feared underlying cause for the symptom. Patients with newly-diagnosed major neurological disease such as multiple sclerosis or motor neuron disease may also develop a reactive depressive illness. In Parkinson's disease and Alzheimer's disease depression is a particularly characteristic and frequent symptom, so much so that it may form part of the disease itself. Depression also frequently complicates stroke.

In all these organic disorders tricyclic antidepressants are effective when given in short courses of 6–12 weeks, but many patients respond to reassurance and explanations of the nature of the underlying cause of their symptoms. The somatic symptoms resolve with the psychological disturbance. Somatic symptoms in depressive illness are especially common in certain cultures, but the reasons for this are not known.

Hysteria

The concept of hysteria is fraught with difficulty for the neurologist. In classical 'conversion hysteria' the physical symptom arises from conversion of an unresolved psychological conflict into a physical disability. The physical manifestation is such that the unresolved conflict is averted, and the patient typically assumes an air of indifference. The latter conceals an underlying torment so that unmasking of the hysterical symptom can safely be achieved only if the underlying conflict is also appropriately brought to the surface, and resolved. Patients developing this form of classical major hysteria show features of the hysterical personality disorder, consisting of immaturity and instability of affect, egocentricity, possessiveness and suggestibility. It is characteristic that the patient thrusts the whole problem onto the doctor, passively accepting advice, investigation and treatment. This form of conversion hysteria is most common among people relatively ill-educated or isolated from the complex world around them.

Contemporary experience of the concept of hysteria is different, and a diagnosis of conversion hysteria in neurological practice is likely to be both wrong and dangerous. Most patients showing hysterical personality traits and exaggerated symptoms or disabilities in fact have an underlying disorder that requires elucidation. The common presentations are paralysis of limbs or parts of a limb, gait disorder, sensory loss, pseudoseizures, involuntary movements, amnesia and blindness. In all these syndromes the diagnosis of hysteria is suspected on clinical grounds by the inappropriateness of the physiological or anatomical features of the clinical disability, by the absence of any demonstrable organic disorder of the nervous system by investigation, and by the presence of a personality disorder, and of an unresolved psychological conflict or problem.

In many patients, however, the situation is more complex. The clinical disorder appears inappropriate, or perhaps exaggerated, but examination and investigation reveal evidence of underlying neurological disease. In these patients recognition of the organic disorder usually results in improvement in the overlying functional component. Sometimes a gradual process of re-education and explanation is necessary, for example, in patients with pseudoseizures (hysterical seizures) superimposed on a background of infrequent epilepsy.

Post-traumatic syndrome

Severe head injuries cause marked disability in relation to the late effects of closed and penetrating injuries (Chapter 8). Minor injuries to the head are a major cause of functional disability, perhaps due to the potent image of the brain and head as a centre for mental activity. The question of the organic or functional cause of 'post-traumatic syndrome' remains unresolved.

The clinical features of this syndrome often appear inextricably associated with litigation; indeed the syndrome is virtually unknown without this association, or without other forms of secondary gain. For example, it is exceptional in sportsmen or boxers after head injury. The syndrome consists of headache, dizziness, difficulty in concentration, double vision, depression and instability of posture and gait, with anxiety and sleeplessness. Sexual function may be disturbed. These symptoms develop a few days or weeks after an injury, even when the injury was apparently trivial and unassociated with loss of consciousness or post-traumatic amnesia. These symptoms persist for weeks or months and become bound up with social problems following failure to return to work so that compensation becomes necessary in order to restore financial equilibrium; the symptoms provide proof of injury. This relation is complex and a decision to return to work or to full activities is critically important in determining functional recovery. It is important to recognize that some features of the post-traumatic syndrome, especially rotational vertigo and positional vertigo, are usually due to damage to the utricle in the inner ear. This can be disabling initially, but usually improves in a few weeks or months. A failed attempt to return to work is emotionally devastating and may result from lack of appreciation of labyrinthine injury.

The prognosis of the post-traumatic syndrome is generally good, although some cases persist, even after financial settlement on favourable terms, suggesting that in these cases there is an underlying organic problem related to the injury. Treatment with antidepressant drugs is often helpful when recovery is occurring, and industrial and social rehabilitation are important aspects of management.

Autonomic and sphincter disturbances

Dysfunction of the autonomic nervous system occurs in primary degenerative diseases of the central pathways, in peripheral neuropathies and with drugs (Chapters 12 and 13). The clinical features reflect involvement of the components of this neural system (Table 1.6).

Table 1.6 *Clinical features of autonomic disorders.*

Postural hypotension
Hypothermia
Disturbed sweating
Disorders of bowel function
  constipation and incontinence
Retention or incontinence of urine
  urgency, frequency and nocturia
Pupillary disturbances
Disturbances of breathing
Loss of libido and impotence

Seizures

The clinical features of seizure disorders are discussed in Chapter 2.

Investigation and management in neurological disease

The understanding and analysis of symptoms and signs in patients with neurological disease is important in planning subsequent investigation and, if indicated, management and treatment. Diagnosis is part of this process. The disorders that affect the nervous system can be classified in similar fashion to those that affect other bodily systems (Table 1.7). The diseases and functional disturbances discussed in the following chapters of this book can be grouped into this classification. Some neurological disorders, such as the management of coma, involve many aspects of the causes of disease listed in Table 1.7, and this approach is therefore useful in everyday practice.

Investigation in neurology is intended to define the clinical problem in order to clarify its underlying cause and, therefore, to aid management and treatment. Various approaches are available.

Table 1.7 *Classification of diseases.*

Acquired
    Inflammatory
    Neoplastic
    Vascular
    Degenerative and demyelinating
    Traumatic
    Toxic
    Metabolic

Congenital
    Genetic
    Developmental

Table 1.8 *Methods of investigation in neurological disease and their use.*

Blood	
haematology	coagulation, anaemia, leukaemia etc.
biochemistry	metabolic disorders
immunological	inflammatory disorders
serological	infections
Imaging	
plain X-rays	trauma
CT scan of head, spine and muscles	CNS, bone and muscle, especially tumours and stroke
MRI	CNS imaging, e.g. multiple sclerosis
myelography	cord and root disease
angiography	vascular disease and tumours
PET scanning	functional metabolic evaluations
ultrasound	Doppler flowmetry in vascular disease
Neurophysiology	
EMG	peripheral nerve and muscle
evoked responses	CNS, root and cord disease
central motor conduction	CNS, root and cord disease
EEG	epilepsy and encephalopathies
CSF	infections and immunological disorders
Ophthalmological	specialized applications
Neuro-otological	
Neuropsychology	dementia, focal brain lesions, epilepsy
Genetic studies	inherited disease
Biopsies	CNS, peripheral nerve and muscle

Disorders affecting the central nervous system require a different approach from those involving the peripheral nervous system, and underlying systemic diseases may have complex clinical effects on the nervous system. The various methods of investigation are listed in Table 1.8, and their relevance in clinical practice is described in the appropriate sections of the text.

2

Fits, Faints and Blackouts

Sudden, transient episodes of loss or alteration of consciousness are a common clinical problem. Patients often describe such attacks as *blackouts*, a term that has no precise diagnostic meaning. Such attacks may be due to epilepsy, vascular disease, syncope, hypoglycaemia, alcoholism, and, perhaps, basilar migraine and vestibular disease. Loss of consciousness may also be a presentation of psychiatric problems. In *narcolepsy* the onset of disturbed consciousness may be abrupt but most sleep disorders are associated with persistent drowsiness, or difficulty awakening or going to sleep. In the *parasomnias* there is abnormal behaviour during sleep, e.g. terror attacks or sleep-walking (somnambulism); these are not epileptic phenomena. In *drop attacks* there is a sudden brief loss of posture, often with transient alteration of consciousness, followed by rapid recovery; the cause of this syndrome is unknown. In some patients, despite intensive investigation, the cause of 'blackouts' remains unknown, and emotional or other intense experiences may be a factor.

In children and young people epilepsy is probably the commonest cause of transient loss of consciousness, although in adolescence and young adults syncope is also frequent. In older populations transient ischaemic attacks from degenerative vascular disease are frequent but many patients with cerebrovascular disease also have epilepsy. Drop attacks, with or without loss of consciousness occur particularly in elderly women.

Epilepsy

Epilepsy is a clinical diagnosis. Recognition is comparatively easy when a fit is witnessed, or described by the patient, but diagnosis in a patient complaining of attacks of altered consciousness or blackouts, without a clear story of certain major features suggestive of epilepsy, may be very difficult. In partial forms of epilepsy an attack may consist of motor or sensory features without change in consciousness, a reflection of the mode of onset, progression and

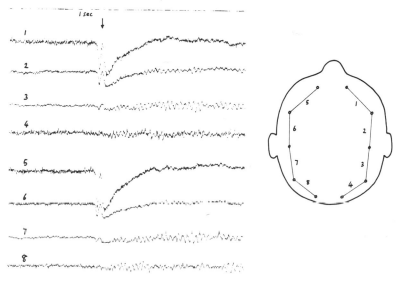

Fig. 2.1 Normal EEG. The electrode placements are shown on the head chart, each line of the EEG tracing representing the potential differences between a pair of electrodes. In the posterior head regions the background activity is at 8–13 Hz (alpha activity). This alpha activity is activated when the eyes are closed. The arrow indicates eye closure artefact.

extent of the physiological abnormality in the brain during the attack. Hughlings Jackson defined epilepsy as 'an occasional, sudden, excessive, rapid and localizing discharge of gray matter'. This definition is as acceptable today as it was in 1873, but the presence of neuronal discharges during the epileptic fit is almost always a supposition, since direct electrophysiological observations are scarcely ever available during seizures; they are, however, commonly available in EEG records made interictally (Figs 2.1 and 2.2).

In some patients recurrent attacks of cerebral dysfunction may occur that may be difficult to distinguish from migraine, or from brain stem vertigo. These phenomena, of uncertain aetiology, were termed 'the borderlands of epilepsy' by Gowers (1907). Any definition of epilepsy must include an exclusion of altered cerebral function due to transient cerebral ischaemic attacks, particularly since clinical phenomena resembling focal epilepsy may be a feature of transient ischaemic attacks and these, like epilepsy, may be recurrent. The term epilepsy implies a tendency to *recurrent seizures*; an isolated seizure does not constitute a diagnosis of epilepsy. However, the probability of recurrence following a first tonic/clonic seizure is 60% in the first year.

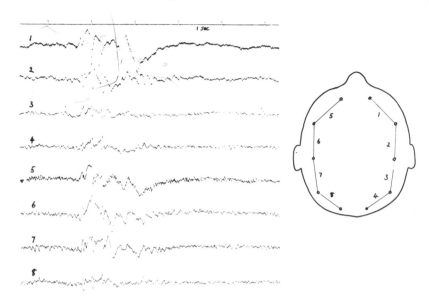

Fig. 2.2 EEG in idiopathic epilepsy. In this EEG generalized bursts containing multiple spikes are seen. The patient had major generalized seizures (grand mal).

Epilepsy is virtually always a manifestation of dysfunction of the cerebral hemispheres. The site of the underlying abnormality in primary generalized epilepsies is controversial, but the development of a generalized seizure probably involves deep central structures, as well as both hemispheres through their callosal connections. This is exemplified by the occurrence of generalized tonic/clonic seizures in patients with focal cortical lesions. Localized abnormalities in the brain stem or cerebellum do not cause epilepsy.

Epidemiology

Epilepsy is a common disorder. The prevalence of patients undergoing treatment for epilepsy is approximately 0.5%. This pool of patients is subject to change in relation to newly diagnosed cases entering it and patients leaving it in remission or from death; the annual incidence of epilepsy varies in different studies from 30 to about 50/100 000 (0.05%). Thus the average duration of epilepsy requiring treatment is about 10 years. However, these figures conceal marked age-related variations. About 2% of children under the age of 2 years have had at least one seizure and about 5% of 8 year olds have had at least one seizure. The incidence of seizures reaches a second peak in adolescence and early life, but declines in maturity.

Table 2.1 *Classification of epilepsy (according to clinical features).*

	Clinical type	Synonyms	Significance
Generalized epilepsy			
	tonic/clonic seizures	grand mal major epilepsy	symptomatic or idiopathic
	absence seizures	petit mal minor epilepsy	idiopathic
	myoclonic seizures	jerks infantile spasms	usually idiopathic
Partial epilepsy			
	simple partial seizures	psychomotor epilepsy	symptomatic or idiopathic
	motor	Jacksonian epilepsy	usually symptomatic
	somato-sensory		usually symptomatic
	visual	focal epilepsies	usually symptomatic
	auditory		usually symptomatic
	autonomic		usually symptomatic
	psychological	psychic seizures	usually symptomatic
	benign focal epilepsy of childhood	Rolandic epilepsy	idiopathic
	complex partial seizures	temporal lobe epilepsy (with altered consciousness)	symptomatic or idiopathic
	focal myoclonus		symptomatic or idiopathic
	reflex epilepsy	reading epilepsy etc.	idiopathic

However, symptomatic epilepsy, due to acquired brain disease, becomes an increasingly important cause with increasing age, especially after the age of 60 years. Mortality rates for people with epilepsy approximate those of the population as a whole, if symptomatic epilepsy, often due to severe or progressive brain disease, is excluded.

Classification

There have been many attempts to classify epilepsy. The terms *grand mal, petit mal, (absence seizures), temporal lobe (psychomotor) seizures* and *myoclonus epilepsy* remain useful as general descriptive terms, and may be well-known to patients.

Currently, the terms *generalized epilepsy* and *partial epilepsy* are used. This classification (Table 2.1) utilizes both clinical and electroencephalographic (EEG) data. In generalized epilepsy the seizure is generalized from the onset, or becomes secondarily generalized from an initial, focal origin. In partial epilepsy the seizure is restricted in its manifestation to one hemisphere, or to part of one hemisphere throughout the attack, or until secondary generalization occurs (Table 2.1). This classification has practical value in relation to the plan of investigation and management. The physician has always to remember that epilepsy may be *symptomatic* or *idiopathic*, depending on whether or not there is an underlying structural or metabolic cause, or whether no such cause can be demonstrated. In symptomatic epilepsy management requires ascertainment and treatment of the underlying cause as well as treatment of the seizures themselves.

Clinical features of generalized seizures

Tonic/clonic seizures. These seizures are the most well-known form of epilepsy. The attack may begin with a poorly characterized subjective sensation, often epigastric in location, or consisting of a feeling of dread. This aura is not of clinical localizing significance, but is probably due to excitation of a small area of the cortex. To the onlooker the patient suddenly loses consciousness, perhaps after a brief moment of confusion or pallor, falling to the ground in a *tonic phase* of extension of the legs and adduction of the arms with flexion at the elbow and wrists. The tonic phase represents widespread excitation of the brain. There may be a loud cry as air is forcibly expired past the tensed vocal cords by contraction of the respiratory musculature. Because the respiratory muscles are tonically contracted, ventilation ceases during this tonic phase and cyanosis develops. Sometimes the eyes roll upwards and the teeth are tightly clenched, causing injury to the tongue. If the bladder is full, urine is expelled by the contraction of the abdominal muscles. Contraction of paraspinal muscles may sometimes be sufficient to cause compression fractures of one or more vertebrae.

This tonic phase is followed by a *clonic phase* of alternating excitation and inhibition causing symmetrical contraction and relaxation of muscles, gradually slowing in frequency during 30 seconds to a minute or two. This is followed by a *post-ictal phase* consisting of flaccid coma with stertorous respiration and salivation, or drowsiness, confusion and headache. Following this the patient will often sleep for an hour or more. During the tonic and clonic phases, and the post-ictal phase of the seizure the patient is unrousable and the plantar responses are extensor; they become flexor when consciousness is regained. Injuries to soft tissues are common in tonic/clonic seizures, and sudden death may rarely occur.

Serial epilepsy consists of recurrent seizures separated by brief periods of consciousness. In *status epilepticus*, a life-threatening event, recurrent or continuous tonic/clonic seizures occur without intervening recovery of consciousness. Status epilepticus may be primarily generalized, or secondarily generalized from a focal onset. This may occur in established epilepsy but it is often a presenting feature of focal brain disease, especially frontal tumours, cerebral abscess and encephalitis.

Tonic/clonic seizures with focal onset. Partial seizures may become secondarily generalized, leading to typical tonic/clonic convulsions. The onset of the tonic/clonic seizure is thus particularly important in defining its underlying cause. Focal motor, sensory, visual or temporal lobe disturbances may occur at the onset of the attack and, especially in the latter, may be prolonged, lasting several seconds or minutes. Thus a prodromal period of disturbed speech (aphasia) is an important indication of left temporal lobe disturbance. However, when there is underlying focal brain disease the pattern of seizure may be variable, some attacks consisting of focal (partial) seizures, and others continuing into a phase of generalization. Focal features developing in the post-ictal phase are of less diagnostic significance, since they may result from the metabolic and circulatory consequences of the seizure discharge. Marked focal disturbances in the post-ictal phase, for example, hemiplegia, are sometimes termed *Todd's (post-epileptic) paralysis*. Such functional disturbances usually resolve in a few minutes; they imply a post-epileptic inhibitory state in cortical neurons rather than metabolic exhaustion.

Absence seizures (petit mal epilepsy). This less dramatic form of generalized epilepsy occurs mainly in children. The attacks consist of sudden brief blank spells without change in posture, often accompanied by pallor or flushing, blinking of the eyelids, pupillary dilatation and slight twitching of the facial and limb muscles. Arrest of thought and activity is characteristic. Recovery is abrupt, but attacks may be repeated and frequent. Behavioural disturbance or learning problems may result from inattention caused by the attacks. Patient and family may be unaware of brief attacks. There is often a family history of this form of epilepsy. Very rarely, attacks may continue for many minutes (*petit mal status*).

Typical absence seizures are most frequent in late childhood and early adolescence, and they only rarely continue into adult life. However, complex partial seizures or tonic/clonic generalized seizures develop in more than half of affected children in adult life. *Akinetic seizures* are a variant of absence attacks in which

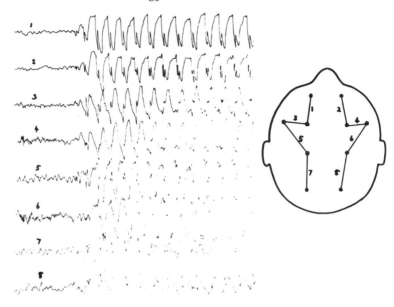

Fig. 2.3 EEG in idiopathic epilepsy of petit mal type. In this primary generalized epilepsy, symmetrical and synchronous bursts of spike and wave discharges occur at 3–3.5 Hz.

the patient may drop abruptly to the ground without tonic or clonic movement.

Absence seizures are accompanied by a characteristic EEG abnormality, consisting of bursts of high voltage spike and slow wave discharges repeated at 3 Hz (Fig. 2.3). Bursts lasting longer than about 3 seconds are associated with the clinical features of the seizure. Overbreathing will often induce the EEG discharge and typical absence attacks.

Myoclonus epilepsy. The word myoclonus is used to describe a sudden jerk of a muscle, limb or of the whole body. Myoclonus occurs in many different diseases of the nervous system, but myoclonus in patients with epilepsy is a feature of absence seizures, and of hereditary and degenerative disorders, especially lipid storage diseases. It is common in idiopathic tonic/clonic generalized epilepsy, especially in the first hour or so after waking from sleep. *Flexion myoclonus* in drowsiness, however, is a normal phenomenon. *Action myoclonus* consists of myoclonus induced by voluntary movement. *Reflex myoclonus* may be invoked by visual, tactile or auditory stimuli.

Salaam spasms (West's syndrome) is a rare form of flexion myoclonic epilepsy, occurring in infants with intractable seizures and associated with mental retardation, and with tuberose sclerosis. The prognosis is poor but sometimes the condition responds to treatment with valproate, pyridoxine or steroids.

Febrile convulsions. Tonic/clonic seizures occurring between the ages of 6 months and 5 years in association with fever greater than 38°C, called *febrile convulsions*, occur in about 5% of children. There is a family history of similar attacks in 50% of cases. The risk of a second attack is about 25%. This dramatic event often leads to the fear of a serious underlying cause, such as meningitis, at least on the first occasion, but investigation reveals no abnormality in the brain.

The risk of development of epilepsy later in childhood or in adult life is dependent on three factors; focal features, repeated seizures during 24 hours, and a long duration of individual febrile seizures (>30 minutes). In the absence of these factors the risk of later epilepsy is about 2.5%, but when two risk factors are present it is 20%, and with all three factors 50%. Thus anticonvulsant drugs probably should be used only in the presence of these adverse clinical features.

Clinical features of partial seizures

Simple partial seizures. These focal epilepsies occur in motor, sensory, psychomotor or compound forms. The clinical manifestations depend on the localization of the causative lesion, but partial epilepsy may also follow childhood epilepsy of idiopathic type. *Motor seizures* originate in the frontal cortex, causing contralateral jerking movements, or Jacksonian march of jerking movement in a limb corresponding to progressive excitation of the motor cortex. The hand or face area is usually affected first, perhaps because of the relative extent of this cortical representation. Adversive eye movements, that resemble nystagmus, are also a feature of frontal seizures. In *benign focal epilepsy of childhood* focal seizures usually occur in sleep. This disorder accounts for 16% of childhood epilepsy. The seizures cease after the age of 13 years. *Sensory* seizures are the sensory equivalent of focal motor seizures. *Visual* seizures consist of hallucinatory experiences, of photopsias (red or orange ball-like images) or, rarely, geometric shapes. *Auditory* seizures are rare.

In *temporal lobe seizures* (psychomotor epilepsy) the attack is characterized by a stereotyped sequence of disturbed perception and awareness. The attack commences with feelings of unreality (*jamais vu*) or undue familiarity (*déjà vu*), and there may be olfactory hallucinations, accompanied by 'tasting movements' of the lips and tongue. Dizziness, vertigo, fear and stereotyped auditory hallucinations, described by Jackson as 'dreamy states' are characteristic. The sense of time may be distorted and there may be visual hallucinations, resembling a remembered scene, macropsia or micropsia. When the left temporal lobe is involved aphasia may be apparent during the attack. Usually only some of these clinical features develop in individual patients, but the attacks are remarkably stereotyped. Olfactory hallucinations are particularly associated with focal lesions, e.g. gliomas, in the temporal lobe.

Complex partial seizures. Simple partial seizures followed by impairment of consciousness, with or without automatisms, are termed complex partial seizures. Impairment of consciousness in the attack implies secondary generalization of the seizure, but the patient does not become comatose. *Automatisms* consist of repetitive, stereotyped, non-purposeful activity or behaviour. They are rarely well-formed, but may consist of complicated behavioural patterns, such as wandering or partial undressing and dressing. Aggressive behaviour may occur if the patient is disturbed, but it is not directed. Psychomotor seizures accompanied by disturbed consciousness are also termed complex partial seizures.

Causes of epilepsy

In idiopathic epilepsy the seizure disorder is associated with a family history of epilepsy; the risk is about 5% in the relatives of an affected person but is higher in febrile convulsions and in absence seizures. It is important to recognize that seizures will occur, given an appropriate stimulus, in all persons; for example seizures can always

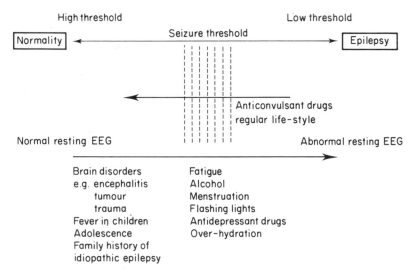

Fig. 2.4 Seizure threshold and epilepsy.

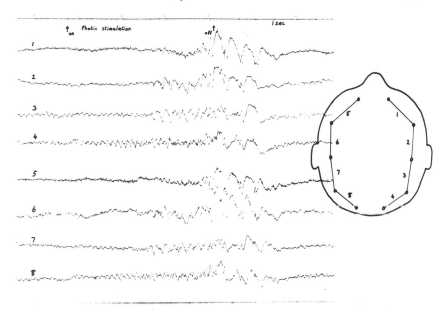

Fig. 2.5 Photosensitive epilepsy. The EEG shows a photoconvulsive response. During flash stimulation at 10 Hz there are following responses in the occipital leads of the EEG which evolve into a generalized burst of spike and wave seizure activity.

be induced by electric shocks applied to the brain and by certain convulsive drugs. However, the seizure threshold (Fig. 2.4) varies in different people, and in response to certain factors, e.g. flashing lights (Fig. 2.5), fatigue, over-hydration, alcohol and drug withdrawal, and the premenstrual phase of the menstrual cycle. The seizure threshold is an inherited property of the brain; when it is low paroxysmal EEG discharges are present in the resting record, consisting of slow waves or spike discharges. Sometimes these are induced only by hyperventilation or sleep.

Epileptiform EEG abnormalities are not necessarily expressed as seizures although they predispose to the occurrence of seizures. Indeed a paroxysmal EEG abnormality is only exceptionally found in people who have never had a seizure, except in relatives of people with idiopathic epilepsy. The interictal EEG record is valuable in the diagnosis of epilepsy since it is a measure of the seizure threshold (Fig. 2.2) and, in addition, it provides information about the localization of underlying focal brain lesions. The type of EEG discharge is also useful in management decisions regarding anticonvulsant drug therapy.

Symptomatic epilepsy occurs because a structural or metabolic brain lesion has caused epileptiform activity in groups of neurons,

Table 2.2 *Causes of symptomatic epilepsy.*

Congenital lesions of the brain
Acquired lesions of the brain
trauma
infection
viral encephalitis
cerebral abscess
meningitis
vascular
tumour
degenerative
metabolic
toxic and drug-induced

leading to partial or generalized epilepsy. The brain may react with seizures to a wide variety of different disorders, including structural disorders of acute or chronic type, and metabolic disturbances, e.g. hypocalcaemia, hyponatraemia and hypoglycaemia. In many instances, e.g. cerebral abscess and hypoglycaemia the prognosis is determined by the underlying causative disorder. Epilepsy may develop months or years after the onset of a brain lesion, e.g. cerebral trauma or infarction, perinatal injury or slow-growing tumour.

Investigation of epilepsy

The diagnosis of epilepsy is essentially clinical. Investigation is designed, first, to delineate more precisely the type of epilepsy in terms of its electrophysiological characteristics as shown by the electroencephalogram (EEG). Secondly, a search for underlying causes (see Table 2.2) is required, especially in late-onset epilepsy, in order to exclude any underlying cause. Since most seizures in childhood and adolescence are febrile seizures, idiopathic (primary epilepsy), or can be related to perinatal or neonatal causes, especially traumatic and hypoxic brain injury, investigation is unlikely to yield any information that will modify management in this age group. A precise definition of '*late-onset epilepsy*' is impossible, but seizures beginning after the age of 20 years generally merit more detailed investigation. When seizures are generalized, there is no neurological abnormality on examination and the EEG shows no focal discharge; investigation yields a causative lesion in only about 4% of cases and most of these will not require specific treatment. Tumours are most likely to be found in subjects in the fourth to sixth decades, and in older subjects vascular and degenerative diseases are common. Thus in most young subjects investigation can be limited, initially, to EEG examination.

Further investigation, when indicated, should include routine blood count and VDRL tests, and blood sugar and calcium measurements may also be considered. A CT brain scan is indicated in late-onset epilepsy and in any patient with partial seizures; in some patients with generalized epilepsy the EEG may disclose an unexpected focal abnormality and, particularly if this is accompanied by slow waves, CT scanning is indicated to evaluate the possibility of focal brain disease. Magnetic resonance imaging is probably of greater sensitivity than CT scanning in evaluating this problem. Additional useful investigations include liver function tests with γGT levels in alcoholism. Further specialized tests are useful in patients with difficult epilepsy, for example combined EEG/video monitoring when seizures are of uncertain type or may be due to hysteria, and ambulatory EEG monitoring.

General medical assessment is required in all patients, and this becomes more important in older patients in whom cardiovascular and cerebrovascular disease may be present. In addition, metabolic disturbances, e.g. Addison's disease, hyperparathyroidism and diabetes may be recognized.

Management and treatment

In general, single seizures do not merit anticonvulsant drug therapy unless there are pressing social or personal reasons for a patient to be free of the risk of subsequent attacks. However, the risk of a second seizure in an adult presenting with a first seizure not due to acquired brain disease, or to alcohol dependency or other drugs, is about 50% in the subsequent year, and 60% in the subsequent 2 years.

The main principle of anticonvulsant drug treatment (Table 2.3) is to use a single drug whenever possible, rather than a combination of drugs. This is effective in most patients, and avoids the potential interaction and unwanted effects of combined drug therapy. The dosage of the drug chosen should be gradually increased during a period of 4–12 weeks until the minimal effective dosage is reached. If seizures continue despite a serum level within the high therapeutic range a second drug should be introduced, and the dosage of the ineffective drug reduced, or withdrawn as indicated. Unfortunately, in some patients drug treatment is unsatisfactory or even ineffective in any combination. Effective treatment, i.e. cessation of seizures, can be achieved in about two-thirds of patients with tonic/clonic seizures and most of the remainder achieve substantial improvement. However, less than 50% of patients with partial seizures achieve remission. Drug level monitoring is only necessary in patients in whom poor control of seizures has been achieved; in these patients it is often an effective means by which to encourage compliance with treatment.

Table 2.3 Commonly used anticonvulsant drugs.

		Indications	Adult daily dosage (mg)	Effective serum levels (mg/ml)	Unwanted effects
1st line drugs	phenytoin	tonic/clonic seizures	200–400	40–80	gum hypertrophy osteomalacia ataxia and nystagmus macrocytic anaemia lymphadenopathy
	carbamazepine	temporal lobe epilepsy complex partial seizures tonic/clonic seizures	200–800	20–40	drowsiness, diplopia, dizziness rash, liver damage blood dyscrasias
	valproate	absence seizures tonic/clonic seizures myoclonic seizures febrile seizures	600–2000	–[a]	liver damage tremor, weight gain hair loss
2nd line drugs	phenobarbitone	tonic/clonic seizures	30–180	45–100	drowsiness and depression ataxia, rash
	primidone	tonic/clonic seizures	250–1000	25–55	nausea similar to phenobarbitone
	ethosuccimide	absence epilepsy	500–1500	300–600	allergies nausea and vomiting blood dyscrasias weight loss
	clonazepam clobazam }	myoclonic epilepsy	1–6 20–60	–	drowsiness ataxia

[a]Valproate drug levels are not useful in determining seizure control.

In certain clinical situations particular care must be taken:

Pregnancy and epilepsy. Anticonvulsant drugs induce hepatic enzymes and cause more rapid breakdown of oestrogen contraceptive medication, thus increasing the chance of pregnancy. This can be obviated by increasing the dose of contraceptive drugs. Pregnancy has no generally predictable effect on epilepsy, although mothers with complex partial seizures often experience more seizures during pregnancy. There is a slightly increased risk of cleft palate in children born to mothers with epilepsy and this risk is doubled if the mother is treated with anticonvulsant drugs; however, the overall risk is only about twice that of normal mothers. Carbamazepine is the safest drug during pregnancy. Phenytoin is particularly associated with cleft palate and ventricular septal defects, and valproate with neural tube defects. Thus carbamazepine is probably the drug of choice in young women with tonic/clonic or partial seizures.

Generalized status epilepticus. This potentially fatal complication of epilepsy arises from poor compliance with treatment, alcoholism, sleep deprivation and intercurrent infections. It may also be a presenting feature of brain disease, especially cerebral tumours (usually frontal in location), meningitis, cerebral abscess and viral encephalitis. Urgent effective treatment of the seizures is essential in order to prevent anoxic brain damage, or even death (Table 2.4). Focal status epilepticus is a less urgent problem. Intravenous anticonvulsants may cause respiratory suppression severe enough

Table 2.4 *Principles of treatment in generalized status epilepticus*

1. Establish airway and administer oxygen
2. Monitor ECG
3. Establish i.v. access with dextrose/saline infusion
4. Check blood sugar; give glucose i.v. if necessary, or even as speculative therapy
5. Stop seizures with medication:
   (a) diazepam i.v. 10 mg given in 1–3 minutes, repeated or given as slow infusion 10–50 mg/h
   (b) chlormethiazole i.v. infusion 100 mg/kg/h may be effective
   (c) paraldehyde 10 ml i.m. (5 ml in each buttock) is very effective and safe
   (d) thiopentone anaesthesia can be used if other drugs fail; 250 mg i.v. followed by 1–2 mg/kg/h, with ventilation in ITU
6. Phenytoin 300–600 mg (13–18 mg/kg) i.v. is useful to 'load' the patient with anticonvulsant drugs if the patient has not previously been treated
7. Consider underlying causation. EEG or CT scan may be required, particularly if clinical examination suggests focal disease. CSF examination is indicated only if CNS infection is suspected, and if the CT scan excludes cerebral mass lesion or herniation.

to require ventilation. *Non-convulsive status epilepticus*, due to absence status or complex partial epilepsy usually responds to diazepam 10 mg i.m. injection. It is not life-threatening but may persist for hours or even days, causing a confusional state.

Febrile convulsions. A first febrile convulsion may be due to a brain disorder, such as meningitis, and children younger than 18 months should be admitted to hospital for investigation. Cooling by sponging is recommended. Rectal diazepam 0.5 mg/kg may be used to stop seizures lasting longer than about 15 minutes in the home situation. In hospital i.v. diazepam is the drug of choice. When indicated, sodium valproate (20–30 mg/kg) or phenobarbitone (5 mg/kg) may be used as prophylactic anticonvulsants for 1–2 years after the last convulsion. Convulsions of less than 15 minutes duration (65% of febrile convulsions) do not require anticonvulsants.

Surgery for epilepsy. In some patients with seizures refractory to anticonvulsant drugs, surgical excision of a discharging cortical focus, localized by EEG, corticography or depth electrodes, may produce a marked reduction of seizure frequency or even remission. This operation is only appropriate in a small minority of patients with epilepsy, particularly those with unilateral temporal lobe disturbances.

Driving and epilepsy. In the UK patients are required to inform the Driver and Vehicle Licensing Centre (Swansea) on recognition of attacks of unconsciousness, or when advised of a diagnosis of epilepsy. A driving licence is revoked until the patient has been free of daytime seizures for a period of 2 years, treated or untreated. Heavy Goods Vehicle and Public Service Vehicle licences usually are not restored. In the case of a single (first) seizure in adult life occurring in the daytime the driving license authority in the UK may, at its discretion, suspend the licence for 1 year. In the case of continuing nocturnal seizures without daytime seizures a period of 3 years of freedom from daytime attacks is required. Many other countries follow similar guidelines. The physician must ensure that the patient understands his responsibilities to himself and to society in this matter.

Other problems of epilepsy. Many people with epilepsy experience personal difficulties coming to terms with the disorder, particularly if seizures occur in public places, or at work. Certain occupations are hazardous, for example working with unprotected machinery, near dangerous chemicals or fires, or on ladders or at heights, and manual workers are particularly at risk of unemployment. Children with seizures should ordinarily attend normal schools, unless their epilepsy is so poorly controlled as to justify special educational arrangements. No sporting restrictions are necessary but unsupervised swimming must not be allowed.

Outcome of epilepsy. The outcome of treated epilepsy is dependent on the type of seizure, the frequency of seizures before treatment and the initial response to treatment. A good prognosis is associated with tonic/clonic seizures, infrequent seizures, a short history of epilepsy and a good initial response to treatment. A poor prognosis is associated with complex partial seizures, with frequent attacks, with associated neurological handicap and with a poor initial response to treatment. Half of all treated patients continue treatment longer than 5 years, and only 30% continue to have seizures 15 years after diagnosis.

In patients whose seizures have ceased for longer than 2 years the question arises as to whether the drugs can be safely stopped. This is a vexed problem, since recurrence may have serious social and personal consequences, e.g. with driving and employment. If a decision is made to withdraw drugs this should be done cautiously during a period of 6 months or more. EEG assessment during this period is of limited value in prognosis.

Differential diagnosis of epilepsy

Epilepsy is usually a characteristic and easily recognizable disorder. A number of other disorders may be confused with epilepsy either because they are paroxysmal, as in migraine and narcolepsy, or because there is a circulatory disturbance with impairment of consciousness or transient focal neurological disturbance, e.g. syncope, transient global amnesia and transient cerebral ischaemia due to cerebral vascular disease, or to cardiac disease. Psychogenic seizures (pseudoseizures) may mimic epilepsy, and cause difficulty in diagnosis, particularly since they frequently occur in patients with well-documented true epilepsy. Hyperventilation may mimic epilepsy and, in children, breath-holding spells may also be mistaken for epilepsy. Video/EEG ambulatory monitoring is very helpful in sorting out these problems.

Psychogenic seizures. Recognition of pseudoseizures requires awareness of the possibility and inquiry from patient, family and friends concerning emotional, personal and social causative problems. Most patients are young women. The attacks consist of tonic/clonic episodes with 'loss of consciousness' of gradual onset. Recovery is abrupt and complete, but the attacks may be prolonged. They never occur during sleep. Self-injury in attacks, including tongue-biting, may be a feature. The EEG recorded during and immediately after an attack is normal; thus a normal EEG in a patient with clinical epilepsy should suggest a diagnosis of psychogenic seizures. The serum prolactin level is elevated 20 minutes after a true convulsion, particularly in patients with generalized attacks, but does not change after pseudoseizures.

Syncope. Fainting is common, particularly in young people. There is a premonitory phase of blurred vision, tinnitus, vertigo, nausea, and of a complex feeling of time suspension, euphoria or even hallucinations that may resemble complex partial seizures. Hyperventilation and pallor develop and the patient slumps into unconsciousness during a period of a few seconds. This is often induced by standing in a warm or crowded environment, e.g. in a train or in soldiers standing at attention. Unlike epilepsy, injury in an attack is rare. In the recovery phase the patient feels weak and nauseated but there is no mental confusion or drowsiness as occurs in epilepsy. If syncope is prolonged a few clonic jerks may be seen, leading to possible confusion with epilepsy, and a true generalized convulsion may occur in some cases.

Syncope results from reduced cerebral perfusion, causing hypoxia of the brain. This is accompanied by slowing of the EEG. The causes of syncope are summarized in Table 2.5.

The common form of vasovagal syncope is *psychogenic or reflex* in origin. This is caused by a sudden fall in cardiac output, pulse rate

Table 2.5　*Causes of syncope.*

Reflex (vasovagal) syncope
   psychogenic fainting
   cough syncope
   micturition syncope
   carotid sinus syndrome
   hypoglycaemia

Cardiac disorders
   arrhythmias, e.g. Stokes–Adams syncope
             atrial fibrillation
             tachyarrhythmias
   valvular heart disease
   other causes, e.g. atrial myxoma, cardiomyopathy

Orthostatic hypotension
   autonomic neuropathy
   Shy–Drager syndrome
   anti-hypertensive medication
   anaemia and hypovolaemia

Cerebral ischaemia due to cerebral vascular disease

and peripheral vascular resistance, induced by emotional, painful or other extraneous stimuli. *Hypoglycaemia*, or irregular meals are common initiating factors. Vasodepressor mechanisms are also important in *micturition syncope*, a disorder exacerbated by fatigue, alcohol and prostatism. Cardio-inhibitory mechanisms are important in carotid sinus syncope, in which the cerebral perfusion is reduced by reduction in cardiac output and cardiac rate is reduced from vagal stimulation. The pulse rate is often raised when measured in the syncopal phase, when recovery is commencing.

In *Stokes–Adams syncope* the initiating event is transient cardiac arrest or extreme bradycardia associated with complete atrio-ventricular block. There is a brief phase of dizziness, absent-mindedness and blurred vision of a few seconds' duration before consciousness is lost. The patient is pale and flaccid, but a few tonic jerks may occur if the attack is long enough to be associated with dilated pupils (a few seconds).

Orthostatic hypotension may cause abrupt loss of consciousness on assuming the erect posture, usually after a brief premonitory phase resembling that of reflex syncope. Attacks are most likely to occur in the morning, when getting out of bed.

The management of syncope is dependent on the underlying cause; Stokes–Adams syncope is managed by cardiac pacing, and reflex syncope can often be prevented by avoidance of precipitating factors, and especially by avoiding 'missed meals'. Coffee, by its caffeine content, is useful in some people; alcohol consumption should be limited.

Hyperventilation syndrome. This consists of overbreathing, either deliberate or associated with tension and anxiety. This causes tingling in the extremities and face, and even tetany. Palpitations, fatigue, headache, giddiness and loss of consciousness may develop, and many such patients are mistakenly diagnosed as epileptic. This syndrome is common. It responds to symptomatic treatment, e.g rebreathing into a paper bag, but psychotherapeutic help may also be required in dealing with the underlying problem in some patients. There is often a history of multiple consultations, and of tranquillizer abuse, and the patient is usually unaware of the hyperventilation.

Narcolepsy

This syndrome consists of four components. *Narcolepsy* itself consists of overwhelming attacks of sleep, up to 20 minutes' duration. *Cataplexy* consists of sudden brief attacks of loss of muscle tone with preserved consciousness, often provoked by sudden emotional stimuli, especially laughter or surprise. Cataplexy may be mild, consisting of brief nodding of the head, rather than collapse. *Sleep paralysis* consists of attacks of complete inability to move, induced on falling asleep or awakening, and lasting a few seconds. *Hypnagogic hallucinations* are vivid visual, auditory or, less commonly, tactile hallucinations occurring on falling asleep or on awakening. These four components of the narcoleptic syndrome do not necessarily occur together; cataplexy occurs in isolation in about 10% of patients. There is a remarkably uniform association with HLA DR2 on chromosome 6, and narcolepsy is often inherited.

The narcoleptic attack is associated with rapid eye movement (REM) sleep. During this stage of sleep muscle tone is reduced, suggesting a possible physiological explanation for the concurrence of cataplexy, sleep paralysis and narcolepsy. The EEG is useful in diagnosis because REM sleep patterns are seen during the initial phase of sleep in narcoleptic subjects, rather than an orderly progression from alertness to light sleep before REM sleep episodes occur. REM sleep is associated with dreaming.

Treatment is difficult. Amphetamine or similar drugs may be effective but are addictive and can cause hypertension. They have largely been replaced by clomipramine 75 mg daily, which is especially useful in managing cataplexy, but is not effective for narcoleptic attacks. Caffeine is sometimes helpful.

Other sleep disorders (parasomnias). The term parasomnia is used to describe motor or autonomic disturbances in sleep resulting from disturbed sleep mechanisms. The commonest is *hypnic jerks*, consisting of jerking of the limbs, especially the legs, sometimes associated with a flash sensation or a dream, occurring at the onset of sleep (sleep-onset myoclonus). These are reported by about 70% of the normal population. *Sleep walking* (somnambulism) is common in children; it usually consists of semi-purposive motor behaviour or utterances, sitting up in bed rather than walking, but occurring during sleep. It occurs in deep, non-REM sleep. *Enuresis* may also be a parasomnic disorder. *Night-terrors* and *nightmares*, consisting of vivid dreams and autonomic outbursts resembling panic attacks, agoraphobia and other mental disturbances in the waking state. They may respond to benzodiazepine and tricyclic antidepressant drugs that suppress deep sleep.

Sleep apnoea is defined as cessation of airflow at nostrils and mouth lasting at least 10 seconds and occurring more than 30 times during a 7-hour nocturnal sleep. Patients with sleep apnoea have prominent snoring, wake frequently during the night and suffer from daytime drowsiness. It is most commonly due to obstruction to the upper respiratory airway, e.g. by nasal septal deviation, adenoid-tonsillar enlargement and congenital deformity. It also occurs in alveolar hypoventilation syndromes, due to muscular weakness or restrictive airway disease. A similar syndrome occurs in massive obesity (Pickwickian syndrome). In multiple system atrophy and Shy–Drager syndrome sleep apnoea is a major problem. The term Ondine's curse has been used to define primary insensitivity of the brain stem respiratory centre, leading to this syndrome. The treatment of sleep apnoea is dependent on causation, and is directed toward maintaining an airway and maintaining adequate oxygenation.

3

Stroke

Stroke, a common clinical problem, is defined as a rapidly developing focal disturbance of brain function of presumed vascular origin and of more than 24 hours' duration. This includes cerebral infarction and haemorrhage, sub-arachnoid haemorrhage, brain stem and cerebellar vascular disease, spinal cord infarction and haemorrhage. Transient ischaemic attacks (TIA) are also a manifestation of cerebrovascular disease, but the focal deficit is reversed in less than 24 hours.

Epidemiology

Stroke is the third commonest cause of death in the UK and in most other affluent countries; only heart disease and cancer rank higher. Approximately 100 000 deaths from stroke occur annually in the UK, and about 1 000 000 in Europe as a whole. About 20% of patients die within a month of the stroke, and 50% of survivors are permanently disabled; 70% show obvious neurological deficit. A third of patients with stroke are younger than 65 years. Of strokes,

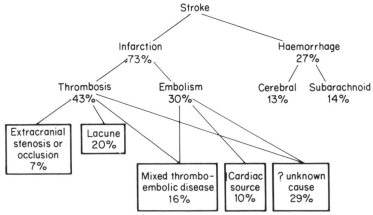

Fig. 3.1 Causes of stroke.

haemorrhage accounts for a quarter, the remainder being due to thrombo-embolic cerebral infarction. Two-thirds of the latter are due to thrombosis, and the remainder to intravascular embolism, often from atherosclerotic vessels (Fig. 3.1). Carotid and vertebro-basilar territory infarcts, and lacunar infarcts occur equally frequently. Of the strokes due to intracranial haemorrhage half are intracerebral haematomas, and half subarachnoid haemorrhage, usually due to ruptured berry aneurysm. These figures vary in different surveys, depending on the method of ascertainment, e.g. clinical data, CT scanning, autopsy results, and the population studied.

The incidence of TIA is difficult to define in relation to completed stroke, but only about 4% of TIAs are followed by stroke. A third of patients with infarction will have another stroke within 5 years. The incidence of stroke is slightly higher in men than in women in all age groups, in contrast to myocardial infarction, which is much commoner in men.

Risk factors for stroke

The most important factor (Table 3.1) for cerebral infarction is age. Most strokes occur in the 65–75 year age group. Hypertension is a factor in 70% of all strokes. Both systolic and diastolic blood pressure levels are important; patients with systolic blood pressure greater than 160 mmHg have a much greater risk than those with a lower systolic pressure. Heart disease is important, especially atrial fibrillation, valvular heart disease, cardiac failure and ECG abnormalities, such as left ventricular hypertrophy. Cardiac surgery may also be complicated by stroke. Ischaemic heart disease, and peripheral vascular disease, are common associations of stroke, indicating generalized atherosclerotic vascular disease. The oral contraceptive pill increases the relative stroke risk 2–3 times, but in a population in which the stroke risk is very low. Hypotension is important in elderly people, many of whom have extracranial and intracranial atherosclerosis. Diabetes mellitus doubles the risk of stroke. Other, less common disorders, such as polycythaemia, leukaemia, bleeding disorders, severe anaemia and vasculitis are also

Table 3.1 *Risk factors for stroke.*

Age
Hypertension
Cardiac disease, including ischaemic heart disease
Diabetes mellitus
Hypotension in the elderly
Oral contraceptive medication

associated with stroke (Table 3.2). Body weight, blood lipids, cigarette smoking, alcoholism, excessive coffee consumption and lack of exercise all show inconclusive associations with stroke.

Since 1950 there has been a striking reduction in the incidence of stroke of all types. Cerebral haemorrhage has decreased in incidence by about 50%, perhaps related to the increasingly effective treatment of hypertension. The incidence of cerebral infarction has decreased by about 50% in the USA, but less in the UK. The reasons for this improvement in incidence and mortality of cerebral infarction are unknown, and cannot be related to changes in the recognized risk factors.

Mechanisms of ischaemic stroke

In most strokes there is focal impairment of blood flow to the nervous system. In *systemic hypoxia*, there is a generalized reduction in oxygen saturation but, even in this situation, there is selective vulnerability of certain parts of the brain, especially the amygdaloid nuclei of the temporal lobes. When the circulation fails, as in severe hypotension or cardiac arrest or dysrhythmia, survival of the brain depends on the autoregulatory capacity of the cerebral circulation. When the mean perfusion pressure falls, the vascular bed dilates to maintain adequate flow. Hypertensive patients are adapted to higher mean perfusion pressures than normotensive subjects, so that blood flow fails at rather higher pressures than in normal subjects. Autoregulation may also fail when there is marked stenosis of a major vessel, especially of an extracranial artery such as the internal carotid artery. This may result in critical flow failure in the terminal parts of this vascular territory (*haemodynamic crisis*). Border-zone infarcts are areas of infarction situated in the anastomotic zones of perfusion of a neighbouring major circulation, e.g. middle and posterior cerebral artery territories. Extracranial major vessel stenosis, especially of the carotid artery (Fig. 3.2), may be detected by the presence of a bruit, but bruits are unlikely with stenosis less than 40%, or more than 90%. High-pitched bruits are associated with tight stenosis.

Thrombotic occlusion is usually extracranial, affecting the common or internal carotid arteries at the carotid bifurcation, and the vertebral and basilar arteries. Thrombosis is usually superimposed on an atherosclerotic plaque (Fig. 3.2), and may be accompanied by embolism of the affected vascular territory prior to the development of complete occlusion. This embolism may present with TIA or with cerebral infarction. The development of infarction implies that the collateral circulation was inadequate so that regional perfusion of the brain was insufficient. The clinical disorder is characteristic in

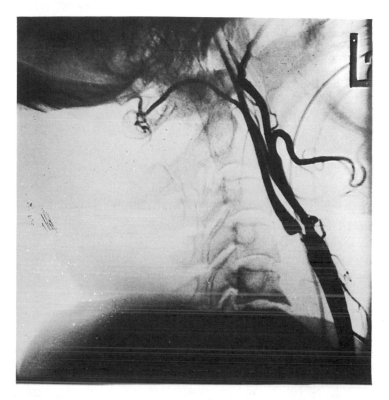

Fig. 3.2 Internal carotid artery stenosis. In this carotid angiogram, there is atherosclerotic narrowing of the internal carotid artery in a short segment close to the carotid siphon, to about 10% of the normal diameter Immediately rostral to the stenosis is a zone of post-stenotic dilation, probably caused by turbulent flow. The adjacent external carotid artery is normal.

individual vascular territories. Primary thrombotic occlusion of intracranial vessels is relatively infrequent, although clots may propagate from an extracranial source.

Cerebral embolism may result from disease of the heart, or of the major vessels. Emboli from vessels consist of atherosclerotic debris, thrombus, calcified material, or platelet/fibrin aggregate. These emboli may briefly occlude a small or medium-sized vessel, leading to TIA, or infarction. Infarction associated with cerebral embolism is often associated with haemorrhage into the margins of the infarcted tissue, occurring during the phase of recanalization of the circulation. Embolism from cardiac disease is particularly associated with myocardial infarction, valvular heart disease, especially aortic and mitral valve disease including mitral valve prolapse, and with arrhythmias.

Table 3.2 *Systemic disorders associated with ischaemic stroke.*

Vasculitis
  polyarteritis nodosa
  rheumatoid vasculitis
  systemic lupus erythematosus
  temporal (giant cell) arteritis
  Takayasu's (pulseless) disease

Septic embolism
  bacterial endocarditis
  septicaemia

Hyperviscosity states
  multiple myeloma and paraproteinaemias

Hypercoagulable states
  thrombocytosis
  polycythaemia rubra vera
  remote effect of cancer (pancreas, stomach, lymphoma)

Haemoglobinopathy
  sickle cell disease

Vascular trauma
  dissecting carotid aneurysm
  Marfan's disease

Other degenerative vascular diseases
  fibromuscular hypoplasia
  Grönblad–Strandberg syndrome
  homocystinuria

Lacunes are small infarcts in the territory of small, deep perforating vessels. They produce characteristic restricted clinical syndromes; the cumulative effect of multiple lacunes may be debilitating. Their cause is uncertain, but they are closely associated with hypertension and with diabetes mellitus and are believed usually to be due to vascular occlusion.

Ischaemic stroke may also occur in patients with systemic disorders (Table 3.2). Despite intensive investigation, including angiography, the cause of ischaemic stroke remains undetermined in about 25% of patients (Fig. 3.1).

Fig. 3.3 *(opposite)* Vascular territories. The territories of perfusion of the major branches of the internal carotid artery are shown in this diagram. The borders of these territories represent parts of the brain in which perfusion may be critically impaired when there is stenosis of a proximal vessel, or systemic hypotension.

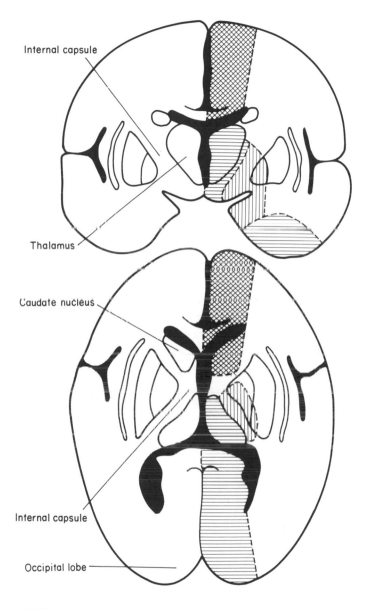

Internal capsule

Thalamus

Caudate nucleus

Internal capsule

Occipital lobe

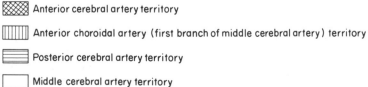

Anterior cerebral artery territory

Anterior choroidal artery (first branch of middle cerebral artery) territory

Posterior cerebral artery territory

Middle cerebral artery territory

Causes of cerebral haemorrhage

Spontaneous intracerebral haemorrhage is usually due to hypertensive haemorrhage, ruptured berry aneurysm, arterio-venous malformations or, less commonly, to haemorrhagic diatheses such as leukaemia or platelet dysfunction. Rarely, intracerebral

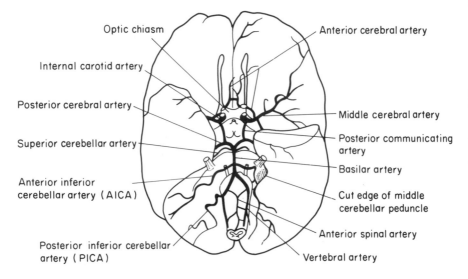

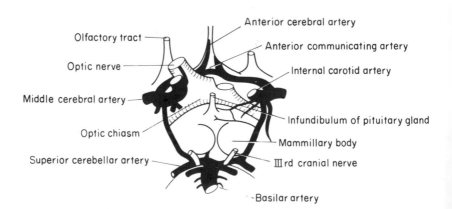

Fig. 3.4 (a) Circle of Willis. The major anastomosis of the carotid and basilar arteries is situated at the base of the brain. Note that the middle cerebral artery arises from the internal carotid artery, and that the posterior cerebral artery arises from the basilar artery, at the origin of the posterior communicating artery.

haemorrhage may be due to bleeding into a cerebral tumour, especially glioma or metastasis. Cranial trauma should always be considered as a cause of intracerebral haemorrhage.

Syndromes of vascular territories

The brain is perfused by two major vascular systems, the carotid arteries and the vertebro-basilar arterial system. The cerebral hemispheres are supplied by the carotid circulation, except for the occipital lobes, posterior parts of the temporal lobes, and the thalami which are usually supplied by the vertebro-basilar system (Fig. 3.3). The brain stem, cerebellum and upper cervical cord form the basilar vascular territory. These anterior and posterior circulations join at the base of the brain to form an arterial anastomosis, the Circle of

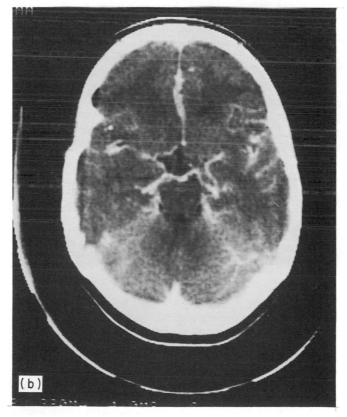

Fig. 3.4 (b) CT scan, enhanced with contrast (given intravenously) showing the Circle of Willis in a normal subject.

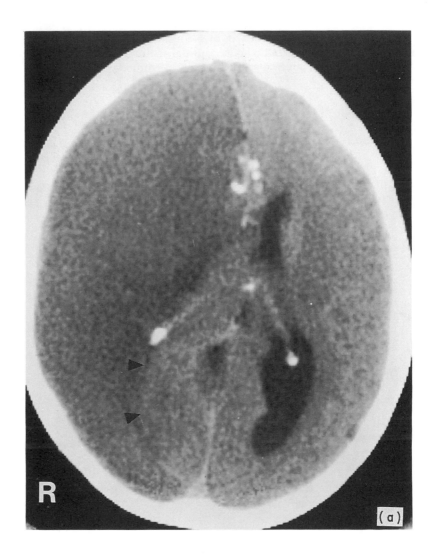

Fig. 3.5 (a) Acute internal carotid territory infarction. There is reduced attenuation in the territories of the right anterior cerebral and middle cerebral arteries. The posterior cerebral artery territory (arrows) is uninvolved. There is marked swelling of the infarcted brain with shift of the midline structures from right to left. This was associated with thrombotic occlusion of the internal carotid artery at the carotid bifurcation in the neck. (b) Middle cerebral territory infarction. There is a large infarct, several months old, shown by the clearly demarcated zone of reduced attenuation in the territory of the right middle cerebral artery. The anterior and posterior cerebral artery territories are uninvolved. The infarct occurred in association with internal carotid artery occlusion.

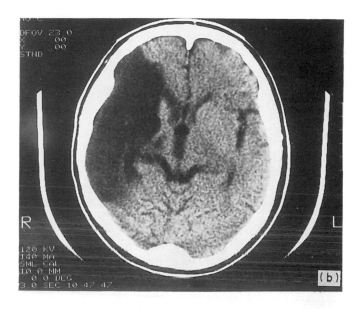

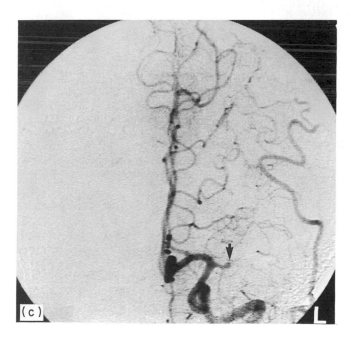

Fig. 3.5 *(continued)* (c) Right hemiplegia and aphasia. There is occlusion of the stem of the left middle cerebral artery (arrow) with an avascular zone in the territory of this vessel.

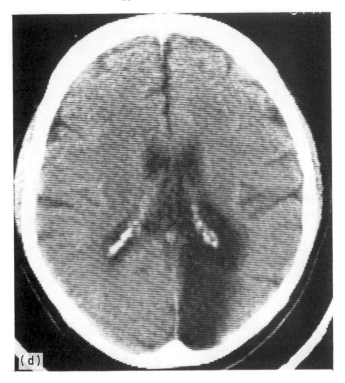

Fig. 3.5 *(continued)* (d) Occipital infarction, in the territory of the left posterior cerebral artery circulation, causing a right homonymous hemianopia.

Willis (Fig. 3.4). This anastomosis allows cerebral perfusion to adapt to changes in flow in one or more of the major vessels caused, for example, by turning the head. This compensatory function may be limited by stenotic vascular disease, or by congenital anomalies in the development of the Circle of Willis. The main branches of the Circle of Willis, i.e. the middle cerebral, anterior cerebral and posterior cerebral arteries, have extensive potential anastomoses in their peripheral territories, both superficially and in the deeper parts of the brain. These peripheral anastomotic zones are termed *watershed areas*; they are especially vulnerable to infarction when autoregulation fails during severe hypotensive/hypoxic crises, e.g. during cardiopulmonary arrest. Some deep perforating vessels are end vessels without access to anastomotic compensatory flow and occlusion of these vessels causes small, lacunar infarcts (see below).

Occlusion or stenosis of major vessels in the neck is frequently asymptomatic but is more typically associated with transient ischaemic attacks or stroke. These variations reflect the competence

Table 3.3 *Carotid territory infarction.*

Right	Left
hemiplegia	hemiplegia
hemisensory loss	hemisensory loss
hemianopia	hemianopia
visuospatial agnosia	aphasia, usually global
constructional apraxia	
neglect of left side (anosagnosia)	

of the anastomotic circulations, the time taken for development of critically severe narrowing or occlusion, and the severity and distribution of embolism from ulcerated atheromatous plaque or from the heart.

Carotid territory infarction

Complete carotid territory infarction (Fig. 3.5) is frequently fatal, and survivors are severely disabled. Both middle and anterior cerebral territories are infarcted and, if the posterior cerebral circulation is derived from the carotid via the posterior communicating artery (10% of normal people) this territory will also be infarcted. Less complete carotid territory infarction is commonly mainly in the middle cerebral territory (Table 3.3). When carotid territory infarction is embolic, e.g. from atheroma at the carotid bifurcation, a stepwise course leading to varying degrees of disability is a characteristic feature. Since the first branch of the internal carotid artery, the ophthalmic artery, supplies the retina, transient ipsilateral loss of vision (*amaurosis fugax*) may be associated with, or occur separately from the contralateral hemiparesis. It is uncommon for this to result in permanent retinal infarction. The major clinical differences between left and right carotid territory infarction relate to the functional differences between the left and right hemispheres. In right-handed people left hemisphere infarction will lead to aphasia and right hemisphere infarction to the spatial disorientation and perceptual disorders characteristic of lesions in the minor temporo-parietal region (Table 3.3).

Middle cerebral and anterior cerebral territory infarction

These vascular territories (Fig. 3.3) represent portions of the carotid territory and, especially in middle cerebral territory infarction (Fig. 3.5), there are close similarities to carotid territory infarction syndromes (Table 3.4). Indeed, in most instances the causative

Table 3.4 *Middle cerebral territory infarction.*

Right	Left
hemiplegia: arm > leg	hemiplegia: arm > leg
hemisensory loss	hemisensory loss
hemianopia	hemianopia
right parietal syndromes	aphasia; expressive > receptive
dressing apraxia	
neglect of left side	
sensory inattention	
loss of geographical orientation	

Table 3.5 *Anterior cerebral territory infarction.*

Unilateral:
  paralysis of contralateral leg, with relative sparing of arm and face
  grasp reflex in affected limb
  expressive aphasia (Broca aphasia) in left-sided lesion
  disturbance of intellect and judgement; emotional lability
  loss of social behaviour

Bilateral anterior cerebral territory infarction:
  dementia with incontinence and apathy
  akinetic mutism
  bilateral grasp reflexes and paratonia
  variably severe corticospinal weakness and gait disturbance

vascular lesion is in the internal carotid artery itself. Anterior cerebral territory infarction (Table 3.5) is often bilateral because flow is dependent on the patency of the collateral flow, especially that through the anterior communicating artery of the Circle of Willis. Mental effects are common and the anterior part of the corpus callosum may be involved, isolating somatosensory cortex in the right hemisphere from the left frontal lobe, resulting in tactile anomia. Typically the leg is weaker than the arm but when the medial striate branch (Heubner's artery) is involved there is weakness of the face and arm without sensory loss, and with sparing of the leg.

Vertebro-basilar territory infarction

The posterior cerebral circulation (Fig. 3.5) is perfused by the vertebrobasilar artery in 90% of normal subjects and, when the basilar artery is atheromatous, or occluded, infarction may occur in this territory causing complex visual and visuo-spatial defects including hemianopia, cortical blindness and visual agnosia (Table 3.6).

Table 3.6 *Posterior cerebral territory infarction.*

Unilateral:
  hemianopia with macular sparing
  visual agnosia and colour agnosia
  right parietal syndrome, including posterior fluent aphasia
  thalamic syndrome

Bilateral ('top of the basilar syndrome'):
  cortical blindness
  visual agnosia with ocular apraxia
  parietal syndrome
  amnesic syndrome with bitemporal infarction
  brain stem (mesencephalic) syndrome, with skew deviation,
    vertical gaze palsy and pupillary abnormalities

Table 3.7 *Vertebro-basilar territory infarction.*

Fatal coma
Ophthalmoplegia and skew deviation
Quadriplegia
Loss of brain stem reflexes
  (survival with locked-in syndrome)

The thalamus may be involved, causing impairment of pain and position sense, and involvement of the mesial temporal lobes may lead to an amnesic syndrome resembling Korsakoff's psychosis and to mood and personality changes. Infarction of a cerebellar hemisphere presents with ataxia of a limb, but often progresses through a phase of mass effect with progressive loss of consciousness, unilateral cranial nerve palsies and long tract signs.

The brain stem vascular territory syndromes described in Tables 3.7 and 3.8 represent the effects of infarction in the territories of long circumferential vessels, e.g. the posterior inferior cerebellar artery, and of perforating and short circumferential vessels. These usually involve infarction of certain cranial nerve nuclei with crossed sensory loss or hemiparesis. These features are particularly characteristic of brain stem infarction. Dizziness, ataxia and diplopia are common symptoms of vertebro-basilar territory ischaemia.

Lacunar infarction

There are many lacunar syndromes, representing small infarcts in the deeper, non-cortical parts of the cerebrum and brain stem. They result from occlusion of the small penetrating branches of the larger arteries, causing small cavities (lacunes) of 3 mm to 2 cm in

Table 3.8 *Brain stem vascular syndromes.*

Posterior inferior cerebellar artery territory
(lateral medullary syndrome; Wallenberg's syndrome)
   vertigo and hiccup
   dysphagia
   ipsilateral Horner's syndrome
   ipsilateral facial analgesia and contralateral limb and trunk analgesia
   ipsilateral cerebellar ataxia and nystagmus
   ipsilateral palatal and vocal cord weakness (IX and X cranial nerves)

Superior cerebellar artery territory
   ipsilateral cerebellar ataxia
   choreiform movements
   contralateral hemianalgesia

Internal auditory artery territory
   unilateral vertigo, deafness and tinnitus

Syndromes of perforating and circumferential brain stem arteries
   Foville's syndrome (medulla)
      unilateral facial (VII) palsy
      paralysis of conjugate gaze to affected side
      contralateral hemiparesis
   Millard–Gubler syndrome (pons)
      unilateral VI and VII palsy
      contralateral hemiparesis
   Benedikt's syndrome (mesencephalon)
      ipsilateral III palsy and gaze palsy
      contralateral tremor and ataxia
      (contralateral hyperaesthesia)
   Weber's syndrome (mesencephalon)
      ipsilateral III palsy
      contralateral hemiplegia

Table 3.9 *Common lacunar infarct syndromes.*

Pure sensory stroke (posterior thalamic infarction)
Pure motor stroke (posterior limb of internal capsule, lower basal pontine or
   peduncular infarction)
Ataxic hemiparesis (basal pontine infarction)
   —hemiparesis with ataxia of whole limbs
Dysarthria—clumsy hand syndrome (usually pontine infarction)
      —facial weakness, dysarthria and dysphagia with slight
         weakness and unsteadiness of one hand

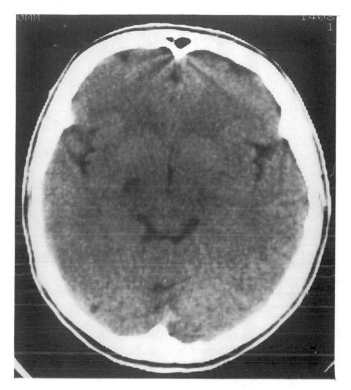

Fig. 3.6 Lacunar infarction in the right internal capsule.

size (Fig. 3.6). The commonest sites are putamen, caudate, thalamus and pons, causing characteristic clinical syndromes (Table 3.9). Most cases are due to hypertension, but diabetes mellitus is also a risk factor for this small vessel disorder. Lacunes are often multiple and may lead to a cumulative and severe neurological disorder, especially when the lesions are bilateral and situated in the basal nuclei and white matter. Incontinence, dementia, a curious, short-stepped shuffling gait (*marche à Petitpas*) and pseudo-bulbar palsy develops in such cases.

Transient ischaemic attacks

Brief attacks of neurological dysfunction, with recovery in less than 24 hours, are termed transient ischaemic attacks (TIA), but the popular terminology 'little stroke' used by patients is probably correct since the risk of stroke after a TIA is about 30% in 5 years (5–6% per year), resembling the recurrence rate of major strokes.

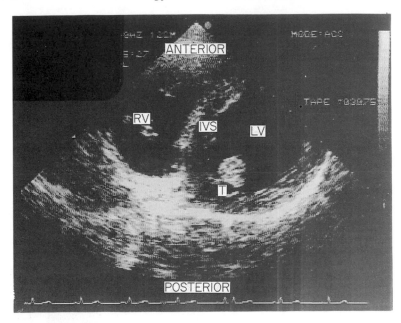

Fig. 3.7 Echocardiogram (transverse view), showing a spherical thrombus (T) in the left ventricle in a patient with a thrombotic trait associated with carcinoma of the pancreas, who presented with stroke. RV right ventricle; LV left ventricle; IVS interventricular septum.

The causes of TIA are the same as those of thrombo-embolic stroke including local vascular factors causing thrombo-embolism, haemodynamic problems associated with vascular stenosis, systemic disorders and cardiac disease, especially arrhythmia. Miller Fisher, who devoted many years to the study of stroke, noted that TIAs rarely last even as long as 1 hour, that recurrent TIAs precede stroke in 90% of patients presenting with stroke but that single TIAs are commonly benign. Carotid TIAs are usually stereotyped but cardiogenic embolism results in variable clinical features depending on the pattern of vascular occlusion. Furthermore, cardiogenic embolism (Fig. 3.7) usually causes stroke-like syndromes of several hours' or days' duration.

In *subclavian steal syndrome*, blood is 'stolen' from the vertebro-basilar circulation into the ischaemic arm. With occlusion or tight stenosis of the left subclavian artery proximal to the origin of the left vertebral artery blood flows up the right vertebral, and down the left vertebral into the distal part of the subclavian artery. This pattern of reversed flow in the vertebral artery is enhanced if the ischaemic arm is exercised, and may lead to brain stem ischaemia with light-headedness, vertigo, visual blurring and diplopia. The blood

Table 3.10 *Syndromes of TIAs.*

Transient monocular blindness (amaurosis fugax)
Transient hemiparesis (with or without sensory loss)
Transient hemisensory loss
Transient dysphasia without other features
Transient diplopia and dizziness
Transient dizziness and ataxia

pressure in the ischaemic arm is 20 mmHg lower than on the normal side, and the pulse is small and delayed. Surgical reconstruction is difficult, and most affected patients have widespread vascular disease; angioplasty may be useful.

The major syndromes listed in Table 3.10 are determined by the vascular territory involved. Isolated syncope, drop attacks and dizziness are often explained on the basis of transient ischaemia but there is little evidence to support this explanation of these symptoms and, in particular, they are not associated with stenotic arterial disease. Similarly, transient disturbances of memory are not clearly associated with vascular disease.

About 50% of patients with typical transient attacks have stenosis of major, extracranial vessels, indicating the importance of this syndrome in planning medical and surgical intervention to prevent major strokes. These patients may have bruits in the cervical vessels.

The major difficulty in diagnosis is distinguishing TIAs from focal seizures, syncope, migraine, unrelated benign systemic illness such as viral infections, hypoglycaemia and anxiety attacks. In seizures convulsive movements precede or accompany the development of hemiparesis or other focal disorder but focal cerebral ischaemia may itself lead to a convulsion.

Amaurosis fugax consists of sudden monocular obscuration of vision, described as a curtain or shade over the eye, lasting for less than 15 minutes. Recovery usually occurs like a blind lifting up across the visual field. Attacks may be recurrent during a few days or weeks, sometimes 30 to 100 times in a few days, but vision is only rarely permanently affected. Hemispheric stroke is a rare complication in patients with amaurosis fugax not associated with cerebral ischaemia, although cholesterol, platelet or thrombotic emboli are sometimes seen, transiently occluding a retinal vessel during ophthalmoscopy.

Transient global amnesia is a sudden loss of recent and immediate memory occurring without clouding of consciousness or disturbance of self-awareness. At the height of the attack the memory disturbance may extend retrogradely for many years. Recovery occurs gradually, with foreshortening of the amnesia, during a period of several hours, leaving the patient amnesic only for the duration of the attack. It is thought that most cases have a vascular aetiology, from ischaemia in the posterior cerebral artery territories involving both mesial temporal lobes, but the syndrome also occurs in partial seizures and in migraine. The syndrome must also be distinguished from *psychogenic amnesia*, a disorder in which there is an amnesic flight from overwhelming personal or social stress (*fugue states*).

Spinal cord infarction: see Chapter 13.

Investigation of thrombo-embolic stroke

The clinical features may suggest intravascular or cardiogenic disease. When the patient is hypertensive, diabetic, is elderly, or suffers from other disabling diseases, e.g. cancer, chronic obstructive airways disease or ischaemic heart disease, investigation will be limited since there is no possibility of interventional treatment but, in younger people, investigation is directed toward finding treatable causes of stroke (Table 3.11). Thus, extracranial vascular bruits should encourage angiography since carotid endarterectomy may be indicated. Significant carotid stenosis (>70% stenosis), when associated with appropriate symptoms of TIA or stroke, is likely to be associated with a bruit, but bruits in asymptomatic people are relatively common and do not require investigation.

CT scanning of the brain is necessary in order to evaluate the presence of single or multiple infarcts, and to exclude intracerebral haemorrhage, arteriovenous malformation or tumour. Angiographic studies are especially likely to be useful when there is a bruit, and have been facilitated by the advent of digital subtraction techniques, utilizing venous injections of contrast medium. Carotid investigation may commence with B mode ultrasound imaging, or with digital

Table 3.11 *Investigation of stroke.*

Clinical examination
  auscultation of neck, chest and heart
  blood pressure
  ophthalmoscopy for emboli, and vascular changes
Haematological assessment, to exclude lymphoproliferative disease,
  hypercoagulable states and vasculitis
Blood test for syphilis
CT scanning of brain (or MRI)
Doppler carotid ultrasound
Digital subtraction angiography (venous or arterial route)
Arch angiography, if indicated

subtraction angiography. Arch angiography is indicated only when proximal disease in the major vessels, i.e. common carotid and subclavian or vertebral arteries is suspected, since it rarely results in surgical or medical treatment. Investigation should always include a test for syphilis, blood sugar and routine haematological tests to exclude lymphoproliferative disease, hypercoagulable states and vasculitis. The fasting blood lipids including cholesterol and triglycerides should be checked. If these tests are negative, and there is no bruit, cardiological assessment including ECG and echo-cardiogram are useful. The latter will reveal mitral valve prolapse and roughened aortic valve cusps.

Management and outcome of thrombo-embolic stroke

In patients with thrombo-embolic stroke there will be a neurological deficit at the time of presentation; most patients with TIA will have recovered by the time a doctor is consulted. In a few patients presenting with stroke some other cause of the neurological disorder will become apparent during the initial clinical evaluation, or following investigation, e.g. cerebral tumour, or subdural haematoma. The aim of treatment in thrombo-embolic stroke is to preserve vital functions, and to limit the extent of the cerebral lesion, and thus the residual deficit. The latter aim is difficult to achieve.

Most patients with severe strokes will be admitted to hospital but it is arguable whether all patients, particularly the very elderly, benefit from hospitalization, especially in the case of mild neurological disability. A poor outcome, either death or failure to

Table 3.12 *Clinical features predicting poor functional outcome or death after an acute stroke.*

Impaired consciousness at presentation
Cheyne–Stokes respiration, or other respiratory abnormalities
Loss of pupillary light reflex
Lateral deviation of the eyes
Bilateral extensor plantar responses

Table 3.13 *Management of acute thrombo-embolic stroke.*

Adequate hydration
Maintenance of airway
Frequent turning in bed
Prevention of urinary retention or incontinence
Bowel care
Skin care
Prevention or treatment of pneumonia
Physiotherapy to prevent frozen shoulder and joint contractures

achieve functional independence, is likely when the patient is somnolent or comatose at presentation (Table 3.12). The combination of hemiplegia, hemianopia and impaired cerebral function also carries a poor prognosis for functional outcome. Brain stem syndromes, particularly with cerebellar ataxia, often recover poorly. On the other hand pure motor or sensory hemi-syndromes often recover. Most deaths from acute stroke occur in the first week after the stroke. The principles of management are listed in Table 3.13.

The blood pressure is often raised after an acute stroke as part of the compensatory mechanism to maintain adequate cerebral perfusion. Antihypertensive drugs should not be used to control this circulatory reaction, although pre-existing antihypertensive therapy should be continued. The head of the bed should be slightly raised in order to reduce intracranial pressure. Lumbar puncture is contraindicated in the acute phase of a stroke, since there may be intracranial brain herniation from the stroke, and CSF examination does not lead to changes in management at this stage. Steroids are of no value in the management of acute stroke, unless there are clinical signs of increasing intracranial pressure and brain herniation. The latter is more characteristic of cerebral haemorrhage, or of other space-occupying lesions such as cerebral tumour, than it is of thrombo-embolic stroke. Anticoagulant drugs have no place in acute thrombo-embolic stroke, with the possible exception of embolism from the heart when the risk of haemorrhage into the damaged brain may be outweighed by the risk of further, major embolic infarction. Low molecular weight Dextran may improve cerebral blood flow but appears not to affect the long term outcome. Cardiac arrhythmias may occasionally result in embolic or haemo-dynamic stroke, and should be managed appropriately by digoxin or calcium channel blocking drugs. Many patients with stroke have other medical disorders, especially diabetes mellitus, anaemia, polycythaemia, leukaemia and autoimmune vasculitis, and these may require treatment.

When the acute phase of thrombo-embolic stroke is over, and the patient is beginning to recover, management resembles that of transient ischaemic attack. The patient needs understanding and reassurance that appropriate measures to promote recovery and to prevent further episodes are in hand, consisting of consideration of medical and surgical approaches. The latter will be determined by the results of CT head scanning, angiographic and cardiological assessments. Heparin or Warfarin anticoagulation may be helpful in patients awaiting surgical endarterectomy, or if there is a very tight stenosis with frequent TIAs, but these drugs are rarely indicated in the long term and they are contraindicated with peptic ulcer, uraemia, hepatic failure, severe hypertension and in the aged. Antiplatelet drugs, particularly aspirin 300 mg (or less)/day, slightly reduce the risk of stroke recurrence, or of strokes following TIAs. Dipyridamole and sulphinpyrazone are no more effective than aspirin alone.

Carotid endarterectomy is a well-established procedure with low morbidity and mortality but the indications for the procedure are not well defined in relation to outcome. Generally, patients with carotid bifurcation disease, especially with ulcerated plaques or tight stenosis, that is related to a clinical TIA or stroke syndrome, are regarded as candidates for surgical treatment. The operation probably halves the risk of subsequent stroke to about 3% per year in the survivors of the operation. Asymptomatic bruits do not require investigation.

In the rehabilitation phase after stroke the attitude of patient and family are of paramount importance. Much depends on the preservation of higher cerebral function, especially speech, language and vision. The aphasic patient is usually devastated by stroke, despite devoted care, and speech therapy. Rehabilitation must include education of family and friends, the provision of aids such as wheelchairs, modification to the home and encouragement of mobility. Physiotherapy is important not only in preventing contractures and frozen shoulder, but in encouraging functional independence. Occupational therapy can be useful in helping a return to independence, self-caring and employment. The physician must recognize depression, a common complication of stroke, and institute treatment with tricyclic drugs, and counselling. Sexual problems after stroke are often neglected and bladder difficulties may be unspoken. Most recovery after a stroke occurs in the first 3 months.

Management of TIA

After one or more TIAs a period of intensive investigation is followed by treatment of the underlying cause (Tables 3.1 and 3.2). Often no cause can be discovered, other than atherosclerotic vascular disease, but in some patients all investigations, including angiography, are normal. It is important to treat hypertension, hyperlipidaemia and diabetes mellitus adequately. Surgical treatment, e.g. endarterectomy, is indicated if there is appropriately located and significant stenosis in a major vessel.

Intracerebral and subarachnoid haemorrhage

Most intracerebral haemorrhages are spontaneous events, usually related to hypertension, but most subarachnoid haemorrhages occur

Table 3.14 *Causes of intracranial haemorrhage.*

Intracerebral haemorrhage	
spontaneous hypertensive haemorrhage	80%
arteriovenous malformations	15%
ruptured berry aneurysm	<5%
other causes, e.g. blood dyscrasias, trauma (see Chapter 7)	<5%
Subarachnoid haemorrhage	
ruptured berry aneurysm	94%
arteriovenous malformations	6%
other causes, e.g. blood dyscrasias, trauma	<5%

from bleeding from ruptured berry aneurysms on intracranial arteries (Table 3.14). About 10% of all intracerebral haemorrhages are cerebellar; positive haemorrhage is less common. Intracerebral haemorrhages most commonly occur in the basal ganglia or in the subcortical white matter.

The mortality of intracerebral haemorrhage is uncertain since CT scanning has revealed an unexpectedly frequent occurrence of small pericapsular haemorrhages in patients with minor stroke syndromes. Major haemorrhages presenting with dense hemiplegia and coma or drowsiness are frequently fatal. In survivors of cerebral

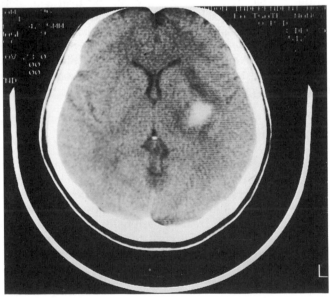

Fig. 3.8 Intracerebral haemorrhage. There is a zone of increased attenuation, representing a resolving haematoma surrounded by a halo of oedema, in the left striatum, involving the internal capsule. This was associated with uncontrolled hypertension.

haemorrhage the clinical outcome is frequently good since, unlike thrombo-embolic stroke, there is little tissue necrosis.

Clinical features of haemorrhagic stroke

Cerebral haemorrhage usually occurs in middle-aged hypertensive patients (Fig. 3.8). There is no history of transient cerebral episodes prior to the stroke. The neurological deficit usually consists of hemiplegia of abrupt or progressive onset during a period of minutes or hours. Vomiting and headache, suggestive of rising intracranial pressure, may occur and consciousness is gradually impaired leading to stupor, coma or even secondary brain stem dysfunction with decerebration and death. The neck may be painful and stiff, and seizures sometimes develop. The diagnosis of primary intracerebral haemorrhage is confirmed by CT scanning, since the intracatoma is characteristically a high density mass lesion, whereas in the first 24–48 hours after thrombo-embolic stroke the CT scan can be virtually normal.

In *cerebellar haemorrhage* the haematoma develops in one cerebellar hemisphere. In the relatively compact posterior fossa this lesion displaces and compresses the brain stem and causes foraminal impaction and obstructive hydrocephalus, thus leading to coma and death with features of progressive brain stem impairment. Thalamic haemorrhage causes coma with gaze palsy, characteristically consisting of skew deviation or lateral gaze deviation. Pontine haemorrhage causes flaccid or decerebrate coma with pinpoint, unreactive pupils; death is almost inevitable.

Management of haemorrhagic stroke

Following diagnosis conservative management, using steroids (dexamethasone 4 mg tds or qds) to control increased intracranial pressure is the initial treatment of choice. In some patients this treatment may need to be continued for several days or weeks before recovery occurs. If the clinical condition deteriorates, particularly if the patient becomes drowsy or develops increasingly severe neurological signs, surgical removal of the haematoma should be considered. This is particularly appropriate with haematomas situated in the basal ganglia, cerebellum and minor cerebral hemisphere.

Arteriovenous malformations (AVM)

Cerebral haemorrhage from AVM (Fig. 3.9) produces clinical features referable to the location of the lesion. Most are wedge-shaped lesions

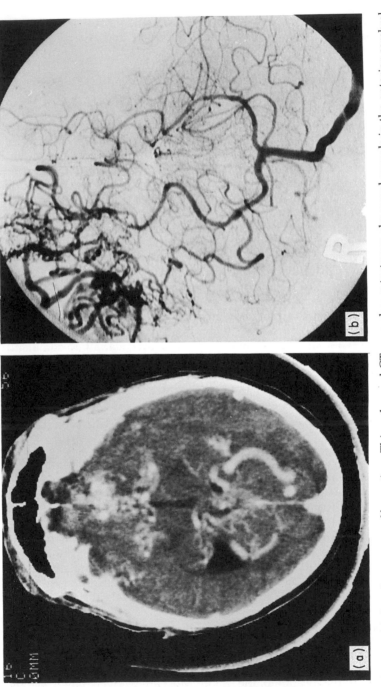

Fig. 3.9 (a) Arteriovenous malformation. This enhanced CT scan shows tortuous abnormal vessels in the anterior cerebral and posterior circulations. There is a large draining vein in the left occipital lobe. (b) Vertebral angiography reveals the details of the abnormal circulation in the right posterior cerebral artery circulation, shown by the mass of tangled vessels.

situated close to the meningeal surface of the brain. They represent congenital malformations but they increase in size with age. Most present as haemorrhage but epilepsy is also a common presentation, and these lesions sometimes cause ischaemic stroke from shunting of blood through the lesion in association with the onset of degenerative vascular disease with increasing age. In infants they may even present as high-output heart failure from this shunt effect. Some AVMs involve the dura or meninges and may cause subarachnoid haemorrhage. Rarely an AVM may cause TIA or migraine-like headache.

Examination may reveal not only focal signs referable to the lesion itself, but a vascular bruit heard best over the eyes or mastoid on the side of the lesion. Occasionally venous engorement in the neck or in the retina may be a clue to the diagnosis. The bruit is evidence of increased flow in major vessels feeding the AVM.

Haemorrhage from an AVM is a potentially serious event. The mortality in the first bleed is 10%, and 20% with each re-bleed. The annual haemorrhage rate is 2–3%. About 60% of survivors are free of symptoms.

Diagnosis and management of AVM

The diagnosis may be suggested by the CT scan appearance. Rarely, there may be speckled or linear calcification in the lesion visible in routine skull X-rays. The CT scan reveals the haemorrhagic mass itself, and draining veins, or a mass of tortuous vessels may be identifiable in the enhanced scan. Selective angiography reveals the pattern of vascular supply and is important in determining surgical treatment.

In some cases the AVM is inoperable by virtue of its size, location or vascularity. Such patients can be treated only with anticonvulsant drugs, if necessary, or by antihypertensive drugs if there is hypertension. It is also possible to reduce the vascularity of surgically inoperable AVMs by selective embolism with fascia or muscle, or by stereotaxic radiotherapy to the lesion. Surgical removal is possible by direct dissection, or by lobectomy in lesions of suitable size and location; this offers the possibility of cure or of substantial reduction in the risk of haemorrhage in the case of partial excision.

Subarachnoid haemorrhage

This is a common problem in neurosurgical practice, accounting for about 15% of all strokes and occurring at an incidence of 17/100 000 per year. In about 10% of cases no cause can be found but in more than 90% of cases in which a cause can be found the haemorrhage

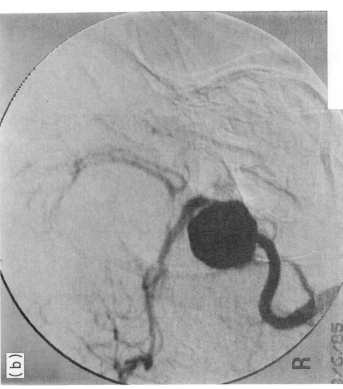

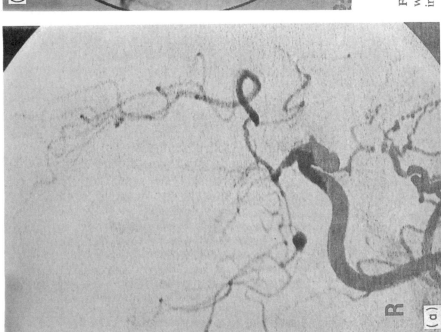

Fig. 3.10 (a) Right middle cerebral artery aneurysm with spasm of the whole middle cerebral artery circulation. (b) Giant aneurysm of the internal carotid artery behind the orbit.

Table 3.15 *Location of cerebral aneurysms.*

Anterior cerebral artery	} 29%
Anterior communicating artery	
Internal carotid artery	} 28%
Post communicating artery	
Middle cerebral artery	23%
Vertebro-basilar artery	5%
Multiple	15%

Table 3.16 *Associated or contributory causes of berry aneurysms.*

Coarctation of the aorta
Ehlers–Danlos syndrome
Type III collagen deficiency
Marfan's syndrome
Fibromuscular dysplasia
Polycystic kidney disease
Pseudoxanthoma elasticum

is due to ruptured cerebral aneurysm. The peak age at risk is the sixth decade, and women are slightly more at risk than men. The risk of recurrent haemorrhage is greater in the first 10 days after a bleed, but is especially great with large (>10 mm diameter) aneurysms. After the initial period of high risk the annual rebleeding rate is about 3%. About 25% of all patients with subarachnoid haemorrhage die within 24 hours of the bleed, often before admission to hospital.

Cerebral 'berry' aneurysms are found at arterial bifurcations (Fig. 3.10); nearly all are situated on the intracranial circulation (Table 3.15). They form at zones of defective media and elastic layers in the arterial wall and thus represent the result of congenital anomalies in the arterial wall. They have been associated with a number of congenital disorders (Table 3.16), as part of a defect in the vascular system or in hypertension. Sometimes, especially in the carotid or vertebro-basilar systems, giant aneurysms may develop, more than 2.5 cm in diameter (Fig. 3.10). These may cause embolism in the distal circulation from intramural thrombus, or present as epilepsy. They may also act as a space-occupying lesion, or cause hydrocephalus. Haemorrhage may also occur.

Clinical features of subarachnoid haemorrhage

The haemorrhage begins abruptly and is usually relatively small, but its effects are characteristic. There is a sudden severe headache, often with abrupt loss of consciousness. If the patient recovers, there is usually drowsiness, confusion, vomiting and meningism with striking neck rigidity. Fever, glycosuria and even pulmonary oedema may develop and hypertension is a feature of the acute stage. Subhyaloid haemorrhages may be seen in the fundi, and papilloedema may develop in the 3–10 days after the haemorrhage, because of impairment of CSF resorption over the cerebral hemispheres. There are profound circulatory effects of the bleeding, leading to cerebral vasospasm and ischaemia of the brain so that hemiparesis, seizures and impaired consciousness may develop or even persist. These are indicators of a poor prognosis and are relative contraindications to investigation and to surgical treatment of the aneurysm.

Most subarachnoid haemorrhages are spontaneous, but bleeds occur also in response to sudden increases in blood pressure as in coitus, straining at stool or lifting heavy weights. Some patients develop the syndrome in association with essential hypertension.

Diagnosis and management of subarachnoid haemorrhage

The diagnosis is often suggested by the characteristic clinical features, but it can be confirmed by lumbar puncture. The CSF is under increased pressure, is uniformly blood-stained, and the supernatant of the centrifuged specimen contains breakdown products of haemoglobin, and appears xanthochromic. The CSF protein content is raised and there is often a mild pleocytosis. Xanthochromia and the elevated CSF protein level may persist for several weeks. The diagnosis is confirmed also by CT scanning which shows blood in the subarachnoid space in the unenhanced scan. Magnetic resonance imaging is also useful at this stage. The aneurysm may be visualized in a CT scan enhanced with contrast, although higher than usual doses may be necessary. Cerebral angiography is required to examine the location and blood supply of the aneurysm more precisely, and to assess the perfusion of the brain and the presence or absence of vasospasm. Other investigations, e.g. EEG and blood flow studies, are not in general use in the management of patients. Spasm of intracranial arteries is frequent (Fig. 3.10), occurring mainly in relation to vessels perfused by the artery affected by the aneurysm. This may be sufficiently severe to impair cerebral perfusion, causing focal neurological signs resembling stroke. Such patients are generally considered unsuitable for immediate surgery because of the risk of permanent neurological sequelae.

The principle of surgical treatment is to isolate the aneurysm from the circulation by placing a clip across its base at its attachment to the arterial circulation. This operation should be performed at the

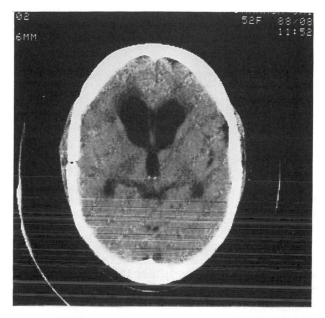

Fig. 3.11 Communicating hydrocephalus following subarachnoid haemorrhage. The lateral ventricles and third ventricle arc dilated and there are small zones of reduced attenuation at the margins of the ventricles in the frontal white matter. The latter are due to diffusion of CSF through the ventricular wall into the brain, associated with breakdown of the blood–brain barrier.

earliest possible moment following the bleed, within the limits imposed by the state of the patient, and of the cerebral circulation, in order to reduce the risk of a potentially fatal rebleed. It is thus essential to expedite investigation. Nimodipine 60 mg orally every 2 hours is effective in reducing vasospasm. In the case of giant carotid aneurysms carotid ligation is sometimes an effective method of reducing perfusion pressure in the aneurysm. The irritant effect of blood in the meninges may cause impaired resorption of CSF leading to communicating hydrocephalus (Fig. 3.11) as a late complication.

Venous infarction

The three main clinical types of venous thrombosis leading to cerebral infarction are cortical venous thrombosis, dural sinus thrombosis and cavernous sinus thrombosis. Blood normally drains from the brain through cortical veins and deep cerebral veins into

Table 3.17 *Predisposing causes of intracranial thrombosis.*

Haematological disorders, e.g. leukaemia, polycythaemia, thrombocytopenia
    and sickle cell anaemia
Systemic diseases, e.g. malignancy, ulcerative colitis, cardiac failure,
    dehydration, Behçet's syndrome
Pregnancy, contraceptive drugs and puerperium
Local factors, e.g. trauma, meningitis, infection, neoplasm

the sagittal sinus and the deep vein of Galen to enter the straight
sinus and then through the transverse and sigmoid sinuses into the
internal jugular veins. Usually one or other side of the venous
drainage system is predominant. The cavernous sinus receives
venous blood from the deep anterior part of the brain and from the
central part of the face, including the nose, and itself joins the
sigmoid sinus. Thrombosis of the cavernous sinus, which usually
follows infection of the face and paranasal air sinuses, is thus often
fatal since a clot may propagate into the sigmoid sinus, causing
obstruction of the venous drainage of a whole hemisphere. In
addition, cavernous sinus thrombosis is often bilateral because the
two cavernous sinuses are in free communication across the midline.

There are a number of recognized predisposing causes of intracranial venous infarction but, in some cases, no cause can be found
(Table 3.17).

Clinical features

Cortical venous thrombosis presents with nausea, vomiting and neck
stiffness, usually associated with focal or generalized seizures.
Hemiplegia may follow the seizures and confusion or altered
consciousness are common. There are often signs of raised
intracranial pressure. In infants cortical venous thrombosis may
present as irritability and weight loss before seizures and coma
supervene.

Dural sinus thrombosis results in raised intracranial pressure, and may
eventually lead to communicating hydrocephalus, from impaired
resorption of CSF over the cerebral convexity and in the arachnoid
granulations. Cranial nerve palsies are common; thrombosis of the
inferior petrosal sinus causes unilateral sixth nerve palsy, and jugular
vein thrombosis may cause ninth, tenth and eleventh nerve palsies.
Lateral sinus thrombosis may present as raised intracranial pressure,
resembling benign intracranial hypertension. Dural sinus thrombosis
is a relatively benign disorder unless the sagittal sinus is thrombosed;
the latter is sometimes rapidly fatal.

Cavernous sinus thrombosis is associated with local infection and the
patient is usually very ill with fever, facial swelling, ocular pain and

external ophthalmoplegia. Proptosis is often marked, and there is involvement of the ophthalmic division of the trigeminal nerve. The pupil is fixed and mid-position.

Management

The diagnosis can be confirmed by CT scanning, which may show haemorrhagic infarction in the brain. Angiography can be used to demonstrate the venous occlusion. CSF examination is important when a space-occupying lesion has been excluded, to exclude meningitis. There is usually a pleocytosis and a raised CSF protein level even without the presence of bacterial or tuberculous infection.

The primary cause, especially infection, must be treated. Epilepsy must be controlled with parenteral anticonvulsant drugs. Raised intracranial pressure may be managed with i.v. mannitol or steroids in the acute phase, or with diuretics and repeated lumbar punctures if it enters a chronic phase. The use of anticoagulant drugs in the acute stage of the illness is controversial; they are probably dangerous in the presence of haemorrhagic infarction but may be life-saving and it is probable that the benefits of this treatment outweigh the potential danger.

4

Dizziness and Vertigo

Definitions of dizziness and vertigo are often difficult to apply in clinical practice. Dictionary definitions of the two words are virtually interchangeable; in medical usage, however, dizziness is defined as a feeling of dazed light-headedness, or a feeling of impending falling, whereas vertigo implies a sense of rotation either of the patient or of the environment, coupled with a sense of imbalance in the head. Vertigo is a symptom of disturbance in the vestibular system, but not all patients with vestibular disorders experience vertigo. Normal posture and balance is dependent on the integration of information from vision, proprioception, including joint position and muscle afferents, and the vestibular system. Incorrect central processing of these inputs, or disturbances in one or other system leads to errors in efferent motor patterns, and a subjective sense of disequilibrium, often termed dizziness by the patient. These patients are uncertain of their position or motion with respect to their environment.

Table 4.1 *Dizziness and vertigo due to localized causes.*

Of sudden onset	acute viral labyrinthitis (vestibular neuronitis)
With focal signs	brain stem ischaemia (TIAs)
	multiple sclerosis
	migraine
	temporal lobe epilepsy
With deafness	Menière's disease
and tinnitus	acoustic neuroma
With tinnitus	acoustic neuroma
With particular	benign positional vertigo
head postures	
With trauma	post-traumatic vertigo
With motion	motion sickness
With drugs	vestibulotoxic drugs, e.g. streptomycin, ethacrynic acid, frusemide, quinine, anticonvulsant drugs, salicylates
With aural	middle ear disease
discharge	

Causes

Dizziness and vertigo may be due to localized disorders within the vestibular system or its connections (Table 4.1) or to generalized or systemic disorders (Table 4.2). Careful assessment of patients with dizziness leads to discovery of a cause in more than 90% of cases. The commonest causes are peripheral vestibular disorders, especially benign positional vertigo, viral labyrinthitis and Menière's syndrome. Psychiatric disorders, including anxiety, panic attacks and hyperventilation syndrome, are almost as frequent. Other causes are relatively less frequent in neurological practice, but brain stem vascular disease must clearly be a common cause of this symptom and the relative frequency of the different causes of dizziness depends on differrent referral patterns, for example to neurological and ENT clinics.

Table 4.2 *Dizziness with generalized systemic and other disorders.*

Postural hypotension
  progressive autonomic failure, autonomic neuropathies
  alcohol
  anaemia, diabetes mellitus, Addison's disease
  syncope
Cardiac dysrrhythmia and cardiac failure
Epilepsy
Cervical spondylosis
Carotid sinus hypersensitivity
Anxiety and panic attacks
  hyperventilation syndrome
  depression
Drugs, especially antihypertensive drugs, diuretics, anti-arrhythmic drugs, anti-Parkinsonian drugs, hypnotics and anticonvulsants. As a non-specific feature of weakness, sensory loss or cerebellar disease

Clinical assessment

The clinical examination is determined by the history. A search for local or systemic causes will be guided, for example, by the occurrence of vertigo, a symptom strongly suggestive of local vestibular disease. Postural hypotension is easily missed unless lying and standing blood pressures are checked. Anaemia, cardiac arrhythmia and other systemic disorders must be considered (Table 4.2). The drug history is important. The history may suggest specific postural or motion-induced factors that can be replicated during the examination. Nystagmus should be sought, and ocular movements, pupillary responses and corneal reflexes assessed.

Table 4.3 *Special neuro-otological tests.*

Positional testing for nystagmus and vertigo
Audiometry
Caloric testing
Brain stem (auditory) evoked responses (BAER)
CT scanning and magnetic resonance imaging

Clinical tests of hearing are important. Fundoscopy is necessary to exclude papilloedema or optic atrophy. Examination of the limbs and posture is important to detect cerebellar ataxia, and the gait and stance must be assessed. Romberg's test, a test of position sense is useful. The head and neck must be examined for limitation of neck movement, and for carotid or subclavian bruits. Peripheral neuropathy and other CNS lesions must be excluded.

Several special clinical tests are important in assessing dizzy patients (Table 4.3). Tests for positional nystagmus are particularly important because they can be carried out at the bedside, without special equipment (see p. 97).

Acute viral labyrinthitis

In this disorder there is an acute onset of severe vertigo, with nausea and vomiting, and great difficulty in standing. The vertigo is worsened by sudden head movement. There is gradual improvement during subsequent days or weeks. Sometimes the disorder may be epidemic. There is marked spontaneous nystagmus with the fast phase to the opposite, normal side. This nystagmus is horizontal but often has a rotary component; there is no vertical nystagmus. The nystagmus is accompanied by vertigo, and is exacerbated by movement of the head. There is no limb ataxia.

Acute viral labyrinthitis usually follows or accompanies an acute viral infection, but a similar syndrome may develop with brain stem infarction, multiple sclerosis, Menière's disease and drug toxicity. Treatment with vestibular 'sedatives', especially betahistine, cinnarizine and prochlorperazine is helpful in suppressing dizziness and vertigo during the recovery phase.

Audiometry is normal, but caloric testing (Fig. 4.1) shows canal paresis, i.e. an absence of nystagmus either to the cold or warm water stimulus on the affected side. The induced convection currents in the semicircular canals fail to stimulate the labyrinth.

Benign positional vertigo

This disorder commences acutely in adults. Most cases are idiopathic, but the syndrome often follows head trauma, often of

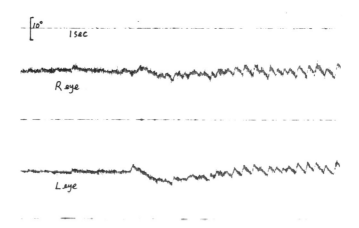

Fig. 4.1 Caloric responses. Perfusion of the right external auditory meatus with cold water induced nystagmus of both eyes to the left, as shown by the fast upward deflection on the electro-oculogram recording. The direction of deflection depends on the polarity of the signal derived from the movements of the eyes. Nystagmus commenced 60 seconds after beginning the infusion. (Upward deflection: eyes to left.)

mild degree. Dizziness and vertigo are not present at rest but follow certain movements or changes of posture of the head, particularly rotary movements, or the assumption of the standing posture. It may occur particularly severely when turning over in bed or, especially, when getting up in the morning. This syndrome is believed to result from damage to the utricle, or from inorganic, gravity-sensitive deposits in the cupula of the posterior semicircular canal. There is a characteristic delay of a few seconds between the head movement and the induction of the vertigo and this forms the basis of clinical testing for *positional nystagmus and vertigo* (Table 4.3).

The patient's response to positional factors is tested by reclining the patient rapidly from a resting, sitting position to a plane such that the head is 30° below the horizontal, with the ear to be tested in the downward position. Nystagmus develops with the fast phase toward the uppermost, normal ear, after a delay of several seconds. The response is brief, is accompanied by vertigo and rapidly fatigues so that often it cannot be replicated. Affected patients are usually aware of the critical position or movement that induces their vertigo and may be reluctant to undergo the test.

Most patients with benign positional vertigo improve spontaneously during several months, or even a year or more. Vestibular suppressant drugs (see above) may be helpful. In some patients the disorder is persistent.

Post-traumatic vertigo

Benign positional vertigo may be a prominent symptom after concussive head injury. This is associated with injury to the utricle, as in idiopathic positional vertigo, or due to rupture of the oval or round window with leakage of perilymph into the middle ear. This results in mild deafness producing a syndrome resembling Menière's disease. In these patients vertigo may be severe. Traumatic haemorrhage into the membranous labyrinth may also occur in head injury and, when there is damage to the cochlea or to the auditory nerve, deafness may be a prominent associated symptom. Many patients with benign positional vertigo describe minor head trauma prior to the onset of their vertigo.

Post-traumatic vertigo usually improves in a period of several months or years, but in some patients ablative vestibular surgery may be necessary to relieve vertigo.

Menière's disease

In this disorder recurrent attacks of vertigo occur, with vomiting and postural instability. These are associated with tinnitus and with progressive sensorineural deafness. The syndrome is usually unilateral, at least in the early stages, and most cases occur after the age of 40 years. Men are slightly more frequently affected than women. The vertigo lasts hours or, more rarely, days, and is associated with horizontal and rotary nystagmus *towards* the affected ear, indicating an irritative lesion in the affected ear. Deafness develops later in the natural history. Positional nystagmus and vertigo may occur in the intervals between attacks.

The cause of Menière's disease is unknown, but there is dilatation of the endolymphatic system of the inner ear. A similar syndrome may occur after trauma, infection or auto-immune disorders, e.g. polyarteritis, involving the inner ear.

Audiometry shows *sensorineural deafness* with selective loss of higher tones, and with *loudness recruitment*. In the latter phenomenon, despite a degree of deafness, there is rapid intensification of perceived loudness with increasing intensity of stimulus so that the intensity to high intensity sounds is similar in the two ears. This phenomenon is indicative of cochlear deafness. Caloric testing shows canal paresis, directional preponderance, or both.

Treatment with diuretics, fluid restriction and abstinence from alcohol are recommended. Labyrinthine ablation may be necessary to relieve recurrent attacks of vertigo in some cases, and selective sacculotomy may preserve hearing. Vestibular sedatives, or anti-histamines such as promethazine 25 mg may be useful in acute attacks, and intramuscular chlorpromazine 50 mg is also effective.

Benign recurrent vertigo

Recurrent attacks of vertigo lasting for minutes or hours occur, often associated with nausea and vomiting, in children or adults. There is often a positional component, and hearing is unaffected. This syndrome has been associated with migraine, and may be prevented by propranolol or pizotifen.

Acoustic neuroma (see Chapter 16)

This tumour arises from the vestibular nerve. It usually presents with progressive deafness or tinnitus, but 20% of patients present with recurrent vertiginous episodes, imbalance or dizziness. When the tumour is large other symptoms arise from pressure or displacement of neighbouring structures in the cerebello-pontine angle, especially facial, abducens and trigeminal nerves. The patient often tends to deviate to the side of the vestibular lesion when walking, and caloric testing shows canal paresis in more than half the patients.

Epileptic dizziness

A sense of dizziness or of vertigo may occur as part of a temporal lobe seizure (partial epilepsy; see Chapter 2) or, less commonly, as the only manifestation of a seizure. The symptom is usually accompanied by an alteration of sense of environment, e.g. of environmental movement or distortion. The EEG shows temporal lobe sharp waves and treatment with carbamazepine is helpful. This symptom may be the presenting manifestation of temporal lobe neoplasm, or other focal lesions, and CT scanning is indicated in late onset cases.

Vertebro-basilar ischaemia

Dizziness and vertigo are relatively common symptoms in vertebro-basilar transient ischaemic attacks, and as a more sustained problem in brain stem infarction (Chapter 3).

Postural hypotension and cardiac dysrhythmias

Syncope (vasovagal attack) is one of the commonest causes of dizziness (see Chapter 2). It is induced by the standing posture and is associated with slowing of the pulse and nausea. Later there is adrenergic stimulation with narrowing of the pulse pressure and tachycardia. In autonomic failure a postural fall in both systolic and diastolic pressures occurs without change in pulse rate (see Chapter 11), a feature indicative of the impaired autonomic response.

Cardiac dysrhythmias may be difficult to detect, but may be suspected by the absence of a postural component in the history; monitoring with 24 hour ECG recordings may be necessary. Carotid sinus hypersensitivity leads to bradycardia or asystole with vasodilatation and hypotension resulting from vagal effects induced by direct pressure on the carotid sinus. Carotid sinus syncope may occur at any age.

Cervical spondylosis

Although cervical spondylosis is commonly invoked as a cause of dizziness and vertigo there is little evidence to support the concept. It is suggested that head turning in the presence of cervical spondylosis may cause temporary occlusion of one or other vertebral artery, leading to transient ischaemia in the vertebro-basilar circulation, and dizziness. Collar immobilization of the neck has been advocated but this is rarely tolerated by dizzy patients. Cervical spondylosis is an almost universal finding in the aged.

Hyperventilation syndrome and psychogenic dizziness

Dizziness, rather than rotational vertigo, is a common feature of anxiety and panic attacks, neuroses, especially agoraphobia and claustrophobia, and depressive illness. This symptom usually forms part of a symptom complex but may be a presenting complaint, particularly when somatic symptoms predominate. Dizziness in the context of anxiety and panic is often associated with hyperventilation. It occurs because hyperventilation lowers the arterial pCO_2, so reducing blood flow and leading to cerebral hypoxia. There are commonly other associated somatic symptoms, such as tingling in the fingers and around the mouth, light-headedness, fullness in the chest, head and epigastrium, palpitations and a sensation of breathlessness. These symptoms can be prevented or relieved by identification of their functional cause and reassurance, rather than by active psychotherapy. The dizziness itself can often be relieved by rebreathing into a paper bag, as a means of maintaining the pCO_2 at normal levels. The process of consultation and medical examination is often effective in showing the patient the underlying problem and suggesting ways of circumventing it. In many cases there are social, sexual, marital or financial problems and when these are dealt with the symptom subsides. Antidepressant or tranquillizing medication, e.g. tricyclic drugs and diazepam, are helpful but should be restricted to courses of 6–8 weeks duration to avoid habituation.

5

Headache and Facial Pain

Headache is a common symptom that scarcely requires definition since nearly everyone has experienced it at one time or another. The term is usually used to describe a persistent symptom located in forehead or scalp, rather than in face or neck, but it may be felt also in the orbits. Headache may take many forms, and diagnosis is dependent mainly on the clinical features and particularly on the patient's description of the symptom. Many headaches are due not to structural disease of the skull or its contents but to the interaction of social and environmental factors with the patient, hence the pejorative use of the terms 'pain in the head' or 'pain in the neck' to describe an unpleasant event, circumstance or person. Facial pain is more likely to have a defined organic cause, and is more likely to be severe and brief in character, but may sometimes be associated with headache.

Causes of headache

It is helpful to consider headache as a functional symptom (Table 5.1) or as a feature of structural disease of the head (Table 5.2). The former predominate; treatment of the latter will relieve the symptom and may prevent the development of more severe disability.

The prevalence of headache is controversial. In one survey 90% of women aged 21–34 years and 75% of men had experienced a headache in the previous year, but with increasing age the symptom was less common so that only 20% of men and 55% of women older than 75 years had experienced headaches in this period. About 70% of all people questioned in this survey said they experienced headache. About 30% of the population have recurrent headaches requiring treatment, usually self-medication. Headache is thus a substantial part of the workload of any neurological clinic, but in the majority of these cases the headache has no structural basis (Table 5.1). Nonetheless headaches of this type are a cause of disability sufficient to cause absenteeism from work and disruption of family and personal life.

Table 5.1 *Functional headache.*

Classical migraine
Common migraine
Tension headache
Cluster headache
Post-traumatic headache
Other functional headaches
   atypical facial pain
   cough headache
   exertional headache
   post-coital headache
   post lumbar puncture headache
   drug, food and alcohol-induced headache

Table 5.2 *Structural headache.*

Raised intracranial pressure
   intracranial tumour, etc.
   benign intracranial hypertension
   hydrocephalus
Meningeal irritation
   meningitis
   subarachnoid haemorrhage
Localized disorders
   sinusitis
   temporal arteritis
   dental disease
   temporo-mandibular joint disease
   orbital inflammation
   glaucoma
   diseases of the skull, e.g. osteomyelitis, secondary carcinoma
   cervical spondylosis
   occipital neuralgia
Accelerated hypertension

Headache of structural cause can often be differentiated from functional headache by its more precisely delineated clinical features, although classical migraine is also well delineated, and by the related features of the structural disorder (Table 5.2).

Headaches may be categorized as acute, new events, occurring in a previously healthy person, or as chronic recurrent headache. This approach suggests a possible diagnostic approach, while preserving the concept of functional or structural headaches outlined in Tables 5.1 and 5.2 (see Tables 5.3 and 5.4), and this is useful in clinical assessment, investigation and management, because it stresses the recognition of treatable underlying causes, whether psychological or organic.

Table 5.3 *Acute headache in a previously healthy person.*

Intracranial infection
Generalized systemic illness, e.g. uraemia
Cranial trauma
Intracranial haemorrhage
Sinusitis
Dental disease

Table 5.4 *Chronic recurrent headaches (see Tables 5.1 and 5.2).*

Structural
   raised intracranial pressure
   glaucoma and uveitis
   sinusitis
   accelerated hypertension
Functional
   migraine
   tension headache
   cluster headache
   atypical facial pain

Functional headache (Table 5.1)

Migraine

Classical migraine is a readily recognized disorder that affects about 10% of people in Britain. The patient describes episodic headache that is usually unilateral and which lasts from 2 hours to 3 days, with total freedom between attacks. The headache is associated with visual or gastro-intestinal symptoms. The visual symptoms consist of scintillating lights or flashes (photopsias), fortification spectra (teichopsia), scotomas or object distortions. Hemianopia may also occur. Fortification spectra consist of jagged, angulated patterns resembling the fortifications of a medieval city. The scotomas and hemianopias of migraine differ from those found in brain lesions in that the zone of abnormality in the visual field appears white, opaque, glistening or scintillating rather than black. The gastro-intestinal symptoms consist usually of nausea and vomiting, but abdominal pain and diarrhoea may be a feature, especially in children. The visual symptoms develop as an aura before the headache commences, and may last 30–40 minutes before the onset of headache. Other focal neurological symptoms, e.g. aphasia, hemi-sensory disturbance, or limb weakness may develop during the aura (hemiplegic migraine). Prodromal symptoms, such as elation, yawning or tiredness, often with food craving may precede the attack. The patient always appears pale in the attack.

The headache of classical migraine is throbbing or continuous and often has a bilateral rather than a unilateral distribution. It may be relieved by cooling, or by pressure on the temporal vessels. Most patients are photophobic and prefer to lie in a darkened room. Movement worsens the headache. The headache is thought to arise from receptors and nerve fibres in blood vessels, and the aura from changes in blood flow caused by vasoconstriction of cerebral vessels, perhaps caused by slowly spreading cortical depression as described experimentally by Leão.

Common migraine is much more frequent than classical migraine, often associated with tension headache and difficult to differentiate clearly from the latter category. Common migraine is said to affect about 20% of the population of the UK. The disorder consists of migrainous headache without aura or prodrome, lasting hours or days. Nausea and vomiting usually develop as part of the attack. Common migraine is not associated with changes in cerebral blood flow.

Migraine variants. There are a number of special syndromes that may rarely be associated with migraine (Table 5.5). In *hemiplegic migraine* a hemiplegia develops during the aura phase, that outlasts the headache. Either side may be affected, and hemianopia or aphasia may occur. Recovery is complete in several hours or, rarely, in a day or more. This variant is often inherited in an autosomal dominant pattern. *Migrainous infarction* consists of cerebral infarction in the territory of an aura. This is an uncommon complication of migraine and it is often associated with coincidental vascular disease. Arterio-venous malformation may sometimes underlie this focal symptom. In *ophthalmoplegic migraine* an extraocular cranial nerve palsy especially of the third nerve occurs, that lasts for 1–2 days from the onset of the headache. The pupil is spared. In *basilar migraine* bilateral loss of vision of cortical origin is associated with brain stem symptoms, especially ataxia, vertigo, dysarthria, tinnitus and facial dysaesthesiae; these symptoms resolve in a few hours but may sometimes occur in subsequent attacks. The headache resolves in a few hours. *Migraine equivalents* consist of auras without headache;

Table 5.5 *Migraine variants.*

Hemiplegic migraine
Ophthalmoplegic migraine
Vertebrobasilar migraine
Retinal migraine
Migraine equivalents

abdominal migraine of childhood is a migraine equivalent that is often followed by classical migraine in adult life.

Tension headache

This syndrome is probably the commonest cause of headache; it may so closely resemble common migraine as to be regarded by some clinicians as part of this syndrome. The headache is typically non-paroxysmal, frequent or persistent, bilateral and described as like a tight band round the head, or a weight pressing down on the head. There is no aura, and visual and gastro-intestinal features are absent. Dizziness is common but most patients with tension headache have difficulty in formulating and describing their symptoms exactly so that the physician feels that the headache has been poorly characterized. There is often a history of domestic, social or occupational stress, and other psychosomatic symptoms may have occurred in the past. The headache usually lasts longer than a week.

There is considerable overlap between the descriptions of common migraine and tension headache. Tension headache is probably due to a combination of common migraine and muscle contraction headache, as is found in anxiety states and depression. It responds poorly to self-medication with common analgesics, although considerable improvement usually results from the reassurance associated with medical consultation.

Cluster headache (migrainous neuralgia)

In this syndrome, which usually affects men, bouts of unilateral headache or pain lasting 20 minutes to 2 hours occur recurrently, even several times daily, for periods of several weeks. The pain is intense, and steady in character, and is located behind an eye and in the cheek. It is often associated with ipsilateral ptosis and Horner's syndrome, lacrimation, and blockage of the ipsilateral nostril. The face may flush in the attack. The incidence of migraine in the families of patients with cluster headaches is similar to that of the population as a whole but, in some patients, classical migraine may precede the development of cluster headaches.

Treatment of migraine syndromes and cluster headache. The management of migraine consists of preventive measures. Certain drug treatments are useful in the prodromal phase, and others in the headache phase. Prevention is the most important aspect, and a number of factors are commonly incriminated as precipitating events (Table 5.6). These are all well-known, and different factors operate in individual patients. Depression is a factor that is often overlooked, and treatment with a tricyclic antidepressant may be very effective.

Table 5.6 *Trigger factors in migraine.*

Missed meals
Chocolate, cheese, alcohol or citrus fruits
Contraceptive drugs
Unusual sleep patterns
Allergies
Environmental stress, e.g. noise, excess light or heat
Unusual exercise
Travel
Depression
Menstruation

Prophylaxis may be achieved, when there are more than two attacks per month, by β blockers, e.g. propranolol, or by pizotifen 1.5 mg daily. Aspirin is also effective, and is contained in many proprietary preparations. In the *aura phase* ergotamine 1–2 mg by mouth, suppository or aerosol is effective in aborting an attack; no more than 12 mg should be administered by mouth in any single week. During the *headache phase* analgesics and anti-emetics may be used, e.g. aspirin or paracetamol with metoclopramide 10 mg.

Cluster headache may respond to ergotamine, but prevention can often only be achieved by methysergide 1–2 mg t.d.s. The latter drug carries a small risk of retroperitoneal fibrosis and should not be taken for longer than 6 months at a time. Ibuprofen (Brufen) is effective in some patients and lithium carbonate given in sufficient dosage to produce blood levels of 1.2 mmol/litre is also effective.

Post-traumatic headache

Headaches that prove surprisingly persistent often occur after minor head injury or concussion. In some patients migraine develops in this context but, in most, there is no evident cause. The relation of psychological to organic factors is controversial. The headache in many respects resembles tension headache in distribution and persistence and, in some cases, resolves when compensation for accidental or industrial injury occurs. It is often associated with irritability, impaired concentration and dizziness, and may be sufficiently severe to prevent return to work. Management is difficult, but treatment with antidepressants and simple analgesics, and reassurance that there is no underlying complication of the causative injury is important.

Other functional headaches

Atypical facial pain is a syndrome of persistent, localized intense facial pain that is usually unilateral, and is associated with depression.

Women are affected four times more frequently than men. No cause can be detected, despite extensive investigation. Treatment with antidepressants may be effective, but the prognosis is often poor. The symptom has usually been present for many months or years and is ingrained into the attitude and behaviour of the patient, who characteristically believes the disorder is organic and may have had many dental and maxillo-facial investigations and minor procedures, without effect.

Cough headache, exertional headache and *post-coital headache* are all associated with movement and exercise, and probably represent functional disturbances associated with activity. Cough headache may rarely be associated with raised intracranial pressure and may be a presentation of posterior fossa or third ventricular tumours.

Post-lumbar puncture headache occurs in about 30% of patients after lumbar puncture. It is due to leakage of CSF after the lumbar puncture and is worsened by standing and relieved by lying flat. It gradually resolves in the week after lumbar puncture, but recovery can be hastened by encouraging fluids, or even by I/M ACTH 10 i.m. daily for 3 days.

Headache is common after alcohol excess, from vasodilation, and the effect of formaldehyde and acetaldehyde metabolites of the alcoholic drink.

Structural headache (Table 5.2)

Raised intracranial pressure

Headache is a characteristic but not invariable feature of raised intracranial pressure. It is particularly likely to occur when there is an acute increase in intracranial pressure and it is not then necessarily associated with papilloedema (Fig. 5.1). It is rare for headache to be the only symptom of raised intracranial pressure.

The headache of raised intracranial pressure arises from stimulation of the basal dura and venous sinuses, and is felt mainly bifrontally or occipitally. It is worse on waking and increased by coughing, exertion, or changing posture. It gradually improves after rising. It is rarely severe, but may be located in the upper neck as well as in the occiput. It tends to gradually increase in severity as the disorder worsens. Vomiting may occur, but this is an uncommon symptom in patients with tumour and is commoner with obstructive hydrocephalus from lesions in the third ventricle, or in posterior fossa tumours and so is a more typical feature of children with raised intracranial pressure. Vomiting is far more characteristic of migraine than of raised intracranial pressure. Focal neurological features are often present, indicating the underlying cause. If untreated, serious

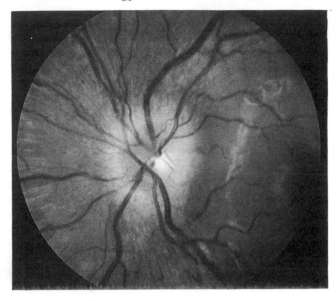

Fig. 5.1 Papilloedema. There is swelling and blurring of the centre and edges of the optic disc; the semicircular white shadow to the right of the disc is due to oedema of the retina in the macular region.

complications, especially blindness, either from occipital infarction or from long-standing papilloedema with retinal infarction, may develop. Ultimately, drowsiness, coma and death may result.

Benign intracranial hypertension. This syndrome presents with the symptoms of raised intracranial pressure, especially headache, blurring or transient obscuration of vision, diplopia or nausea and vomiting. Transient visual obscuration is due to retinal ischaemia consequent on the circulatory changes due to the raised pressure in the retina, and diplopia is commonly the result of sixth nerve palsies. The physiological blind spot is usually enlarged, a non-specific effect of the papilloedema. The syndrome is especially common in obese women, and tends to occur at menarche. It has been associated with tetracycline therapy and with withdrawal of steroid treatment and a dyshormonal cause has long been suspected but never demonstrated. Cases associated with middle ear disease are due to lateral sinus thrombosis, from extension of infection into the petrous bone, sometimes called otitic hydrocephalus.

In benign intracranial hypertension there is increased water content in the brain, without oedema on CT scanning, but with small ventricles and an effaced pattern of cerebral sulci. Diagnosis is made by exclusion of other causes of raised intracranial pressure, such as tumour, hydrocephalus, chronic meningitis and venous sinus thrombosis. It thus requires CT scanning and, in some cases, angiography. It is particularly important to exclude bilateral subdural haematomas.

Treatment is directed towards reducing the intracranial pressure. This can be done by repeated lumbar punctures, on a daily basis if necessary at first, which allows the CSF pressure to be checked, or with dexamethasone 2–4 mg q.d.s. in the acute stages. In the longer term acetazolamide 100 mg t.d.s and especially weight reduction are effective measures. If vision is at risk surgical incision of the optic nerve sheath may be necessary to prevent irreversible optic nerve damage.

The visual fields and acuity should be assessed frequently during follow up. Sometimes an unsuspected underlying cause for raised intracranial pressure becomes evident during these later assessments that invalidates the original diagnosis.

Meningeal irritation

Headache is a major feature of meningitis, whether bacterial or viral, and of subarachnoid haemorrhage. The headache is severe, and fronto-occipital. It is often associated with fever and almost invariably with signs of meningeal irritation, especially neck stiffness on passive neck flexion, and Kernig's sign. Vomiting is common, and other features of cerebral illness, e.g. seizures, confusion, drowsiness, coma and focal neurological signs are often present. In meningitis these features develop in a few hours or days, except in chronic meningitides, such as tuberculosis in which a course of several weeks is common. In subarachnoid haemorrhage the onset is abrupt.

Other inflammatory causes of headache

Focal infection within air sinuses (Fig. 5.2) causes localized headache with local inflammation and, if severe, fever. Sinusitis usually follows upper respiratory tract infection, and it is accompanied by nasal stuffiness, catarrh, change in the voice, and impairment of the sense of smell. The headache is usually worse in the supine or prone position and is alleviated by rising to the erect posture. There may be local tenderness over the affected sinus, and a green or yellow nasal discharge, sometimes haemorrhagic, is usually present. The infection may be confirmed by opacification of air sinuses on X-ray or CT scan, and by bacteriological investigation, if indicated. Treatment with antibiotics is rapidly effective. Chronic sinusitis may lead to cerebral abscess by direct invasion of the frontal lobes.

Dental and periodontal infections cause local pain and swelling, but sometimes the pain may extend into the face. In *temporomandibular*

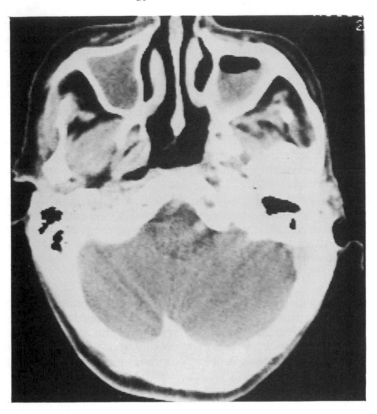

Fig. 5.2 CT scan of sinusitis. There is fluid filling the right maxillary sinus, and an air/fluid level is seen in the left maxillary sinus.

joint disease, particularly when jaw occlusion is abnormal, persistent aching pain may occur in the temporalis region. It is usually worse with chewing and talking and can often be elicited by pressure of the temporomandibular joint during jaw movement. Appropriate maxillo-facial treatment to restore dental alignment is often effective. *Local disease of the skull*, e.g. with metastatic cancer, myeloma or osteomyelitis may present with cranial pain and headache. *Ocular disorders*, especially glaucoma and iritis, may cause local pain in an eye and in the adjacent forehead; vision is usually affected and the eye may feel tense and show conjunctival infection.

Temporal (giant cell) arteritis. This is common in the elderly, but is virtually unknown in people younger than 55 years. It is a disease of medium-sized arteries containing elastic tissue, and so it particularly affects temporal, occipital, external carotid and vertebral arteries, but it may also involve other arteries of the head and neck (*cranial arteritis*). There is granulomatous inflammation, which is often nodular and palpable on clinical examination. The affected vessels are tender and local and generalized headache is a prominent symptom. There may be ischaemic symptoms in the distribution of the affected vessels, thus causing transient or even permanent blindness, claudication of the muscles of mastication, ischaemic scalp ulcers, and stroke. *Polymyalgia rheumatica* is more common than the syndrome of cranial arteritis, but the pathology of the two disorders is identical, and most patients with cranial arteritis also complain of muscle pain. The ESR is typically raised (>40 mm/h), and there is a polyclonal increase in serum globulins. In untreated patients retinal infarction, stroke or myocardial infarction may develop.

The diagnosis is confirmed by temporal artery biopsy, or by muscle biopsy in patients with prominent muscular symptoms. Treatment with steroids, initially in high dosage, produces immediate relief of symptoms, especially of headache. Maintenance therapy with small doses of prednisolone may be necessary for many years, even indefinitely.

Neuralgias

Neuralgic pain differs from headache by its sharp, brief and lancinating quality. It is due to disease of sensory nerves in the face and scalp (see Chapter 18).

6

Infections of the Central Nervous System

Infections of the central nervous system may involve the meninges, the brain or the spinal cord. In *meningitis* the infection is limited to the pia and arachnoid; the term *encephalitis* is used to describe infection of the brain itself. *Subdural* and *extradural abscesses* occur when there is bacterial infection of these potential spaces. Bacterial infection in the brain may cause *cerebral abscess*. Infections of the CNS may be due to one of several classes of organism, including bacteria, mycobacteria, fungi, yeasts, spirochaetes, protozoa, helminths and amoebae. In addition, viruses and virus-like infectious agents may invade the nervous system or its meninges.

Epidemiology

Bacterial meningitis (Table 6.1) is predominantly a disease of the very young, especially neonates and infants. Very old and immuno-compromised people are also at greater risk. Meningitis often develops in the context of chronic sepsis near the meninges, e.g. in the presence of middle ear disease (Table 6.2), and epidemics of bacterial meningitis, especially meningococcal meningitis, occur particularly when people are living close together, or in impoverished conditions. Such epidemics may be associated with nasal colonization of healthy carrier subjects by the organism. Overall, bacterial meningitis occurs in about 5/100 000 of the population per year in developed countries.

The incidence of viral meningitis is more difficult to determine since it is often very mild, frequently accompanies childhood exanthems such as measles, and is usually a benign, self-limited illness. Many cases are due to enteroviruses. Viral encephalitis is a more serious but infrequent illness that may occur in epidemics, as in St Louis encephalitis, or sporadically as in most British cases. Viral encephalitis may be due to direct viral invasion of the nervous system, e.g. in mumps, or it may follow the infection representing a post-viral or

Table 6.1 *Causes of acute bacterial meningitis related to age and other factors.*

Neonates
  Coliform bacteria
  Group B streptococcus
  Staphylococcus
  Listeria monocytogenes

Infants
  Meningococcus (*Neisseria meningitidis*)
  Haemophilus influenzae
  Pneumococcus (*Streptococcus pneumoniae*)

Children and adults
  Meningococcus
  Pneumococcus
  Others: *Mycobacterium tuberculosis*
          brucellosis
          leptospirosis
          syphilis
          acanthamoeba
          Lyme disease (Borrelia)

CSF shunts
  Staphylococcus aureus
  Staphylococcus epidermidis
  (other organisms)

Table 6.2 *Source of infection in bacterial meningitis.*

Haematogeneous (with bacteraemia)
  pulmonary infection
  bacterial endocarditis
  septicaemia

Direct invasion of meninges
  mastoiditis and middle ear infections
  sinusitis
  skull fracture or neurosurgical operation

Congenital or acquired sacral sinus

allergic encephalitis. Sporadic viral encephalitis is infrequent but may be a serious or even fatal illness as in Herpes simplex encephalitis (Table 6.3).

Bacterial meningitis

In most patients the typical features of pyogenic meningitis develop during 24–72 hours. During this time the patient develops a high

Table 6.3 *Causes of acute viral (aseptic) meningitis and meningoencephalitis.*

Sporadic
H. simplex
H. zoster
mumps
measles
varicella
infectious mononucleosis
lymphocytic choriomeningitis
cytomegalovirus
rabies
Epidemic
Enteroviruses
poliomyelitis
coxsackie viruses
echoviruses
Adenoviruses
Arboviruses
Equine (Eastern and Western)
Japanese B virus
St Louis
Russian spring/summer

fever, severe headache, vomiting, photophobia, confusion and altered consciousness. Seizures and focal neurological signs indicate involvement of the brain itself either from direct spread or from arteritis and circulatory changes. In very young children and the elderly the typical features of meningism may be absent, but neck stiffness and limitation of straight-leg raising (Kernig's sign) are invariable features in most other patients. Neck stiffness may be slight or so marked that the head appears retracted and hyper-extended. In children with non-specific fevers meningism may be present without true meningitis. In adults, alcoholism, diabetes mellitus, malignancy, pregnancy and immunosuppression may be predisposing factors. The causative organism varies according to age (Table 6.1), an important consideration when planning treatment.

In neonates coliform organisms are acquired from the mother during childbirth. *Haemophilus influenzae* is often found in the nose, nasal air sinuses and middle ear, and N. *meningitides* is spread by nasal droplets from carriers, or from animals, and is thus endemic to a community with sporadic and epidemic cases. In meningococcal meningitis the organism spreads through the blood stream to involve skin, lungs and joints as well as the CNS. The skin rash is characteristic, with petechiae from which the organism can sometimes be cultured. Meningitis resulting from pulmonary

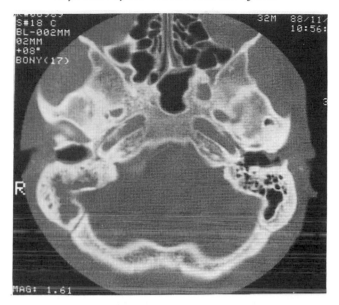

Fig. 6.1 CT scan using 'bone window' settings to show bony detail in a patient with right-sided chronic mastoiditis, admitted with acute bacterial meningitis. There is destruction of the mastoid air spaces, with involvement of the inner ear, and erosion of the medial surface of the petrous temporal bone allowing pus to gain access to the extradural, subdural and subarachnoid spaces.

infection or bacterial endocarditis is usually found in children; adults tend to develop cerebral abscesses from these causes, or from right to-left shunts in the lung or heart. Meningitis following open skull fractures is likely to be staphylococcal, but may be due to multiple organisms. When sinus infections, or mastoiditis (Fig. 6.1), cause meningitis, *H. influenzae*, *S. pneumoniae*, staphylococci or anaerobic organisms may be responsible. *Listeria* monocytogenes causes meningitis in infants, and in immunocompromised adults; it may involve the brain stem, and a curious presentation with fever, confusion, cranial neuropathy and cerebellar dysarthria has been noted in the latter group.

Diagnosis. The diagnosis is confirmed by lumbar puncture, which reveals turbid CSF, under increased pressure, with raised protein, a polymorphonuclear cellular reaction and a low glucose level (Table 6.4). The ratio between CSF and blood glucose in bacterial meningitis is always less than 0.5. Lumbar puncture is always indicated in the diagnosis of bacterial meningitis and should only be deferred if there is clinical suspicion of an expanding focal lesion,

Table 6.4 *CSF changes in infections of the CNS.*

Disease	Appearance	cytology cells/μl	protein g/litre	glucose mmol/litre	Pressure
Normal	clear and colourless	lymphocytes <5	<0.4	2.5–4.2 (>50% blood glucose level)	80–160 mm CSF
Bacterial meningitis	yellowish and turbid (purulent)	usually >1200 >60% polymorphs	raised >0.8	reduced <2.5 (<50% blood glucose level) may be absent	raised
Tuberculous meningitis	colourless, viscous	0–400 mainly lymphocytes	raised >0.8 may be very high, e.g. up to 4.0; fluid may clot on standing	reduced <2.5 (<50% blood glucose level) may be absent	raised
Fungal meningitis	clear or cloudy	<400 mixed lymphocytes and polymorphs	raised usually <1.5	reduced <2.5	normal or raised
Viral meningitis	clear or cloudy	10–1000 mainly lymphocytes	normal or slightly raised	normal (may be low in measles)	raised
Cerebral abscess	clear or purulent	normal or raised, usually <200	slightly raised usually <1.0	normal or low	raised

e.g. cerebral abscess. Only then should CSF examination be deferred pending urgent CT brain scanning. CSF cultures are positive in 85% of untreated patients but only in 50–60% of partially treated patients. Many patients fall into the latter category but Gram-staining of CSF sediment remains a worthwhile investigation. Other methods for rapid bacteriological diagnosis are available that detect bacterial antigen in CSF. In complicated cases, with focal signs or with cerebral infarction the same principles of diagnosis apply.

Treatment. Appropriate antibiotic therapy is essential. When turbid CSF is found at lumbar puncture intrathecal benzylpenicillin 6 mg can be given. Intravenous treatment is then begun. Since the causative organism will not be known initially, or perhaps for several days, broad-spectrum therapy is necessary at first. In adults with bacterial meningitis of undetermined origin intravenous benzylpenicillin 1.2 g 4-hourly with chloramphenicol 1 g stat, then 500 mg 6-hourly i.v. or i.m. is appropriate. If a diagnosis of meningococcal meningitis is established by Gram-staining of CSF or, later, by culture, benzylpenicillin 1.2 g 4-hourly remains the treatment of choice. This organism is also sensitive to chloramphenicol and, usually, to sulphonamides; the latter are relatively little used, however, because of the likelihood of bacterial resistance and the small risk of sulphonamide-sensitivity reactions. Pneumococcal meningitis responds to high-dose i.v. penicillin and *Haemophilus influenzae* to chloramphenicol. The combination of chloramphenicol and penicillin is thus the treatment of choice in purulent meningitis. *Haemophilus influenzae* also responds to treatment with ampicillin 200 mg/kg/day in divided doses, and ampicillin is also effective in *Listeria* meningitis. Thus i.v. ampicillin should probably be added to i.v. benzylpenicillin and chloramphenicol in the initial treatment plan of purulent meningitis of uncertain origin. Intravenous treatment by 4-hourly bolus is essential in order to establish high concentrations of antibiotic in the CSF and CNS.

Alternative drugs are available in patients sensitive to one or more antibiotics in the conventional regimen described above, or when it is known that the infecting organism is resistant. These include cephalosporins, e.g. cefuroxime and cotrimoxazole. Gram negative organisms such as *E. coli* and *Pseudomonas aeruginosa* are likely to be resistant to sulphonamides and trimethoprim. Gentamycin and colomycin may be useful but are relatively toxic.

General principles of management, especially fluid balance, and glucose homeostasis are important. Inappropriate ADH secretion may lead to hyponatraemia which may be controlled by fluid restriction. Steroid therapy is not indicated in bacterial meningitis, unless disseminated intravascular coagulation develops.

Sequelae. The mortality of bacterial meningitis remains significant, in the range 5–15% for the common forms. In survivors, cranial nerve palsies, deafness, hydrocephalus, seizures, venous sinus thrombosis, hemiplegia and visual impairment with optic atrophy may be problems. Pneumococcal meningitis carries the highest mortality and morbidity. Communicating hydrocephalus may develop months or years later. During treatment subdural empyema or effusion may require drainage.

Protection of contacts. Family members and others in close domestic or occupational contact with patients with meningococcal meningitis may be at risk, especially when the disease is endemic. The risk is about 0.4% (500 times the general population). Sulphonamides are the most well-tried and effective drug, but many strains are resistant and oral ampicillin (250–500 mg q.d.s.) or rifampicin (600 mg b.d.) are also used for 2–4 days.

Cerebral abscess

Abscess within the brain results from haematogeneous or direct invasion (Table 6.5). Abscesses (Fig. 6.2) are most commonly found in the frontal or temporal lobes or in the cerebellar hemispheres. In the temporal lobe or cerebellum they are often due to middle ear disease, and in the frontal lobe they result from infection spreading from the paranasal air sinuses. These abscesses follow chronic suppuration rather than acute infections, since the infection must involve the skull (osteomyelitis of petrous temporal bone) before penetrating the meninges. Rarely, in haematogeneous cerebral abscess, there is an acute, stroke-like illness at the onset of the illness with malaise, fever and leucocytosis. In direct invasion from sinusitis there is also a brief phase of meningeal reaction prior to the development of the abscess itself. This acute phase is followed by

Table 6.5 *Causes of cerebral abscess.*

Middle ear disease (40%)
Sinusitis
Penetrating wounds
  e.g. compound skull fractures
Haematogeneous
  chronic pulmonary infection (20%)
    e.g. empyema, bronchiectasis
  congenital heart disease (with R–L shunt) (10%)
  osteomyelitis
  bacterial endocarditis
Idiopathic (15%)

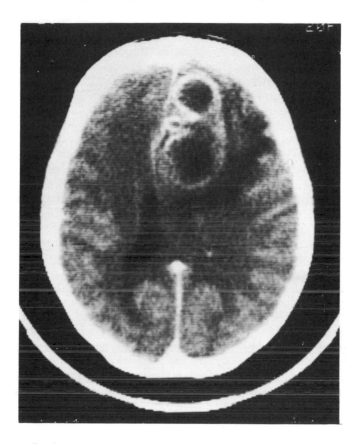

Fig. 6.2 Cerebral abscess. In this contrast-enhanced CT scan there is a multi-locular cerebral abscess in the left frontal region, with prominent surrounding oedema, compression of the left lateral ventricle and shift of the mid-line structures towards the right.

a relatively quiescent phase in which the patient appears well and relatively symptomless or recovering from the initial illness, before the abscess enlarges producing signs of raised intracranial pressure and of focal brain involvement with focal signs and focal seizures. If undiagnosed, the abscess may rupture into the ventricle or meninges causing sudden meningeal irritation, and coma or death. As the abscess expands and nears the meningeal or ventricular surface of the brain meningeal inflammation develops with neck stiffness, recurrent fever and a polymorphonuclear exudate in the CSF (Table 6.4). The CSF protein is raised and the glucose level normal. Rarely the cell count may approach 1000/mm^3 and an erroneous diagnosis of pyogenic bacterial meningitis is tempting but the glucose is either normal or only slightly low and prominent focal neurological features should then suggest abscess. The temporal course of brain abscess is variable, depending on coincidental antibiotic therapy, host resistance, the site of the abscess and whether or not there are multiple abscesses. The clinical course often mimics that of cerebral tumour.

Treatment. The diagnosis is established by CT brain scan, which shows the characteristic ring-like enhancement around a hypodense or isodense lesion in the contrasted scan. The CT scan has replaced CSF examination as the major step in diagnosis; indeed the latter should be avoided if the diagnosis is considered. The CT scan can be used to follow progress during antibiotic treatment and surgical aspiration of pus. Aspiration of pus is useful since it reduces the size of the mass lesion, and provides material for bacteriological examination. Antibiotics can be instilled into the abscess cavity (e.g. benzylpenicillin 6 mg; chloramphenicol 1–2 mg). Systemic antibiotic therapy consists of benzylpenicillin 1.2 g 4–6 hourly i.v., chloramphenicol 500 mg 6-hourly i.v., and metronidazole 500 mg 8-hourly i.v. The latter is used because of its effectiveness against anaerobic organisms in otogenic abscesses. Gentamycin and fucidic acid are also useful when staphylococcal infection is present. Steroid therapy is useful when there is raised intracranial pressure. Since seizures occur in more than half the patients anticonvulsant therapy is also indicated (phenytoin 200–400 mg daily). Surgical excision of the abscess cavity can be avoided in many patients by continued high-dose antibiotic therapy with CT scan monitoring of the size of the abscess, probably reducing morbidity, but the overall mortality is 30%, a figure similar to that of MacEwen in Glasgow, who first attempted surgical treatment of cerebral abscess 100 years ago.

Sequelae. The major problems are epilepsy, which develops in about 70% of survivors and which may be severe, and permanent neurological disability. The latter occurs in 40% of patients and consists of hemiplegia, visual field deficits, the effects of communicating hydrocephalus, speech disorders and changes in personality from frontal lobe damage.

Extradural and subdural empyema

Extradural abscess arises from penetrating trauma or from contiguous spread from chronic infection of paranasal air sinuses. Subdural empyema results from sinus infections, especially from acute ethmoidal or frontal sinus infection. Half the patients are younger than 20 years. The illness begins with fever, headache, irritability and confusion followed by the rapid development of hemiplegia, focal or generalized seizures and altered consciousness. If the abscess ruptures into the subarachnoid space there is an abrupt clinical deterioration with meningeal features and coma. Thrombosis of dural sinuses and a rapidly progressive cortical thrombophlebitis may also complicate the illness, causing seizures, cerebral infarction and haemorrhage, and focal neurological deficits.

Treatment. The diagnosis must be suspected early if a good result is to be obtained by prompt surgical evacuation of pus and broad-spectrum antibiotic therapy. Sometimes there is a boggy tender swelling of the scalp with signs of raised intracranial pressure. CT scanning is diagnostic, revealing the sinus infection or fracture, and subdural pus over the convexity and in the interhemispheric region. The outcome of treatment is good if begun early, but an overall mortality of 30% is common even in the best centres.

Other specific infections

Tuberculosis of the CNS

Infection of the meninges, brain or spinal cord with *Mycobacterium tuberculosis* is a serious illness that, like other forms of extra-pulmonary tuberculosis, leads relatively frequently to residual disability despite eradication of the infection. There are several clinical syndromes (Table 6.6). In the UK there is a marked susceptibility for tuberculosis of the CNS to occur among immigrants, particularly in people from the Indian subcontinent and South east Asia. CNS tuberculosis is also commoner in the malnourished, in alcoholics and in immunosuppressed patients. Unusual forms of CNS tuberculosis have been recognized increasingly among Asian peoples.

Tuberculous meningitis

This is the commonest form of CNS tuberculosis. The disease is nearly always secondary to rupture of a tuberculous focus in the

Table 6.6 *Tuberculous infection of the CNS.*

Meningitis
Tuberculoma
Tuberculosis of the spine
Other forms
   spinal arachnoiditis
   tuberculous encephalopathy

meninges into the CSF (Rich's focus). The Rich focus itself is probably of haematogeneous origin. The illness begins insidiously with fever, lethargy, loss of appetite and night sweats. This prodromal phase usually lasts 2 or 3 weeks and is followed by a phase of confusion, or by the development of meningeal features, with headache, vomiting and photophobia. Neck stiffness and a positive Kernig's sign may not be prominent at this stage, but become more evident when the disease is more florid, 3–6 weeks after the onset, when other features, such as cranial nerve palsies, hemiplegia, seizures and extensor plantar responses may be found.

Miliary tuberculosis, or hilar lymphadenopathy are found in about 30%, but other pulmonary signs of tuberculosis occur in about 75% of patients with tuberculous meningitis. Features of extrapulmonary involvement occur in some patients. Fundoscopy may reveal choroidoretinal tuberculomas. In some patients the disease may be more indolent and, in these, communicating hydrocephalus with drowsiness and papilloedema is frequent. The ESR is raised in 75% of patients. The tuberculin skin test is usually positive but a negative test does not exclude the diagnosis.

The diagnosis is made by examination of the CSF. There is a lymphocytosis (10–1000 cells/ml) with raised CSF protein and a low, often very low, glucose level. Simultaneous blood glucose measurement is essential (Table 6.4). The CSF protein level ranges up to 10 g/litre, and the CSF may clot on standing. In some patients there may be some polymorphs in the CSF but mononuclear cells always predominate. Acid-fast bacilli may be found by Ziehl–Nielsen staining of the CSF sediment, or of the clot itself but in many cases they cannot be demonstrated and cultures must be set up. Unfortunately, cultures of *M. tuberculosis* grow only very slowly and several weeks elapse before a result is available.

The CSF features of tuberculous meningitis overlap with those of partially treated bacterial meningitis, cerebral abscess, fungal meningitis and viral meningoencephalitis. These infections, however, can usually be excluded by microbiological examination of the CSF; and neoplastic invasion of the meninges should be recognized by cytological studies of the CSF.

CT scanning of the brain is important because it may reveal an enhancing basal exudate, best seen in the cerebral cisterns around the upper brain stem, and because communicating hydrocephalus is a common feature that requires monitoring during treatment. Communicating hydrocephalus develops when there is impairment of circulation of the CSF through the basal and convexity meninges, from adhesions and exudate. It may lead to raised intracranial pressure, and to tentorial herniation and, if severe, requires CSF shunting. This is important in the management of the disease. Tuberculous arteritis, centred on the vessels passing through the basal exudate may cause cerebral infarction, a serious and life-threatening complication.

Serous tuberculous meningitis. This probably represents a mild or early phase of tuberculous meningitis; the CSF shows a mild lymphocytosis with raised protein count and normal or borderline glucose level. The meningitic reaction may subside spontaneously, but cases have been recorded in which typical tuberculous meningitis develops weeks or months later.

Tuberculoma

Focal, nodular caseation in meninges or brain itself may be the sole manifestation of tuberculous involvement of the brain. The lesions may be solitary or multiple (Fig. 6.3), involving cerebrum or subtentorial structures, including spinal cord. They are well demonstrated in CT scans. This is a rare form of CNS tuberculosis in the UK. Most cases occur in Asian immigrants, and tuberculomas are much more common in the Indian subcontinent where nearly

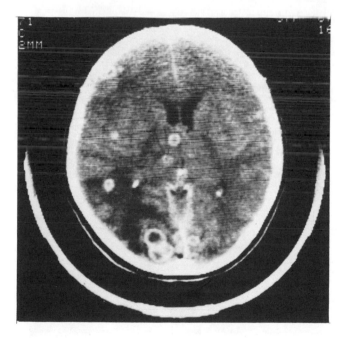

Fig. 6.3 Tuberculomata. There are multiple small loculated lesions, each with an enhancing rim, and a larger right occipital lesion surrounded by oedema. The patient responded slowly to treatment with anti-tuberculous chemotherapy.

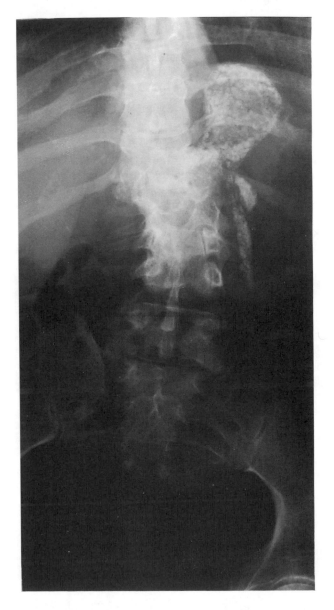

Fig. 6.4 Pott's (tuberculous) disease of the spine. There is angulation and deformity of the spine at the T12 to L2 levels, with a calcified left paraspinal and psoas abscess.

50% of intracranial mass lesions are tuberculomas. Epilepsy, progressive focal neurological deficits and raised intracranial pressure are the commonest presenting features. The clinical course may be relapsing; some lesions are found by chance as calcified, non-symptomatic lesions.

Tuberculosis of the spine

Spinal tuberculosis (Fig. 6.4) is less common than formerly (Pott's paraplegia). The infection commences in the intervertebral region, involving the disc and extending subdurally and then into the meninges to involve the spinal cord and roots. It then causes local pain and deformity before spinal and root compression develops. Sudden paraplegia may develop from sudden vertebral collapse, or from tuberculous arteritis involving vessels supplying the spinal cord, and in these patients the outlook for functional recovery is poor. Tuberculous meningitis may develop when the infection penetrates the meninges but this is often relatively indolent and localized, although the lumbar CSF shows typical features of tuberculosis (Table 6.4). Spinal tuberculosis may be the primary manifestation of the disease, or follow miliary infection. In lumbosacral spinal tuberculosis psoas abscess may be a diagnostic feature.

Tuberculous spinal arachnoiditis

In this condition, reported almost entirely in people from Southern India, but also noted in immigrants to the UK, there is an indolent progressive lumbosacral radiculopathy with root pain. The CSF shows features consistent with tuberculous infection but *M. tuberculosis* can not usually be isolated. A therapeutic trial with antituberculous drugs results in improvement.

Treatment. In pulmonary tuberculosis treatment schedules have been shortened and simplified in recent years, but clinical experience of CNS tuberculosis has shown that treatment of this form of the disease is more difficult than that of pulmonary tuberculosis and that the outcome is often not entirely free of disability. Treatment is therefore usually begun with four antituberculous drugs: rifampicin 450–600 mg/day (10 mg/kg in adults), isoniazid 300 mg/day, pyrazinamide 2–3 g/day (20–30 mg/kg) and ethambutol 1.5 g/day (15 mg/kg) or streptomycin 0.75 mg twice daily. Streptomycin crosses the blood/brain barrier relatively less well than the other drugs and is toxic to the labyrinth and cochlea, but has been a mainstay of treatment for many years and is still in common use. It should be given for 1–3 months only. It can be given by the intraventricular or intrathecal route in very ill patients (20–50 mg) on a daily basis for 10–14 days. Corticosteroids are of dubious value but are indicated in the management of raised intracranial pressure or of cerebral oedema. Pyridoxine 20–50 mg/day is essential in patients given isoniazid in order to prevent isoniazid neuropathy in slow acetylators of the latter drug. Rifampicin, isoniazid and pyrazinamide should be continued for 9–12 months; it may be possible to stop the third drug after 6 months.

Progress must be closely monitored by clinical observation and by CT scanning to assess ventricular size. If communicating hydrocephalus develops, CSF shunting may be necessary and this route can then be used for the administration of streptomycin directly into the ventricles. CSF examination should also be repeated to assess progress, but if there is rapid clinical improvement frequent lumbar punctures are unnecessary. Adequate nutrition is an essential part of treatment of this debilitating disease.

Treatment of forms of CNS tuberculosis other than tuberculous meningitis is identical. Tuberculoma of the brain should be suspected by the clinical and CT scan appearance and antituberculous treatment, rather than surgical excision, is indicated. Surgical removal may be followed by the rapid development of tuberculous meningitis. In tuberculoma the lesions may expand during the early phase of treatment, perhaps representing necrosis or an immune response, and this may lead to an initial deterioration with raised intracranial pressure.

Outcome. The survival rate in tuberculous meningitis is 80–90%, but many patients are left with disability, including optic neuropathy, deafness, spinal cord syndromes, hydrocephalus, seizures and encephalopathy. The prognosis is dependent on early diagnosis and treatment. Drug resistance is more common among Asian patients and this factor is probably also important in determining prognosis. In a proportion of patients tuberculous meningitis or tuberculoma may recur after the cessation of treatment. Drug-induced disability, especially deafness and disequilibrium from streptomycin, optic neuropathy from ethambutol and peripheral neuropathy from isoniazid treatment are all potentially preventable.

Neurosyphilis

Neurosyphilis developed in about 20% of untreated patients with syphilis, but became much less common with the advent of antibiotic therapy, especially penicillin. In the *primary stage* of acute infection by *Treponema pallidum* there are no neurological manifestations, although there may be a mild lymphocytosis in the CSF. This stage is marked by the primary chancre. The *secondary stage* of syphilitic infection consists of dissemination of the infection. There is fever, malaise and lymphadenopathy, with a characteristic maculo-papular rash involving skin and mucous membranes, including palms and soles. The rash is pruritic. There may be involvement of the liver and a meningitic illness with headache, neck stiffness and malaise may be a feature. The CSF shows a lymphocytosis with a slightly raised protein; the CSF glucose may be slightly reduced. Secondary syphilis occurs about 6 months after the primary infection. Signs of invasion of the CNS itself are rare at this stage.

Tertiary syphilis develops later. *Meningovascular complications*, consisting of an obliterative endarteritis affecting large and medium sized arteries, with infiltration by lymphocytes, plasma cells and macrophages represents a hyperimmune response to the infection. It develops 5–10 years after infection, rarely occurring earlier. Meningovascular syphilis presents as hemiplegia, resembling stroke, or as a diffuse subacute meningitis with cranial nerve palsies and signs of involvement of the CNS including aphasia, focal signs, confusion, memory impairment, optic atrophy, incontinence, apathy and anxiety. Argyll-Robertson pupils (see below) are usually present. The CSF shows raised pressure with a mononuclear cellular exudate and a raised protein (0.5–1.5 g/litre) level. The CSF IgG and IgM content is increased. There may be hydrocephalus and cerebral infarction may be seen on CT scans. Cranial nerve palsies in meningovascular syphilis are associated with syphilitic leptomeningitis. Rarely, large granulomatous meningeal lesions (gummas) may develop causing compression of the brain and mimicking cerebral tumour, cord compression (pachymeningitis cervicalis hypertrophica) or radiculitis.

Tabes dorsalis is characterized by lancinating pains in the legs, abdomen or pelvis, with ataxia. The syndrome develops 8–12 years after primary infection. Examination shows loss of the pupillary light reflex with preserved accommodation and small irregular pupils (Argyll-Robertson pupils). There is loss of position sense in the legs and to a lesser extent in the arms. Vibration sense is markedly impaired and there is impaired deep pain sensation, e.g. to Achilles tendon compression. The ataxia is thus due to the deficit in position sense, associated with the posterior column lesion. There is a characteristic, high-stepping, stamping, wide-based gait, and Romberg's test is positive. Incontinence and impotence are common; the bladder may be atonic. Optic atrophy and sensory-neural deafness occur. The plantar responses are often extensor. This syndrome is often associated with Charcot's joints; i.e. painless subluxation and arthropathy of joints in the legs, spine and, to a lesser extent, upper limbs, and trophic perforating ulcers of the feet. The mental state is normal.

In *general paralysis of the insane* (GPI) there is a progressive dementia, sometimes accompanied by tabetic signs, with a characteristic, hesitant dysarthria and dysphasia. There is a progressive dementia often commencing with impaired concentration, memory and judgement. Extreme anxiety and delusions, often of grandeur, may be prominent features. Epilepsy is a feature in about half the cases. GPI develops 10–15 years after primary infection. The CSF shows changes similar to those of tabes dorsalis; i.e. mononuclear cells (up to $70/mm^3$) with slightly raised protein. Tests for syphilis are positive in blood and CSF.

The term *latent neurosyphilis* is used to describe patients in whom there are no clinical signs of neurosyphilis but the immunological tests for syphilis in the CSF are positive; these tests are positive also in the blood. These abnormalities are sometimes discovered on routine investigation in patients presenting with stroke or with epilepsy.

Treatment. The treatment of choice for neurosyphilis is benzylpenicillin 300 mg i.m. 6-hourly together with probenecid 0.5 g by mouth 6-hourly for 17 days, or procaine penicillin 1.2 g i.m. once daily with probenecid 0.5 g orally 6-hourly for 17 days. This latter regimen is preferred for out-patients. Prednisolone 10 mg tds orally is usually advised for 24 hours prior to steroid treatment, and during the first 48 hours of steroid treatment. In patients allergic to penicillin erythromycin 500 mg qds orally for 3–4 weeks, or doxycycline 100 mg tds may be used.

Follow up at 3-monthly intervals should include lumbar puncture to assess disease activity. The cell count should be less than $15/mm^3$ at 6 months; the protein and IgG levels gradually fall but the TPI test remains positive indefinitely. If there is doubt about the effectiveness of treatment the course of penicillin/probenecid should be repeated.

Progression of optic neuropathy and deafness may occur despite treatment and this has been treated with some success with intermittent courses of high-dose prednisolone. Dementia may also progress. The lightning pains of tabes dorsalis do not respond to antibiotic treatment but may improve with carbamazepine 300–1000 mg daily. The prognosis of stroke in meningovascular syphilis is good but little recovery can be expected from tabes dorsalis or from GPI; indeed, some progression may continue despite treatment.

Lyme disease

This summertime zoonosis, caused by the spirochaete *Borrelia burgdorfi*, is transmitted by the bite of infected ticks found in woodland

Table 6.7 *Protozoal and metazoal causes of meningoencephalitis.*

Toxoplasmosis
Malaria
Trypanosomiasis
Schistosomiasis
Amoebiasis
Echinococcus
Cysticercosis
Trichinosis

in temperate countries. A chronic migratory erythema develops, with recurrent arthritis, myocarditis and fever. Neurological manifestations may occur without the skin rash, consisting of lymphocytic meningoencephalitis, Bell's palsy, peripheral neuropathy and transverse myelitis. Immunofluorescent tests are available for diagnosis. Treatment with penicillin or tetracycline is effective.

Tropical infections and infestations (Table 6.7)

Although these disorders are rare in temperate countries they are well-known causes of disability in tropical countries. Neurological syndromes result from invasion of the brain or meninges by the causative organism. In some, neurological involvement occurs only at a particular stage in the life cycle of the organism or parasite. In *malaria*, haemorrhagic encephalitis is a serious and often fatal complication of *P. falciparum* infection. *Toxoplasmosis* causes subacute or chronic meningoencephalitis, with a lymphocytic CSF, but it may also present as a localized parenchymal granuloma with focal signs or seizures. It is particularly common in immunocompromised or malnourished people. African trypanosomiasis (*T. rhodesiensis*) causes an encephalopathy, with seizures, lassitude and sleepiness leading to coma (African sleeping sickness). *Schistosomiasis* may involve the conus medullaris, presenting with incontinence and a cauda equina syndrome, or with a transverse cord lesion. The ova or larva stages of infestations with metazoa are characterized by dissemination through many organs, including the brain, causing meningitis, seizures and hydrocephalus. Ruptured cysts in *amoebiasis* may cause a severe, even fatal chemical meningitis.

Fungal infections

Most cases occur as opportunistic infections (Table 6.8) in patients with impaired immune responses or in whom there is an open route

Table 6.8 *Opportunistic infections of the CNS.*

Bacterial infections
  Gram negative bacilli
  Staphylococcus aureus
  Listeria monocytogenes
  Streptococcus
  Nocardia asteroides
Fungal infections
  Candida albicans
  Cryptococcus neoformans
  Aspergillus fumigatus
  Mucormycosis
Viral infections
  Herpes zoster
  Herpes simplex encephalitis
  Measles
  Papova viruses; progressive multifocal leucoencephalopathy
  Cytomegalovirus

Table 6.9 *Causes of opportunistic infections of the CNS.*

Surgical operations on the brain
CSF shunts
Leucopenia
Leukaemia, lymphoma
Cytotoxic drug and steroid therapy
Multiple antibiotic therapy
Splenectomy
Other immunocompromised states, e.g. organ transplantation
Hypogammaglobulinaemias
HIV infection (AIDS syndrome)
Malignant disease

of infection (Table 6.9). *Cryptococcal* infections represent 50% of CNS fungal infections. Signs of meningism may be accompanied by features of invasion of the brain, with focal symptoms and signs, and drowsiness or coma. The illness may be prolonged and diagnosis difficult. Specific antigen detection tests are available for CSF and blood samples, and the organism can often be detected with special stains in CSF sediment. The cellular response in the CSF is predominantly lymphocytic, the CSF protein is raised, and the CSF glucose level is lowered.

Cryptococcus infection has varied neurological manifestations, often without prominent meningism or systemic reaction. In *candidiasis* CNS involvement is common but may be undetected, although abscess formation, meningitis and vascular invasion may occur. *Aspergillosis* is associated with corticosteroid therapy, malignancy or multiple antibiotic therapy, but spread to the CNS is haematogeneous. Vascular involvement is frequent, causing a stroke-like course. Despite the infection the CSF glucose may be normal. *Mucormycosis* invades the brain from infection in the nose or nasopharynx. There is always a predisposing cause (Table 6.9). Major vessels at the base of the brain are invaded, leading to hemispheric infarction and death. The orbits are often also involved.

Fungal infections can often be effectively treated with amphotericin B or 5 fluorocytosine. These drugs have been used in combination (amphotericin B 20 mg/day by i.v. infusion with 5 fluorocytosine 150 mg/kg/day orally in four divided doses).

Mollaret's meningitis and other meningitic syndromes

Recurrent lymphocytic meningitis with fever, without detectable cause, is extremely rare. Suspected cases are usually later shown to be due to a recognizable infection. *Leptospirosis* and *brucellosis* may also cause recurrent lymphocytic meningitis, although in these conditions other systemic features are usually prominent.

Viral infections

Viruses (Table 6.3) may cause meningitis, encephalitis, a mixed clinical picture (meningoencephalitis) or spinal cord involvement (myelitis) The peripheral nervous system is involved in H. simplex or H. zoster infections and it is the route of infection in encephalitic rabies. Enteroviruses commonly cause acute aseptic meningitis, arboviruses and H. simplex usually invade the brain causing encephalitis or a mixed meningoencephalitis, and mumps, an infection known only in man, may cause meningitis or encephalitis.

Acute aseptic meningitis

This is usually a benign, self-limited disease of acute onset or with a prodrome of a few days fever and chills. Headache, fever, malaise and neck stiffness are the main features, although the latter may be unimpressive in relation to that characteristic of bacterial meningitis. The headache is usually frontal or retro-orbital and is often associated with photophobia. Drowsiness may be noted, and there may be abdominal pain and vomiting. The CSF is under increased pressure, contains lymphocytes in increased number, but shows normal protein and glucose levels (Table 6.4). Recovery occurs in a few days and antiviral therapy is not required.

The syndrome of aseptic meningitis frequently accompanies mumps infection, developing a week or more after the parotitis. This is probably the commonest cause of aseptic meningitis, but coxsackie virus and echovirus infections are also common.

Viral encephalitis

In viral encephalitis there is invasion of the brain by the virus; the meninges are frequently also involved but this may be subclinical. Involvement of the spinal cord (myelitis) may also be evident in some cases. The illness may be acute or subacute, with fever, headache, photophobia and drowsiness. These features of meningeal involvement are accompanied by focal neurological deficits, e.g. hemiplegia, aphasia, seizures or confusion. Coma, a feature suggesting a poor prognosis, may supervene. Examination may show features of generalized illness, e.g. a skin rash or lymphadenopathy, and focal signs are often found. There may be neck stiffness. Papilloedema is not a feature.

The peripheral blood may show a lymphocytosis. The EEG is usually abnormal, with diffuse slowing of background rhythms. Focal, temporal lobe abnormalities with periodic discharges are common in H. simplex encephalitis. The CT scan is frequently normal, but may show areas of decreased attenuation, especially in the temporal lobes in H. simplex encephalitis, or localizing swelling. The CSF shows a moderate increase in protein content, with a lymphocytosis, but with normal glucose levels. Serial complement-fixing titres for viral antibodies are positive in only about 60% of cases and therefore are not generally useful in diagnosis and management. Sometimes the CSF cell count shows a pleocytosis with both lymphocytes and polymorphs.

Management. Patients with mild viral encephalitis do not require specific treatment. Seriously ill patients need supportive management with fluid balance, control of secondary infections, treatment of seizures with anticonvulsant drugs and general nursing care. Herpes simplex encephalitis is particularly serious, and carries a high mortality; indeed, it is probably the commonest form of fatal encephalitis in the UK and USA. Treatment with acyclovir (5 mg/kg i.v. given over 1 hour, at 8-hour intervals, for 7 days) has greatly improved the prognosis, improving survival from <30% to >80%. The clinical diagnosis of H. simplex encephalitis is difficult and, since acyclovir is relatively free from toxic effects, it is reasonable to treat all patients with severe viral encephalitis, i.e. those in coma, or with rapidly advancing disability, with the drug for a 5-day trial period.

The outcome of severe viral encephalitis is variable. Almost 50% of patients have residual disability, with hemiparesis, perceptual problems, personality change or seizures, and prolonged rehabilitation may be required. Some forms of viral encephalitis, however, are always mild, without residual problems, as in the case of mumps. Conversely, H. simplex encephalitis is frequently accompanied by residual disability in survivors. Steroid therapy is not indicated when there is direct viral infection since it seems to increase morbidity.

Post-infectious encephalomyelitis

In this syndrome an illness resembling acute viral encephalitis develops 1–2 weeks after an acute viral infection. In most cases the syndrome follows measles infection, but it was also a well-recognized complication of smallpox vaccination. The illness consists of an acute onset of headache, vomiting, confusion and coma, often developing in a few hours during the week following measles infection at a time when the fever is resolving. Focal neurological signs and seizures may develop, and there may be striking perceptual problems, including deafness or blindness, or signs of spinal cord involvement. The CSF usually contains both lymphocytes and polymorphs with an increased protein level and a normal glucose level. In measles, this complication occurs in 1/1000 cases; of these 95% have encephalomyelitis, 3% myelitis and 2% polyradiculitis.

Treatment is empirical, but steroids reduce the mortality, although survivors are often handicapped by motor, sensory, perceptual, psychological or personality deficits, or by epilepsy. In the acute phase antibiotic therapy for secondary infection and seizure prevention are important in preventing secondary brain damage.

The term *acute disseminated encephalomyelitis* probably refers to the same condition, this term has often been used to refer to para-infectious complications of measles, German measles, mumps, chicken pox or vaccination against rabies or influenza. Post-infectious encephalomyelitis and acute disseminated encephalomyelitis differ from acute viral encephalitis in that there is demyelination of white matter in addition to involvement of grey matter, and that the disorder results from a hyperimmune reaction to challenge by a viral agent.

An acute cerebellar syndrome may develop some 1–3 weeks after chicken pox infection. This syndrome is of uncertain pathogenesis.

Other specific viral infections

Poliomyelitis

This enterovirus involves the motor system. The infection spreads from the gut through viraemia into the nervous system, causing a lymphocytic meningitis. The infection specifically involves anterior horn cells and motoneurons of the somatic efferent cranial nerve nuclei causing acute flaccid paralysis with lower motor neuron signs. Recovery is slow and incomplete. There is a tendency for muscles that were active during viraemia to be more severely affected. When there is bulbar involvement the mortality approaches 50%. Since the advent of nationwide immunization programmes the disease has become rare in the UK.

H. zoster

Endogeneous reactivation of latent varicella infection results in the syndrome of H. zoster infection. This reactivation may occur in healthy adults but commonly indicates a decreased immune response, e.g. in patients with Hodgkins disease, during steroid therapy, in the elderly and during immunosuppressive therapy. The infection is commonly manifest by localized cutaneous involvement within the distribution of one or more sensory dermatomes. The vesicular, painful rash may be preceded by malaise, fever and hyperaesthesia or itching in the affected skin; when the rash develops the skin may be analgesic but spontaneous pain may develop and this can be a persisting problem. The virus is latent in the dorsal root ganglion and this distribution of sensory abnormalities reflects reactivation of virus spread in cutaneous nerves within the dermatome and replication in epidermal cells. Thoracic dermatomes are most commonly involved but H. zoster also affects the trigeminal ganglion, often appearing in the ophthalmic division, leading to the risk of corneal involvement, and to persistent upper facial neuralgic pain.

Involvement of motor roots may accompany severe episodes so that radicular weakness develops. In the thoracic region this is not important but in the arm or leg there is potentially severe disability since recovery is almost always incomplete. Rarely, cranial nerves may be affected, most commonly the second, third or seventh. Thus, involvement of the facial ganglion may cause facial palsy with vesicles in the external auditory meatus (Ramsay Hunt syndrome). The eighth nerve may sometimes be involved.

Generalized zoster may complicate leukaemia, or occur in immunosuppressed patients; it may also develop after segmental H. zoster infection.

Meningitis, encephalitis, myelitis or polyneuritis are infrequent manifestations. The prognosis for recovery from the neurological disability is relatively poor without specific antiviral therapy.

Treatment and outcome. Without specific antiviral therapy recovery from the neurological effects of H. zoster infection is usually incomplete. Segmental H. zoster infections, including cranial nerve infections, are frequently followed by intractable post-herpetic neuralgia. This consists of a continuous aching, deep pain with sharp lancinating and very severe jabs of pain in response to contact. The patient may refuse to touch, wash or even dress the affected part and treatment with analgesics, carbamazepine, antidepressants or even psychotropic drugs, or with neurostimulation therapy is frequently ineffective.

Antiviral therapy with oral acyclovir 800 mg five times daily for 7 days is effective in healing the vesicular lesions and in reducing pain during the acute phase. It is most effective if given within 24–48 hours of the appearance of the rash. In addition, early treatment seems to limit the severity of post-herpetic neuralgia.

Rabies

This infection results from inoculation by a penetrating bite from an infected mammal, usually a dog, fox or bat. The virus multiplies in the wound and migrates along nerves to enter the CNS after an incubation period of 1–3 months. Shorter incubation periods are characteristic of facial bites. A phase of vague illness, consisting of malaise, fever, anxiety, depression, irritability or psychosis is followed by laryngeal spasm and terror when disturbed (hydrophobia probably implies hyperexcitability when encouraged to drink?). In 20% of cases there is an ascending flaccid paralysis.

All forms of rabies are fatal once the disorder is established. However, treatment with human rabies immunoglobulin has resulted in survival in a few recent cases. During the incubation phase immunization with human diploid cell strain vaccine is effective if given before there is CNS invasion. Immunoglobulin is given intramuscularly and to the wound site at the same time as the course of vaccine is commenced. The active disease is often complicated by seizures and spasms, and anticonvulsants are useful. Steroids should be avoided. Death often occurs from cardiac arrhythmia. Advice on treatment can be obtained from the Rabies Control Officer through the Public Health Laboratory Service in the UK.

Persistent viral infections

Viruses have the propensity for chronic, latent and slow or persistent infection, as well as acute infection of the nervous system. In *chronic infections* virus replication continues over a long period. The virus

Table 6.10   *Persistent viral infections.*

Conventional viruses
   subacute sclerosing panencephalitis
   progressive multifocal leucoencephalopathy
   cytomegalovirus
   congenital rubella
   Herpes zoster
   Herpes simplex
   HIV infection

Unconventional viruses
   Kuru
   Creutzfeldt–Jakob disease
   Gerstmann–Straussler syndrome

infection may be partially controlled by the host immune system so that only a few cells may be damaged at any given time. Examples include congenital rubella and cytomegalovirus infections, in which there is a long phase of active viral infection.

In *latent infections* virus persists in nervous tissue in an undetectable and inactive form. During this phase the host immune system is inactive and the patient is asymptomatic. The infection may become reactivated, often in response to extraneous factors, such as steroid treatment, malignancy and changes in immune competence; when this occurs infectious virions are produced and active clinical infection develops.

In *slow or persistent infections* (Table 6.10) there is often an initial acute infection but this is followed by a latent period or a period of slow progression leading to an illness that may not resemble the initial syndrome. Alternatively, a chronic progressive illness may develop without a history of initial infection. Persistent infections may develop with certain *conventional viruses*, e.g. rubella, H. zoster, H. simplex, cytomegalovirus, measles, Epstein–Barr virus, papova viruses (JC virus) or retroviruses such as human immunodeficiency virus (HIV). *Unconventional viruses*, which are transmissible, filtrable 'viruses' that do not evoke an inflammatory response and are relatively resistant to sterilization, may also cause persistent infections, as in kuru, Creutzfeldt–Jakob disease and Gerstmann–Straussler syndrome.

Conventional viruses

In these syndromes (Table 6.10) there is often a history of acute infection, followed by a phase of gradual progression.

Subacute sclerosing panencephalitis (SSPE)

This is a rare (1 per million cases of measles) late manifestation of measles virus infection. The disease begins in children or young adults, with an insidious onset of behavioural disturbance and intellectual decline, followed by clumsiness, apraxia, regular myoclonic jerks, seizures and, eventually, a state of decorticate mutism. Death occurs 1–3 years after the onset, but longer survival may occur. Boys outnumber girls 3 to 1. The CSF protein is slightly raised and contains high levels of IgG, which shows high titres of reactivity against measles antigen. The EEG shows characteristic periodic complexes occurring every 5 seconds corresponding to the myoclonic jerks. Measles virions can be detected in the brain at autopsy. Treatment with antiviral agents is not effective, although isoprinosine may slow progression of the disease; steroids may lead to more rapid deterioration. The disease can be prevented by measles immunization.

Progressive multifocal leucoencephalopathy (PML)

This disease is due to infection with a polyoma virus (JC virus). It occurs only in immunocompromised subjects, especially when there is a lymphoproliferative disorder, and in the acquired immunodeficiency syndrome (AIDS). The initial infection may cause mild respiratory symptoms, but is often unnoticed. There is a subacute progression leading to ataxia, incoordination, dysphasia, dysarthria, hemianopia, personality changes, dementia and, sometimes, brain stem disturbances. The disease is usually fatal in less than a year. The CT scan shows non-enhancing, low density lesions in the brain, usually at grey/white matter junctions. The diagnosis is confirmed by brain biopsy, in which stacked virus particles can be demonstrated by EM or by immunofluorescence. The CSF is normal. There is no effective treatment.

Cytomegalovirus infection

This virus particularly affects the subependymal lining cells of the ventricles in newborn infants causing failure of brain growth with periventricular and intracerebral calcification. In severe cases there is mental retardation, spasticity, seizures, deafness and microcephaly. This is the commonest known cause for mental retardation, affecting 1 in 1000 newborns. The virus can be isolated from the faeces and from urine.

Congenital rubella

This infection is acquired by the fetus during maternal infection. The syndrome is characterized by congenital cataract, mental retardation, microcephaly, deafness and spastic diplegia, or by any combination of these. In some infants an encephalitic syndrome resembling SSPE (see above) may develop during infancy. The syndrome can be prevented by prior immunization against rubella.

HIV infection and AIDS

HIV is a retrovirus with cytopathic effects which is related to lentiviruses. The latter group includes visna and caprine arthritis/ encephalitis virus, both of which may cause neurodegenerative disease in sheep and goats. HIV 1, the commonest retrovirus infection in humans, is related to a simian T cell lymphotropic virus (STLV III) which produces a simian AIDS syndrome, with encephalitis. HIV 2 is a related human retrovirus first isolated in West Africa.

Acute infection usually results from homosexual contact or from contact with blood products, as in haemophiliacs, and by shared needles amongst drug addicts. Heterosexual transmission is less common in Western countries, although this mode of infection appears common in Africa. The acute seroconversion phase is accompanied by a glandular fever-like illness including fever, rash

Table 6.11 *Classification of HIV infection (Centers for Disease Control; 1986).*

Group 1
Acute infection;
a 'flu-like illness, with seroconversion for HIV antibody, sometimes associated with aseptic meningitis.

Group 2
Asymptomatic infection;
latent phase

Group 3
Persistent generalized lymphadenopathy;
lymph nodes 1 cm or bigger at two or more sites for 3 months or more without other cause.

Group 4
Other HIV-related disease:
a) constitutional disease, with fever, weight loss and diarrhoea without other cause.
b) neurological disease, with dementia, myelopathy or peripheral neuropathy.
c) secondary infections.
d) secondary cancers, especially Kaposi's sarcoma and primary cerebral non-Hodgkin's lymphoma.
e) others, e.g. chronic interstitial pneumonia.

and lymphadenopathy. Encephalopathy, meningitis, myelitis or neuropathy, including the fifth, seventh and eighth cranial nerves, may occur at this stage, but these features are uncommon. This phase persists for about a week.

Lymphadenopathy, typically symmetrical, firm, discrete and non-tender without hilar enlargement, may persist for many months. Kaposi's sarcomas are characteristic skin lesions. Acute inflammatory polyneuropathy, resembling Guillain-Barré syndrome, but with a CSF lymphocytosis may occur in this phase.

The HIV virus is neurotropic and persistent infection of the CNS is therefore almost invariable. The acquired immunodeficiency syndrome (AIDS) consists of evidence of HIV infection, opportunistic infections, weight loss and features of CNS involvement, with altered T cell immunity (Table 6.11).

About 30% of patients with AIDS develop subacute encephalitis and about 10% present with neurological problems. This AIDS encephalopathy presents with forgetfulness, loss of concentration, apathy and psychomotor retardation with loss of balance and difficulty walking. Examination reveals dementia with gait ataxia

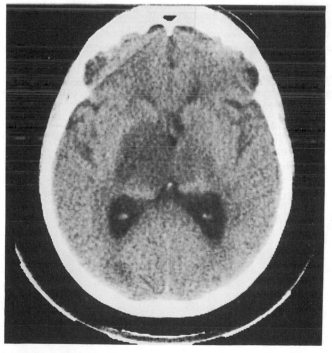

Fig. 6.5   AIDS and cerebral toxoplasmosis. There is a large, ill-defined, low attenuation lesion in the deep central region of the brain, and another smaller lesion in the right occipital lobe.

leading to a wasted, demented state with incontinence within a year of the onset. The CSF shows a mild lymphocytosis with increased protein level, and the EEG shows slowed background rhythms. Seizures may occur. The CT scan shows cerebral atrophy with dilated ventricles. This syndrome is usually due to HIV infection of the brain, but it may be mimicked to some extent by other infections to which these patients are susceptible, e.g. atypical mycobacterial infection, fungal infection, subacute sclerosing panencephalitis, progressive multifocal leucoencephalitis, H. simplex encephalitis, cytomegalovirus or toxoplasmosis infections, listeriosis, *Cryptococcus neoformans* and *Pneumocystis carinii* infections. These infections often pursue a more rapid course and may be identified by focal features, as in toxoplasmosis (Fig. 6.5), and by their CT scan or MRI, and CSF manifestations. The fundi are often abnormal in patients with AIDS because of the multiplicity of opportunistic infections that may develop.

A quarter of patients with AIDS develop a subacute paraplegia with incontinence, often associated with progressive dementia. This syndrome is thought to be due to HIV infection in the spinal cord causing a vacuolar change at pathological examination.

Intracranial lymphoma is a common complication in people with AIDS who have developed lymphoma in other organs, but it may also occur as a primary intracerebral space-occupying lesion.

Management. Opportunistic infections should be treated with appropriate antibiotic drugs or chemotherapy. Intracranial lymphoma may respond to radiotherapy, but recurrence is usual and may occur very rapidly. AIDS encephalopathy and myelopathy cannot be treated satisfactorily with current antiviral agents, but it is possible that specific antiviral treatment against the HIV retrovirus, e.g. with zidovudine (Retrovir) may prevent the development of AIDS in HIV-positive patients. Seizures should be managed with anticonvulsant drugs. Repeated investigation of patients with AIDS encephalopathy is not helpful, but the appropriate treatment of opportunistic infections during the early stages of this complication may result in clinical improvement. Standard precautions to prevent cross-infection from body fluids and blood should be used in assessing such patients, as would be used in patients with hepatitis B.

Unconventional viruses

Infection with this class of agents, presumed to be viruses but sometimes classified separately as prions (proteinaceous infectious particles thought to be derived from genome proteins of the cell), was first recognized in kuru, a disease found in certain isolated tribes in New Guinea. This disease consisting of a progressive cerebellar ataxia and dementia was transmitted by cannibalism. Similarities between the pathology of this disorder and Creutzfeldt–Jakob disease were recognized and transmission of the latter disease by contact with brain tissue and other tissues of infected patients was recognized after transmission from man to ape by brain inoculation experiments. This work led to recognition of the whole class of persistent viral infections of the CNS. Scrapie, an encephalopathy of sheep and bovine spongiform encephalopathy are similar diseases.

Creutzfeldt–Jakob disease

This disorder consists of a progressive encephalopathy that most commonly develops in the fifth or sixth decades. It begins with fatigue, minor gait problems, blurred vision and impaired memory. This phase continues for several months; rarely subacute hemiparesis may develop. Dementia is inexorable and rapid and is associated with ataxia, myoclonus, cortical blindness, incontinence, spasticity and amyotrophy. The latter is prominent in some cases. Death occurs in a year in 80% of cases. The EEG shows generalized periodic complexes at 1 Hz. The CSF is usually normal, although the protein level may be slightly raised. The CT scan shows cerebral atrophy. Familial cases have been recognized, perhaps implying intimate contact with the infectious agent rather than vertical transmission.

At autopsy there is vacuolar, spongiform degeneration of the cortex. This is due to extensive vacuolation of the neuropil with a reactive gliosis and neuronal loss. In the amyotrophic form anterior horn cells are lost and widespread spongiform change is not prominent

Management. There is no treatment for the condition. Since it is transmissible, tissue such as cornea should not be used for transplantation. Contamination of nursing and medical staff with body fluids and blood should be avoided by simple barrier nursing precautions. Brain biopsy is not required for diagnosis; surgical instruments require sterilization by prolonged heat sterilization or by treatment with 0.5% sodium hypochlorite.

Gerstmann–Straussler syndrome

This is a rare familial and transmissible disorder, clinically resembling Creutzfeldt–Jakob disease but with more prominent spasticity and without myoclonus. The brain shows amyloid plaques.

---7---

Coma and Brain Death

In *coma* the patient is unrousable and unresponsive to all external stimuli. Other terms in common use to describe patients in whom consciousness is disturbed refer to less severe states of altered consciousness. In *stupor* the patient can be roused only by vigorous external stimuli, and arousal is brief and often incomplete. *Obtundation* is a word often used to refer to a state of abnormal drowsiness, often found in patients with space occupying or metabolic brain diseases before stupor or coma supervene. The patient can be woken easily from what appears to be sleep, but drifts off again during conversation or examination; while awake the patient may be confused. *Acute confusional states*, in which there is global intellectual impairment in a setting of clouding of consciousness, are also termed *delirium*, a term that usually implies reversibility with appropriate treatment. *Consciousness* itself is a state of normal brain activity in which the patient is aware of self and environment; *sleep* is a normal state of altered consciousness from which arousal to normal consciousness occurs in response to internal or external stimuli.

Causes of coma (Table 7.1)

Coma may be due to metabolic or structural disease of the brain; rarely it may be psychogenic. Coma results from lesions affecting the brain diffusely or multifocally, or from large lesions in the pons, midbrain or diencephalon; i.e. in deep mid-line structures. Supratentorial mass lesions, such as tumours or haematomas, may damage diencephalic and brain stem structures, while subtentorial mass lesions may directly damage the upper brain stem, and therefore the reticular activating system. In metabolic disorders, such as hypoglycaemia, hypnotic drugs or hypoxia, coma results from widespread depression of brain function. The clinical features of these three types of disorder differ. In addition, the prognosis of coma due to subtentorial mass lesions is far worse than that of coma with supratentorial mass lesions or metabolic disorders.

Table 7.1 *Causes of coma; metabolic and diffuse structural disorders.*

Metabolic	Structural
Drug overdose (including alcohol)	Meningitis
Hyperglycaemia	Encephalitis
Hypothyroidism	Other infections, e.g. cerebral malaria
Hypoxia	Subarachnoid haemorrhage
Hypothermia	Epilepsy
Diabetic coma	Severe closed head injury
Cardio-respiratory failure	
Hepatic encephalopathy	
Uraemia	

Metabolic coma

Metabolic encephalopathies have certain common features. In particular there is a progressive deteriorating course during a period of hours or days from an alert state, through clouding of consciousness and delirium, to stupor and coma. During the intermediate phase, periods of irritability with visual hallucinations, and less commonly auditory hallucinations, and seizures may occur before increasing drowsiness and unresponsiveness supervene. Careful clinical observation may indicate the likely cause of metabolic coma. In *hepatic encephalopathy* there may be signs of chronic liver disease with jaundice, telangiectasia, liver enlargement and tenderness, and hepatic fetor, and a characteristic slow, irregular flapping tremor of the outstretched hands and fingers may be seen. In *renal failure* the skin is pigmented, there may be a uraemic frost and fetor, and urine output may be negligible. The fundi show uraemic/hypertensive changes with haemorrhages and exudates, there is metabolic acidosis with deep sighing hyperpnoea, and a distal flap with myoclonus is present. In *hyperthyroidism* the characteristic diurnal features of myxoedema are present, with slowly reactive and slowly relaxing tendon reflexes. In *diabetic keto-acidotic coma* there are signs of acidosis, with deep rapid ventilation and tachycardia, and the urine contains glucose and ketone bodies. In *hyperosmolar diabetic coma* acidosis is not a feature but frequent multifocal seizures occur, often with focal neurological signs. *Hypothermic coma* should be recognized by the low core temperature; a special low-reading rectal thermometer may be necessary to document this. The heart rate is slow and ventricular arrhythmias may be found on ECG recordings. It often occurs in the elderly and in hypothyroid patients. *Hyperthermic coma* may complicate neuroleptic medication, or may develop in parkinsonian patients treated with anticholinergic drugs, when bacterial infection occurs.

In *hypoglycaemia* the patient may present with flaccid unresponsive coma, with stroke-like syndromes, e.g. hemiparesis, and with seizures. As a clinical rule, any patient in undiagnosed coma should have blood and urine sugar estimations immediately, and if any suspicion remains after instant bedside testing (not waiting for the laboratory test) 40 g glucose should be given intravenously. The consequences of untreated coma-producing hypoglycaemia are so serious, with permanent diffuse brain damage, that treatment forms the basis of diagnosis in this condition. Diabetics may develop severe hypoglycaemia without typical warning features, because an associated diabetic neuropathy prevents the aura of fear, hunger and anxiety that would occur in otherwise normal subjects.

Drug overdosage is probably the commonest cause of metabolic coma. The diagnosis may be suspected by the patient's family or friends, or by the ambulance service and a search of the patient's clothing or home may be rewarding. Sedatives such as barbiturates, benzodiazepines, phenothiazines and alcohol directly depress brain activity and produce flaccid coma, with depressed respiration, hypotension and depressed vestibular function. In the early phase, nystagmus, ataxia and dysarthria are prominent. Doll's head eye movements are preserved until deep coma supervenes, when doll's head and caloric-induced eye movements become depressed. However, except in glutethimide poisoning, the pupillary light reflexes are preserved. The tendon reflexes are not increased, although the plantar responses are usually extensor. Poisoning with opiates causes coma with pinpoint pupils (Fig. 7.1) and respiratory irregularity, often with hypoventilation. The combination of alcohol and sedative or opiate overdosage is often overlooked and blood alcohol levels should be checked when this is suspected on social grounds. A blood alcohol level of 25–100 mg/dl is associated with euphoria, nystagmus and inco-ordination, 100–200 mg/dl with excitability, ataxia, dysarthria, hypoalgesia and confusion, 200–300 mg/dl with drowsiness, diplopia, marked ataxia and pupillary dilatation, and levels greater than 300 mg/dl with analgesia, hyperventilation, severe dysarthria, stupor or even coma. It must be remembered that chronic alcoholics, accustomed regularly to high blood alcohol levels, may tolerate a blood level of 150 mg/dl without clinical effects, and this feature is used as one component of a working definition of chronic addition to alcohol.

Structural coma

Coma with structural brain disease may be due to diffuse (Table 7.1), supratentorial or subtentorial lesions (Table 7.2).

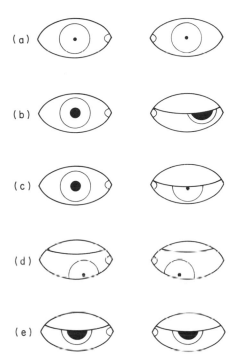

Fig. 7.1 Pupillary anomalies. (a) Bilateral pinpoint pupils occur with brain stem lesions, opiate and other drug intoxications and with pontine infarction. (b) Left third nerve palsy. There is ptosis, dilatation of the pupil with absence of the light reaction, and slight lateral deviation of the eye. (c) Horner's syndrome. There is ptosis and a small, reactive pupil. (d) In thalamic haemorrhage the eyes tend to 'look towards the tip of the nose', and the pupils are small; later they become large and unreactive as upper brain stem involvement develops. (e) When brain stem death occurs the mid brain disturbance is manifest by mid-position, fixed (unreactive) pupils, with eye closure.

Table 7.2 *Causes of coma: focal structural lesions.*

Supratentorial lesions	Subtentorial lesions
Intra-cerebral haemorrhage	Cerebellar haemorrhage
Cerebral infarction	Pontine haemorrhage
Subdural haematoma	Upper brain stem infarction
Extradural haematoma	Tumours
Cerebral tumours	Cerebellar/brain stem abscess
Cerebral abscess	Trauma
	Brain stem encephalitis

Diffuse structural causes of coma (Table 7.1)

These disorders cause dysfunction in the brain as a whole and therefore present with coma as a major manifestation. The underlying cause is recognizable from specific features of the history, and by clinical examination. Thus, when the meninges are inflamed by *infection*, or from the presence of *subarachnoid blood*, there is headache at the onset or during the progression of the illness, often with vomiting, drowsiness, fever and signs of meningism, especially neck rigidity. In addition, papilloedema, or sub-hyaloid haemorrhages, may be seen in the fundi. Focal signs may also be present, consisting of focal seizures, hemiparesis, and cranial nerve palsies, especially third (Fig. 7.1) and fourth nerve palsies. *Epilepsy* itself is recognized usually by the history, since most seizures occur prior to medical intervention. *Trauma* is usually evident from the circumstances but sometimes, as in criminal trauma, it may be concealed and careful examination of the head, neck, external auditory meati, face and nose is always indicated. In most of these diffuse structural disorders focal neurological signs are evident on examination.

The diagnosis can be confirmed by CT scans of the head, and by EEG in the case of epilepsy and encephalitis, but CSF examination is mandatory when bacterial or viral meningitis, or encephalitis is suspected, and also in most cases of subarachnoid haemorrhage. In comatose patients with fever, meningitis should be suspected even in the absence of neck rigidity, provided that a space-occupying lesion has been excluded.

Supratentorial (focal) structural causes of coma (Table 7.2)

Expanding supratentorial lesions, whether *extracerebral*, e.g. extradural haematoma, subdural haematoma, or extracerebral tumours, or *intracerebral*, e.g. intracerebral tumour, abscess or haemorrhage, or focal cerebral oedema, produce coma by involvement of midline diencephalic structures or, secondarily, from reticular dysfunction due to brain stem displacement.

There are two major clinical patterns of brain shift from supratentorial lesions that may impair brain stem function and result in coma. These are central or transtentorial herniation of the diencephalon and uncal herniation. Both cause vascular and obstructive complications that endanger life, but may be reversible with appropriate treatment.

Transtentorial herniation of the diencephalon (*central* herniation) is due to downward displacement of the basal nuclei, caused by pressure transmitted from above, e.g. with parietal, frontal and occipital lesions such as tumours, abscess or haematoma. The basal ganglia and diencephalon are displaced caudally towards the midbrain, resulting in oedema and haemorrhage in the pretectal area and in the upper midbrain. In this syndrome focal signs may be present initially from the causative lesion, but in extracerebral mass lesions no such signs may be present. These features are superseded by a phase of drowsiness and irritability, with irregular breathing and occasional deep yawns. Roving eye movements may be present, but the pupils, although small (Fig. 7.1), react normally to light. There is a full range of oculocephalic and caloric eye movements. Paratonic (generalized) resistance to passive movement of the limbs is a feature. Later, respiration becomes Cheyne–Stokes in type (periodic breathing), the pupils become smaller and upward gaze may be impaired to dolls-head testing. Bilateral corticospinal signs develop, to be followed by neck stiffness and decorticate or even decerebrate rigidity. At this terminal stage the pupils dilate and become unreactive (Fig. 7.1) and respirations become irregular, with loss of ocular movements. This syndrome is often accompanied by papilloedema.

This syndrome of transtentorial herniation can be categorized into an early diencephalic stage, an intermediate mesencephalic phase and a late pontine phase. Death results when medullary dysfunction develops. Recovery is unlikely when there are signs of mesencephalic or pontine dysfunction. Herniation of the cingulate gyrus on the side of the lesion may precede the development of transtentorial herniation. Although this is usually asymptomatic it results in secondary vascular problems in the hemispheres and may precipitate the diencephalic syndrome of transtentorial herniation. Its importance is that it may be recognized on CT scanning in patients with supratentorial lesions, and its presence should indicate the need for treatment of rising intracranial pressure, by neurosurgical removal of the mass lesion.

In the syndrome of *uncal herniation* the pattern of clinical deterioration is different. A space occupying lesion situated laterally in the middle fossa, or in the temporal lobe displaces the uncus and the hippocampal gyrus, i.e. the medial portion of the temporal lobe, towards the midline and over the lateral edge of the tentorium. This is a typical complication of temporal lobe tumours, abscess or haematoma, or of extracerebral masses such as subdural haematoma or extradural haematoma. A characteristic sequence of clinical events follows uncal herniation leading to irreversible complications if the causative mass is not removed. The herniated temporal lobe directly compresses the ipsilateral third nerve against the free edge of the tentorium; this causes initial constriction of the pupil followed by pupillary dilatation and then by the development of a complete third nerve palsy with ptosis. At the latter stage the patient is often stuporose or in coma due to midbrain compression but in chronic lesions a complete third nerve palsy may occur without other features of herniation (Fig. 7.1). The initial constriction of the pupil, due to irritation of the third nerve is often missed since it is transient. The temporal lobe lesion itself may cause contralateral hemiparesis.

Increasing uncal and hippocampal herniation leads also to compression of the ipsilateral posterior cerebral artery causing ischaemia and infarction in the occipital lobe, and thus contralateral hemianopia. Eventually the brain stem itself is compressed and displaced causing distortion of the opposite cerebral peduncle which becomes compressed against the opposite tentorial edge (*Kernohan's* notch refers to the groove in the cerebral peduncle found at autopsy); this may produce a hemiparesis ipsilateral to the mass lesion, and to the third nerve palsy (Fig. 7.1). Compression of the upper brain stem itself causes drowsiness, stupor or coma, often with hyper-ventilation and, later, Cheyne–Stokes respirations. Decerebrate posturing of the limbs develops in this late, preterminal stage; both pupils dilate and become unresponsive to light, and both plantar responses are extensor. The clinical features at this stage are indistinguishable from those of the central syndrome of transtentorial herniation described above.

Clinical management of rising intracranial pressure syndromes

The combination of careful nursing observations, using the Glasgow coma scale (Table 7.3), or its equivalent, based on level of consciousness, limb movement and eye opening, together with observations of the pupillary light responses, the pattern of respirations and the pulse and blood pressure, enable the clinician to ascertain the clinical course. Deterioration in coma scale assessments with specific features of increasing neurological deficit and, particularly, features of the central transtentorial herniation syndrome, or of uncal herniation are indications of the need for radiological and neurosurgical reappraisal. Inadequate ventilation from brain stem dysfunction will lead to cerebral hypoxia and an

Table 7.3 *Glasgow coma scale (maximum score 15, minimum score 3).*

Eye opening		Verbal response		Motor response	
Spontaneous	4	Oriented	5	Obeys command	6
To speech	3	Confused	4	Localizes pain	5
To pain	2	Inappropriate words	3	Withdraws from pain	4
None	1	Incomprehensible sounds	2	Flexion to pain	3
		None	1	Extension to pain	2
				None	1

Table 7.4 *Reversible additional factors causing raised intracranial pressure in patients with mass lesions.*

Hypoxia
Hypercapnia
Hyperpyrexia
Seizures
Hyponatraemia
Cerebral venous obstruction
Meningitis
Straining against a ventilator

intensification of the intracerebral disorder. Further, uncal herniation leads to changes in cerebral circulation and increasing brain swelling. Other causes of increasing intracranial pressure that are remediable are shown in Table 7.4.

Modification of these factors by steroids (dexamethasone 4 mg qds), i.v. mannitol (40 g of 40% solution by rapid intravenous infusion 8 hourly (0.25 g/kg)), positive pressure ventilation to induce hypocapnia, and control of seizures, hyperpyrexia and hyponatraemia are essential in management. Patients in whom the Glasgow coma scale is 8 or less require urgent investigation and neurosurgical assessment.

Persistent states of altered consciousness

In patients who survive coma some remain indefinitely in a sleep-like state in which periods of wakefulness occur, when their eyes open and move. Their responsiveness is limited to primitive postural and reflex responses with eye-opening and grimacing, sucking, chewing, swallowing and tooth-grinding movements implying an alerting response, or wakefulness without awareness of self or environment. They never speak or otherwise communicate and their cognitive state cannot therefore accurately be assessed. These patients have long periods of wakefulness but never show evidence of a functioning or communicating mind. At postmortem there is extensive damage to the cortex and forebrain, but the brain stem is spared.

These *persistent vegetative states*, or non-cognitive states have been increasingly recognized after ischaemic or traumatic brain injuries since the advent of effective resuscitative measures in patients who fail to make satisfactory recovery from coma. About 1% of patients in coma remain in a persistent vegetative state for some days, weeks or longer before death occurs from intercurrent infection, malnutrition or cardiorespiratory failure.

The term *coma vigil* (*akinetic mutism*) is a relatively ill-defined syndrome of wakefulness interspersed with sleep. In the waking periods the patient appears alert and may follow people or objects with his eyes and appear to be on the verge of speech, but no communication occurs. No limb movement is possible but grimacing mouth and tongue movements, and swallowing occur. This state has been associated with deep, medially-placed frontal lobe lesions, e.g. after anterior cerebral artery territory infarction or haemorrhage associated with anterior cerebral artery aneurysms. Bilateral cingulate gyrus lesions are also associated with this syndrome.

The *locked-in syndrome* is probably a form of de-efferentation such that mental function, including cognition, is preserved but no voluntary movement apart from vertical eye and eyelid movement is possible. Some jaw movement may also occur. The patient can communicate only by vertical eye movement and blinking but remarkable examples of sophisticated communication by these means have been described in patients surviving many months or even years. The lesion is usually infarction of the pontine tegmentum but other lesions, e.g. pontine tumour, pontine haemorrhage, head injury and central pontine myelinolysis (Chapter 9) may produce this syndrome. Sensation is preserved and these patients can see and hear, so that they are aware of their environment and, of course, of the conversation of their nurses and doctors. The EEG is normal,

Table 7.5 *Criteria for diagnosis of brain death in UK.*

Nature and duration of coma:
  known structural disease, or irreversible systemic or metabolic cause
  absence of drug intoxication or hypothermia (including muscle relaxants and respiratory depressant drugs)
  persistence of condition for 24 hours

Absence of cerebral function:
  no behavioural or reflex response to noxious stimuli above foramen magnum level

Absence of brain stem function:
  pupils fixed in mid-position or dilated
  no oculo-vestibular responses to ice-water caloric testing
  absent dolls-head eye movement
  absent gag, swallowing and coughing reflexes
  absent spontaneous respirations: respirations should be absent during a 10-minute period, following 100% oxygenation, during which the $PaCO_2$ is at least 8.0 kPa (60 mm Hg)—oxygen is given by endo-tracheal catheter during the test

Purely spinal reflexes may be present, e.g. tendon reflexes and plantar responses, and decerebrate postures do not invalidate a diagnosis of brain death

The clinical findings must be independently verified by two clinicians, one of more than 5 years' experience a feature that differentiates this state from the more global defects of cerebral function characteristic of persistent vegetative states, coma vigil and other syndromes of diffuse cerebral damage. In the locked-in syndrome REM sleep is abnormal or absent.

Brain death

With the advent of effective cardiopulmonary resuscitation and intensive care it has become necessary to define criteria for death based on the absence of brain function, rather than absence of heart beat and circulation. This enables diagnosis of death to be made on neurological criteria even when the circulation is intact, a diagnosis that is important in clinical practice not only for decisions regarding the selection of organ for transplantation but, more importantly, to avoid mechanically ventilating a patient with a dead brain but a beating heart.

Certain criteria are essential in the diagnosis of brain death (Table 7.5). In some countries other criteria, such as absent auditory evoked potential responses and even absence of cerebral blood flow have been required for the diagnosis of death, but these do not add further information to the criteria outlined above. The EEG criteria themselves, although useful when this investigation is available, are not strictly necessary in UK practice since it is accepted that EEG activity may be present from cortical function even when the brain stem is totally infarcted and life cannot be sustained.

8

Head Injury

Head injuries are common. They vary in severity from trivial bumps on the head to catastrophic injury resulting in immediate death. There are important demographic trends in head injury that imply the possibility of prevention.

Epidemiology of head injury

About half of all head injuries occur in people aged less than 30 years (Figs 8.1 and 8.2). However, there is an increased predilection for head injury in the elderly. Head injuries arise from road traffic accidents (50%), domestic accidents (16%), industrial accidents (14%), assaults (13%), sporting injuries (3%) and a number of miscellaneous causes. There are about 5 000 deaths each year from head injury in England and Wales, and about 50 000 in the USA. Thus the relative incidence in the UK is about a third of that in the USA; striking variations are found in other countries reflecting local factors. In England and Wales 2 000/100 000 people attend casualty every year with head injury, and 250/100 000 are admitted (125 000 admissions/year). The mortality is 9/100 000. Of these deaths, half occur before reaching hospital, and 30% of those reaching hospital who die do so in the casualty department. In the 15–24 year age group head injuries are the commonest cause of death, a trend that is most marked in males (3 : 1).

Alcohol intoxication is an important factor in road traffic accidents, despite the laws concerning permissible levels of alcohol in the blood of drivers. In about 50% of road traffic accidents one driver has greater than 80 mg/100 ml in his blood, and in 30% of accidents involving pedestrians the pedestrian is drunk. Admissions to hospital for head injury follow a pattern consistent with the importance of alcohol intoxication, since they cluster between the hours of 5 p.m. and midnight, reaching a peak on Friday and Saturday nights. Head injuries are commoner in social classes IV and V, reflecting a number of factors, e.g. the use of motorcycles, unskilled occupation, and alcohol abuse. In children, and in the

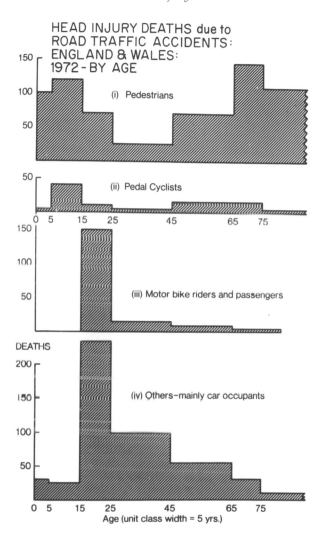

Fig. 8.1 Deaths from head injury in pedestrians, pedal cyclists, motor cyclists and passengers, and car occupants in England and Wales in 1972. Note the risks to pedestrians in childhood and adolescence, and in old people, and the risks to young motor cyclists and to young car occupants.

aged, head injuries sustained in accidental falls are particularly important.

Overall, about 85% of head injuries are minor; severe injuries constitute only about 5% of all head injured patients coming to the casualty department.

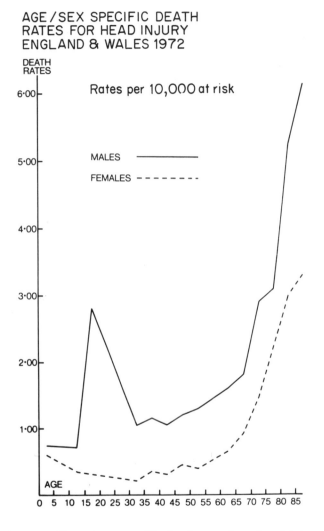

Fig. 8.2 Age-specific and sex-specific death rates from head injury; note the relative risk in young males.

Clinical syndromes of head injury

Recognition of clinical syndromes of head injury is important in determining management.

Minor head injury

This term is used to describe the commonest clinical syndrome of cranial trauma. There is no loss of consciousness, or only a brief period of loss of consciousness with rapid return of normal alertness and mental function. There are no clinical or radiological features of other complications, such as skull fracture. Sometimes higher mental function may be impaired for several hours after recovery of consciousness, so that the patient has no memory both for the period of unconsciousness, and for a subsequent period of several hours (*post-traumatic amnesia; PTA*). *Retrograde amnesia* is impairment of memory for a period of seconds, minutes or, less commonly, hours prior to the injury itself; it is always accompanied by post-traumatic amnesia. Because of the relative reliability of its assessment ('what is your first memory after the accident?') the post-traumatic amnesia is often used as a measure of the severity of the injury. Generally, the longer the PTA the more severe the cerebral effects of the cranial trauma, and the longer the period of recovery and rehabilitation needed.

Concussion is an imprecise term that implies reversible impairment of consciousness of brief duration. It may or may not be associated with cerebral damage. Loss of consciousness in minor head injuries reflects absorption of the energy of impact within the brain, especially in the cerebral neurons and in the deep white matter of the cerebral hemispheres and upper brain stem. Axonal injury occurs in the white matter from streaming of the brain around relatively rigid internal structures, such as blood vessels, and this is not inevitably recoverable. These shearing forces account for the permanent deficits found in patients with more severe, closed head injuries (see below).

Severe head injury

In severe head injury there is prolonged and deep loss of consciousness, or potentially life-threatening complications are present (Table 8.1). Management of the patient with a severe head injury consists of initial assessment of the severity of the injury, and of the presence or absence of injuries to other body parts, followed

Table 8.1 *Severe head injury syndromes.*

Severe closed head injuries (with or without skull fracture)
Cerebral contusions
Intracerebral haemorrhages (including subarachnoid bleeding)
Subdural haemorrhage
Extradural haemorrhage
Open head injuries, with communication between intradural compartments and atmosphere
Head injuries with depressed skull fractures

by evaluation of the clinical syndrome. The latter requires continuous assessment in order to recognize the development of complications, e.g. intracranial haematoma, metabolic disturbances or seizures. The mortality of severe head injuries, excluding acute subdural haematoma, is about 30%.

Assessment of severely head-injured patients. The factors that lead to permanent sequelae after cranial trauma, apart from *injury to brain caused by the trauma itself,* are *intracranial haematoma, seizures, meningitis, hypoxia* and *hypotension.* The initial and continuous assessment of patients with head injury is intended to discover and quantify these problems.

General assessment: It is of cardinal importance to ensure the maintenance of vital functions, especially the patency of the airway, the adequacy of ventilation and the state of the circulation. The airway should be examined and if necessary an oral airway or intubation carried out. Sometimes the comatose patient will have inhaled material leading to pulmonary insufficiency and, later, infection. The movements of the thorax must be assessed to exclude fractured ribs and to consider the possibility of cervical or thoracic spinal injury. The cervical spine should not be passively moved until it is clear, from the presence of spontaneous or reflex movements and, if necessary, by radiological examination that there is no unstable fracture of the cervical spine. Brief assessment of the abdomen, including the genito-urinary system, and of the limbs to exclude major fractures, haemorrhage or occult blood loss into the tissues from soft tissue injury is essential. Haematuria may indicate renal, bladder or urethral injury.

Consciousness: The level of consciousness should be assessed using the Glasgow coma scale (Chapter 7), which depends on verbal responses, eye opening responses and motor responses. An alert patient will have a score of 15 (the maximum) but a patient with a severe head injury will have a score of 7 or less. The presence of seizures should be noted.

Signs of cerebral impact: The scalp will show bruising or lacerations at the site of injury. Fractures of the skull bone are often accompanied by bleeding from the nose or pharynx, and from one or both ears. There may be bruising of the mastoid area or pinna (battle sign). CSF may be recognized by its appearance and glucose content, leaking from nose or external ear. Fractures of the skull may be palpable, visible or occult; the latter are rarely clinically significant. Bleeding in the extradural space may produce a soft or tense boggy swelling in the region of the temporalis muscle. Facial and orbital lacerations and fractures should be carefully assessed since early repair of the latter is likely to lead to the best functional results.

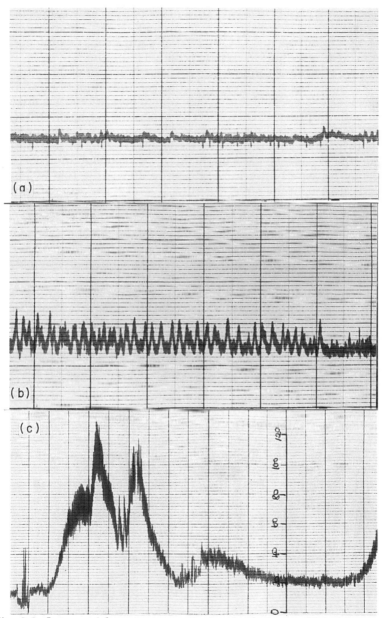

Fig. 8.3 Intracranial pressure monitoring (scale in mm Hg); (a) normal awake tracing. (b) B waves; sleep tracing showing regular oscillating increases in pressure. (c) A waves; in raised intracranial pressure intermittent waves of very high pressure occur that may be greater than the mean perfusion pressure of the brain.

Specific signs of brain injury: Cranial nerve palsies, for example facial or oculomotor nerve palsies, may be present, usually indicating skull base or orbital fractures. Other focal signs, e.g. hemiplegia or diminished response to sensory stimulation on one side, are indicative of cerebral compression by haematoma, or of direct injury or contusion. These features should be carefully quantified so that progress can be assessed during subsequent observation. Meningism is sometimes present when there is subarachnoid haemorrhage.

The features of raised intracranial pressure are rarely present initially but develop during the first 3 days after injury (Fig. 8.3) in about 50% of patients, particularly those with cerebral contusion and oedema. Increased intracranial pressure during the first 24 hours is indicative of intracranial or intracerebral haemorrhage. Later, hydrocephalus may also produce raised intracranial pressure. In the comatose patient this can be recognized clinically only by deteriorating consciousness, or by the development of papilloedema with or without signs of focal brain involvement indicative of cerebral herniation (see Chapter 7 and below). Cerebral infection is not likely in the early stages of head injury.

Investigations: In the initial assessment a chest X-ray and cervical spine X-ray are often worthwhile to ensure adequate ventilation, to assess the ribs and to exclude cervical spine fractures. CT scanning is invaluable in assessing the brain injury itself and should never be deferred. At this stage a number of other base-line studies, including haemoglobin, electrolytes and blood urea, blood sugar and, perhaps, blood alcohol levels should be obtained. Access to the circulation by intravenous line is invaluable in later management.

Continuous assessment: The Glasgow coma scale (see Chapter 7), simple nursing observations and assessment of neurological deficits should be used at 15–30 minute intervals during the initial critical few hours or days, since changes will determine the necessity for re-investigation by CT scanning or other tests and, therefore, for medical or surgical intervention. In some patients, when there are features of increasing intracranial pressure, monitoring of the pressure in the subdural or subarachnoid space by implanted transducers can be useful in determining the effectiveness of medical or surgical means of managing intracranial pressure (Fig. 8.3).

Clinical syndromes of severe head injury (Table 8.1)

Severe closed head injury syndrome. The term 'closed' head injury is used to denote an injury in which there is no communication between intradural compartments and the atmosphere. However, this does not exclude the presence of a skull fracture, whether depressed, hairline or undisplaced. In minor head injuries there is only brief unconsciousness, or post-traumatic confusion, usually of less than 15 minutes and 60 minutes duration respectively. When these features are of longer duration, especially if there is unconsciousness for more than an hour and confusion or disorientation for more than 24 hours, it is likely that there has been some cerebral damage and recovery is likely to be delayed or incomplete. In addition, complications such as cerebral contusion or intracranial haemorrhage are likely to develop only in those patients with severe closed head injuries. All patients with severe head injury should be admitted to hospital and preferably assessed by CT scanning of the brain.

Diffuse brain damage and contusions. When there has been diffuse brain damage from head injury, associated with shearing stresses within the brain, the patient will be comatose or even decerebrate, often without focal cerebral or brain stem signs. Seizures may occur in about 5% of patients in the first week. The development of pupillary asymmetry or dilatation and loss of the light reaction on one or both sides (third nerve palsy) with slowing of the pulse, increase in blood

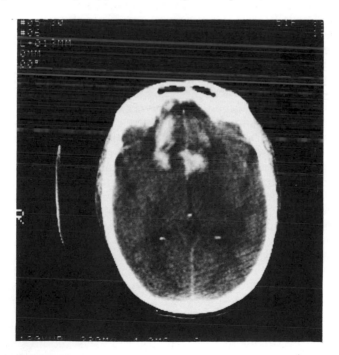

Fig. 8.4 Cerebral contusion. There are extensive patchy bifrontal intracerebral haemorrhages. The brain is oedematous with obliteration of the sulcal pattern, and compression of the lateral ventricles.

pressure and hyperventilation or, later, Cheyne–Stokes respiration, suggests rising intracranial pressure. This is a common complication of diffuse brain damage in closed head injury. The main value of CT scanning in severe closed head injury syndrome is the early recognition of brain swelling, shown by effacement of the gyral pattern in the cerebral hemispheres, smallness of the ventricles and oedema of the brain. Often tiny, punctate haemorrhages can be seen in the white matter and sometimes a zone of grey/white matter haemorrhagic contusion can be recognized at the surface of the hemisphere opposite the injury (Fig. 8.4); the contre-coup lesion due to the shock wave following the impact dissipating at the brain/skull interface opposite the site of injury. There may also be bleeding near the ventricles or within the subarachnoid space and ventricular system. Effective management of raised intracranial pressure, with careful monitoring of the clinical syndrome, is important in determining survival and prognosis (see below). Generally, the longer the period of unconsciousness and subsequent confusion, the worse the prognosis.

Extradural haemorrhage. Haemorrhage in the extradural space (Fig. 8.5) usually arises from arterial or venous bleeding associated with skull fracture and laceration of a major vessel, e.g. the middle meningeal artery in the temporal region. Most extradural haemorrhages are found in the middle fossa but they may also occur occipitally and frontally. This complication of severe head injury is of major importance because it may lead to brain compression in a few hours, yet treatment is relatively simple.

In extradural haemorrhage in the temporal region the injury may not be severe in itself. In half such patients the initial injury is not severe enough even to cause unconsciousness; in 15% the patient recovers from an initial brief period of unconsciousness before lapsing again into coma from cerebral herniation associated with the mass effect of the lateralized haemorrhage. The syndrome presents with headache, irritability and then drowsiness. Later, usually in a few hours, stupor develops in association with ipsilateral pupillary dilatation. The latter progresses to fixation of the dilated pupil and oculomotor palsy, followed by deep coma, bilateral fixed dilated pupils and death. The haematoma is nearly always associated with a fracture of the squamous part of the temporal bone and this should be visible on plain skull X-rays or CT scan. The haematoma itself can sometimes be detected as a firm, boggy swelling beneath the temporalis muscle. The haemorrhage almost invariably progresses, increasing gradually in size, and thus always requires surgical evacuation and haemostasis. With early evacuation of the haematoma the prognosis for complete recovery is excellent, but any delay is potentially fatal, especially when there are signs of incipient

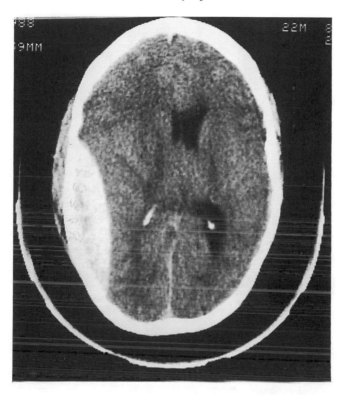

Fig. 8.5 Right extradural haematoma. There is soft tissue swelling in the right temporal region of the scalp. The extradural haematoma is seen as a biconvex, high-attenuation mass beneath the skull on the right. There is marked shift of the brain to the left, with compression of the right lateral ventricle. The patient was comatose with a left hemiplegia and a dilated right pupil; rapid improvement occurred when the haematoma was evacuated.

cerebral herniation, e.g. ipsilateral third nerve palsy, contralateral hemiplegia and papilloedema. Extradural haematoma may also complicate severe head injuries in which there is diffuse brain injury and contusion; it should then be evacuated as part of the initial management.

Subdural haematoma. Bleeding into the subdural space may be an acute or chronic disorder (Fig. 8.6). Acute subdural haematomas are a feature of 25% of all severe head injuries and in more than a half there is associated intracerebral haematoma or contusion. Chronic subdural haematomas are much less frequent and may present weeks or even months after injury, or even after injury has been

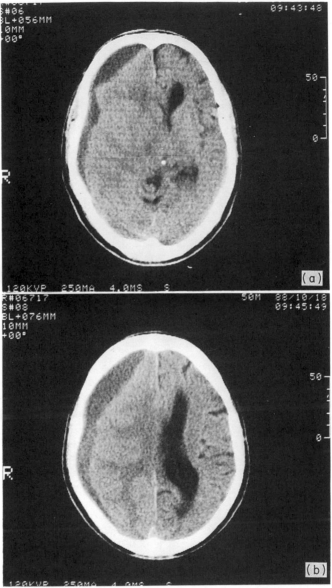

Fig. 8.6 Subdural haematoma. (a) The subdural haematoma is seen as a peripheral zone of reduced attenuation (fresh subdural haematomas may be isodense with the brain and difficult to detect). The frontal horn of the right lateral ventricle is compressed and displaced to the left, and the pineal gland is similarly displaced. (b) The haematoma is clearly seen. The left lateral ventricle is enlarged due to obstruction of its outlet (the foramen of Luschka) from distortion caused by the side to side herniation of the brain.

forgotten. The injury may be relatively trivial, and need not cause loss of consciousness.

Acute subdural haematoma. This is a complication of severe blows on the head, with unconsciousness from the onset, or with rapid deterioration in the first few hours after injury. Even at presentation more than a half of patients with acute subdural haematomas are decerebrate with fixed dilated pupils and, in these cases, the outlook is almost hopeless. There are often associated skull fractures and cerebral contusions and signs of diffuse injury may be present at autopsy. The mortality in patients diagnosed and operated on within 4 hours of the head injury is 30% and delayed diagnosis results in a mortality of 90% or more. The diagnosis should be considered in any patient comatose longer than an hour; in all these patients prompt evaluation by CT scanning is necessary.

Subacute and chronic subdural haematoma. Subacute subdural haematomas present 2–14 days after injury, usually with a history of trauma. In subacute subdural haematoma there are usually prominent symptoms and signs of raised intracranial pressure with headache, vomiting, confusion and papilloedema. Focal signs are uncommon but ipsilateral partial third nerve palsy (dilated pupil) and contralateral hemiparesis may be present.

Chronic subdural haematomas present weeks or even months after injury, often following relatively mild injury. Skull fracture is relatively uncommon (10%). Chronic subdural haematomas (Fig. 8.6), like subacute subdural haematomas, are due to venous bleeding in the subdural space, from rupture of small veins bridging this space. The blood is contained within a thin arachnoidal membrane medially and a thicker dural layer of granulation tissue laterally. The latter is itself vascularized and recurrent small haemorrhages into the haematoma may occur, thus causing the haematoma to slowly expand. In addition, osmotic changes within the degenerating material in the haematoma may also cause slow swelling of the mass and thus slow progression of the clinical syndrome. About 15% of chronic subdural haematomas are bilateral.

Chronic subdural haematoma results not only from trauma, but also from ruptured aneurysm, in patients with a haemorrhagic diathesis due to liver disease, leukaemia, thrombocytopenia or anticoagulant drug therapy, in alcoholics (presumably from recurrent head injuries), in patients with whiplash injuries to the neck, and after haemodialysis. Subdural haematoma may also develop as a complication of surgical craniotomy or burrhole procedure. Thus not all subdural haematomas are due to trauma.

Small haematomas, less than 50 ml volume and occupying only a thin rim over the cortex, are usually symptomless, but larger subdural collections displace and compress the brain thus causing distant and local symptoms. About 80% of patients have headache but there are two major presentations. Firstly, there may be local symptoms from cerebral compression, and irritation, e.g. hemiparesis, hemisensory impairment, focal epilepsy, hemianopia. Secondly, a generalized disturbance with diffuse mental change, fluctuating drowsiness and confusion may develop. This second syndrome is associated with raised intracranial pressure but there is only rarely papilloedema (20%), probably because the haematoma increases in size only very slowly. Signs of third nerve compression on the ipsilateral side may develop when brain displacement becomes critical and sixth nerve palsies may also develop. The variable level of consciousness is associated with spontaneous fluctuations in intracranial pressure. Hemiparesis is a feature in about 40% of patients; it may be contralateral (60%) or ipsilateral (due to brain stem compression from uncal herniation). Pupillary changes, reflecting the terminal stages of the disorder, are relatively uncommon (5%).

Drainage of the haematoma by burrhole or craniotomy with removal of the membrane is associated with full recovery in 90% of patients. The prognosis is good, even in comatose patients.

The diagnosis of chronic subdural haematoma is often difficult. The disorder presents in many different clinical guises, and there is often no known history of trauma, although this may later become evident. The CT brain scan is almost always diagnostic, provided that intravenous contrast enhancement is used, but plain skull X-rays may reveal pineal displacement, indicating a laterally-placed mass lesion, in 16% of cases. Unenhanced CT brain scans may not reveal the lesion in some cases because the haematoma is isodense with the brain, but the diagnosis should be suspected if the gyral pattern is effaced in one hemisphere compared with the other. Bilateral subdural haematomas (15%) are particularly difficult to recognize since there are then no features of lateralization or ventricular displacement. Enhanced CT scans will reveal the membrane limiting the haematoma. Angiography is now little used in the investigation of suspected subdural haematoma, but can provide evidence of an avascular mass in the subdural space. Isotope brain scans may also reveal the haematoma in 80% of cases.

Intracerebral haemorrhages. Bleeding into the cerebral or cerebellar hemispheres with head injury is usually associated with very severe injuries, and in most cases the presence of an intracerebral haematoma is not the only cause of unconsciousness. However, in a few cases surgical removal of a temporal lobe haematoma in the non-dominant hemisphere results in clinical improvement by relief of the mass effect and, therefore, of brain displacement.

Open head injuries. Communication between the intradural compartment and the atmosphere is due either to major destructive accidental trauma, with compound skull fracture, or to penetrating wounds by foreign bodies such as bullets. In these instances not only is there a risk of infection, but it is likely that there has been local and shock-wave induced brain injury. The latter is particularly likely with high-velocity bullet wounds from modern military weapons. Surgical triage with primary closure and antibiotic treatment is the preferred method of management, but healing by granulation of large open wounds may be necessary.

Depressed skull fractures. Skull fractures that are depressed do not necessarily require surgical elevation. Only those deeper than 1 cm, or associated with local neurological abnormality, or that are compound, need treatment. If the depressed fracture is on the forehead and is unsightly, surgical treatment is also indicated.

Management of severe head injury

The mainstay of successful management is careful clinical assessment and monitoring (see above). In the initial period associated injuries, especially soft tissue injuries to abdominal organs, fractures of limbs or pelvis, neck injuries and injuries to the thorax that might impair ventilation, are of cardinal importance. The initial CT scan will determine management of surgical problems such as acute subdural haematoma or extradural haematoma. Intracerebral haematomas should be managed conservatively in the initial period. Seizures should be treated with anticonvulsant drugs and in compound fractures or open head injuries antibiotic cover will be required. If clinical or CT scan features suggestive of rising intracranial pressure and cerebral oedema develop during the first few days after a severe head injury i.v. mannitol is probably the treatment of choice. Steroids, although usually used, are relatively ineffective. Controlled mechanical ventilation can be used to cause hypocapnia and so reduce intracranial pressure. CSF examination is only indicated if meningitis is suspected. Inappropriate ADH secretion with hypo-osmolar states is occasionally a problem and this should be managed with fluid restriction.

Late complications and outcome of severe head injury

The survivors of severe closed or open head injury suffer from various disabilities and these are often severe enough to prevent return to work or to ordinary activities. Small children recover relatively better but often show marked personality change and learning difficulties.

About 5% of patients with closed head injuries develop *epilepsy;* open head injuries carry a much greater risk (about 40%). In most patients the epilepsy commences in the first 2 years after injury. Epilepsy is a rare complication when the post-traumatic amnesia is less than 48 hours.

Communicating hydrocephalus may develop weeks or months after the injury; in some cases it may be delayed for many years. The disorder presents with the triad of dementia, incontinence and gait disorder. There is dilatation of the whole ventricular system, including the fourth ventricle and temporal horns, and CSF shunting results in improvement. The CSF is often, but not invariably, under increased pressure. Generalized atrophy may mimic communicating hydrocephalus, but CSF shunting has no effect; atrophy is a common finding in patients with mental impairment after a severe closed head injury.

The *mental effects of severe head injury* are often of paramount importance. Recovery is slow, but usually reaches a peak by 2 years after the injury. Personality change with irritability, shallow affect, lack of insight and poor judgement, a change in sexual behaviour, sleeplessness, lack of concentration amounting to distractibility, poor memory for recent events and names, and other subtle, focal defects such as aphasia, apraxia and specific recognition defects may be disabling. These deficits lead to profound psychosocial problems, such as marital breakdown, depression and morbid anxiety. These matters are often important aspects of medico-legal assessment for the purposes of litigation.

A small proportion of survivors are left with *severe focal neurological deficits,* such as severe aphasia, hemiplegia, quadriplegia or decerebrate coma, akinetic mutism and persistent vegetative states. Most patients in the latter situation fail to survive, but a few linger on for many years, requiring continuous care. A *post-traumatic dementia* may also be recognized in severely injured patients, necessitating continuous psychiatric care.

Persistent effects of minor head injuries; post-traumatic syndrome

Many people with minor head injuries complain of persistent effects sufficient to impair the quality of life. These usually consist of non-specific headache, dizziness, irritability, poor concentration and impairment of recent memory. Depressive symptoms such as lack of confidence and drive, insomnia and impaired sexual drives are also prominent. This syndrome generally improves with time, and is often most prominent when the injury occurred in the context of the possibility of litigation, as in road traffic accidents. There has been much controversy as to its cause, but the weight of evidence favours an underlying organic basis for the syndrome.

Spinal injuries, nerve root and plexus injuries

See Chapters 13 and 14.

9

Multiple Sclerosis and other Demyelinating Diseases

The term 'demyelinating disease' is used to refer to a group of diseases characterized by damage to or loss of myelin in the central nervous system. This may be focal or diffuse; multiple sclerosis is by far the commonest of these diseases (Table 9.1). Demyelination also occurs in the leucodystrophies, a group of diseases in which there is abnormal myelin metabolism, and these disorders are therefore sometimes termed 'dysmyelinating diseases'.

Demyelination of peripheral myelin is much better understood than demyelination of central myelin. Since the biochemical and immunological characteristics of central and peripheral myelin differ, there is no clinical association between demyelinating diseases of the CNS such as multiple sclerosis and demyelinating diseases of the peripheral nervous system. Only in sulphatide (metachromatic) leucodystrophy and in systemic lupus erythematosus is there any association between central and peripheral demyelination.

Table 9.1 *Demyelinating diseases.*

Multiple sclerosis
Devic's disease
Acute transverse myelitis (see Chapter 13)
Acute disseminated encephalomyelitis (see Chapter 7)
Central pontine myelinolysis
Progressive multifocal leucoencephalopathy (see Chapter 6)
Schilder's disease
Leucodystrophies (see Table 9.3)
Lupoid encephalopathy

In the CNS myelin is formed by oligodendrocytes; demyelinating disorders are therefore associated with disease of these cells. In cell-mediated allergic demyelination, as in certain viral infections (Chapter 7) demyelination occurs as a 'bystander' effect associated with the immune process. Remyelination is usually effective in such disorders but in the common, major demyelinating disease in humans, multiple sclerosis, remyelination is characteristically ineffective, accounting for the poor recovery and progressive course of the disease. Unlike oligodendrocytes, the Schwann cells of the peripheral nervous system have an excellent capacity for regeneration and repair.

Multiple sclerosis

Multiple sclerosis is a disease characterized by the occurrence of symptoms and signs of neurological dysfunction in more than one site in the central nervous system. Thus, lesions are said to be disseminated in time and place. About 75% of patients have a relapsing and remitting course in the early stages of the illness, but later a progressive course is common. Relapses are not accompanied by any feature suggesting systemic illness. Most cases are aged 16–60 years, with a mean age of onset of 29–33 years. Women are affected slightly earlier than men and the incidence in women is 1.8 times that in men.

Clinical features

The disease is characteristically variable in its presentation and course. In advanced cases weakness, spasticity, fatiguability, ataxia, sensory loss or paraesthesiae and urinary incontinence are almost always present and visual difficulty is also common. Most patients, however, do not progress to such severe disability.

The initial symptoms consist of weakness in one or more limbs (40%), optic neuritis (22%), paraesthesiae (21%), diplopia (12%), vertigo (5%) and disturbance of micturition (5%). These symptoms are frequently not associated with major abnormality on examination. Thus, fatiguability, a common symptom in the disease, may not be a feature of a definite corticospinal syndrome, although there may be subtle reflex asymmetry. Similarly, paraesthesiae are not usually associated with definite sensory changes; indeed, well-defined sensory loss is an infrequent early feature of the disease. During the initial stages of the disease symptoms occur in isolation often without clinical evidence of additional lesions, but careful clinical examination may reveal other abnormalities, thus suggesting the diagnosis. Involvement of higher cerebral function is unusual in the initial stages of the disease.

Motor symptoms are common, consisting usually of weakness of one limb, clumsiness of a hand, or of weakness of both legs. Patients are often not fully aware of the distribution of weakness, tending to present with symptomatic weakness of the most severely affected limb so that the full extent of disability is revealed by observation of gait and by clinical examination. Weakness is usually accompanied by signs of upper motor neuron lesion, including spasticity, hyperreflexia and extensor plantar response. Muscular atrophy is unusual, except in the terminal phase.

Optic neuritis is particularly common in younger patients. It is due to demyelination in the optic nerve. Loss of vision develops rapidly during a period of a few days, or up to 2 weeks, and then gradually improves during the subsequent 1 to 3 months. Central vision is severely affected but peripheral vision may be relatively spared. The eye is painful on palpation and during movement. The optic disc is swollen in about 50% of patients but haemorrhages are uncommon (in arterial or venous occlusion swelling, haemorrhages and exudates are common). Most cases are unilateral but the opposite eye may be involved subsequently in some patients, and subclinical involvement is frequent. The risk of the subsequent development of multiple sclerosis approximates that following any single episode of demyelination and, in the UK, is about 50%. In many patients examination at presentation with optic neuritis will reveal other abnormalities indicating a diagnosis of definite multiple sclerosis (see below).

In the acute stage the pupil is moderately dilated and the Gunn phenomenon characteristic of an afferent pupillary defect is present; the pupil shows rhythmic constriction and dilatation (hippus) with continuous illumination, and then slowly dilates (swinging light test) after first illuminating the opposite eye. During recovery the optic disc becomes pale, sharply demarcated and atrophic (primary optic atrophy) and there is often a residual central, paracentral or arcuate scotoma to colour testing. The visual acuity may not return to normal. The visual acuity may decrease slightly, leading to blurred vision, after body heating (e.g. a hot bath) or exercise (Uhthoff's phenomenon). During the acute phase phosphenes, consisting of brief random flashes in the impaired visual field, may be noted during eye movement, resembling showers of sparks. These derive from cross-talk between damaged, demyelinated fibres in the optic nerve induced by movement.

About 10% of patients with multiple sclerosis show primary optic atrophy, but in many there is no history of optic neuritis.

Cerebellar disturbances are common, ranging from mild ataxia of one limb, clumsiness of a hand, or mild dysarthria to severe gait ataxia. It is often difficult to distinguish cerebellar ataxia in patients with mild corticospinal signs. The presence of moderately severe cerebellar ataxia has a poor prognosis since it is unlikely to recover, unlike corticospinal weakness which often recovers, and usually implies brain stem involvement. Limb ataxia is often accompanied by nystagmus and some patients experience vertigo, indicating a brain stem origin of the cerebellar dysfunction, at the onset.

Ocular movements are often abnormal, although in many patients there is no diplopia, representing functional accommodation to the ocular disturbance. Diplopia occurs in about a third of patients, usually due to a sixth nerve palsy or to *internuclear ophthalmoplegia*. In the latter disorder there is limitation of adduction, with nystagmus of the abducting eye, during lateral conjugate gaze. This is usually best seen during rapid gaze movements in the lateral plane when there appears to be a dissociation between the velocity of movement of the two eyes, the adducting eye moving more slowly. The syndrome is due to a lesion in the medial longitudinal fasciculus interrupting the connections between the third and sixth nerve nuclei and the pontine lateral gaze centre. It is almost always due to multiple sclerosis and may be unilateral or bilateral. Paresis of lateral conjugate gaze or other complex supranuclear ocular movement disorders are uncommon. Nystagmus on lateral gaze is frequent and correlates with cerebellar pathway lesions.

Facial myokymia, consisting of continuous, rapid flickering and undulating movement of one side of the face, is a rare sign that is particularly characteristic of multiple sclerosis. *Trigeminal neuralgia* in a young person is also characteristic of the disease, and may be bilateral. *Tonic seizures*, consisting of momentary stiffening of one side, thought to be due to demyelination in motor pathways (a positive symptom) also occur in the disease and, like trigeminal neuralgia, usually respond to treatment with tegretol.

Clinical syndromes of multiple sclerosis

Certain clinical syndromes, correlating with the location of lesions and with their natural history, can be recognized. A progressive course is commoner in older-onset cases. *Progressive spastic paraplegia* may occur without other clinical features and pathological examination shows lesions restricted to the cervical cord, and to the cerebellum. Mild ataxia in the upper limbs may be a feature. Brown-Sequard syndrome may develop in young people with the disease, but usually evolves to paraplegia. *Optic neuritis* may precede overt multiple sclerosis by many years. *Recurrent sensory symptoms* with mild posterior column signs are often relatively benign; but a chronic progressive paraplegia may develop in later life. *Generalized involvement* with optic neuritis, oculomotor abnormalities, ataxia, dysarthria, paraplegia, sensory abnormalities and personality change occurs in the severe relapsing and remitting form of the disease found in young people. *Brain stem features* may occur in isolation, with involvement of long tracts. *Acute multiple sclerosis* is usually severe, and has a poor prognosis for functional recovery.

Outcome

Life expectancy is reduced by a mean of 10 years for men and 14 years for women; 25 year survival is about 75% compared with 85% in an age-matched control group. Fifteen years from the onset 15% of survivors are able to work normally and 40% can do some useful work. Long term survivors tend to have mild, non-progressive disease. About 70% of survivors are moderately or severely disabled 15 years after the onset. In assessing prognosis and outcome the standardized Kurtzke disability scale is often used (Table 9.2). Although not linear, this scale is easy to use and does not require specialized medical knowledge.

Table 9.2 *Kurtzke disability scale.*

0	Normal including neurological examination
1	No disability; minimal signs, e.g. extensor plantar response
2	Minimal disability; slight weakness or gait disturbance
3	Moderate disability but fully ambulatory
4	Relatively severe disability, but still self-sufficient and socially active
5	Disability preventing full-time work
6	Requires assistance for walking, e.g. sticks
7	Restricted to wheelchair but can transfer to bed etc. without assistance
8	Restricted to bed but can use arms effectively
9	Helpless, bed-bound
10	Terminal or dying

Improvement is more likely to follow acute relapses (onset of a symptom in < 72 hours) than when there has been a slow progressive onset during several weeks. The greater the degree of recovery from a relapse, the greater the degree of recovery in the next relapse. Symptoms remaining for 6 months recover in only 10% of patients; symptoms of 2 months duration have a greater chance of recovery. Remission never occurs after 8 years of progressive or static disease. In Kurtzke's series 86% of patients with symptoms of a week or less prior to hospital admission improved, but only 64% of patients with symptoms of 8–14 days duration and only 36% of patients with symptoms of 15–31 days duration improved. Most patients with multiple sclerosis who improve, relapse subsequently (525 of 586 cases in McAlpine's series); 25% of these relapsed in the first year, and 50% within 3 years. A progressive course is much commoner in patients with an older age of onset, especially when this is after the age of 40 years. However, the course cannot be predicted in individual patients, although once the pattern has been established the prognosis is more reliable. Some cases pursue a 'malignant' course, death occurring within 5 years of onset. 'Benign' multiple sclerosis has also been recognized in about 15% of patients; in these there are few relapses, complete recovery occurs after each relapse and there is no significant disability 25 years after the onset.

Relapses

Despite the dramatic nature of the relapsing course of the disease no clear cause has been ascertained for relapses. Patients are often convinced that extraneous factors such as minor trauma, viral infection, fatigue and emotional stress have induced their relapse but these factors are common in everyday life and it is difficult to prove their relevance. However, there is clinical evidence that infections precede relapses more frequently than by chance, and immunization has also been associated with an increased risk of relapse. There is also an increased risk of relapse during the puerperium, but not during pregnancy itself; this risk is about 50% greater than for comparable periods. In some women particularly severe exacerbations develop at this time. Surgical operations and anaesthesia also seem to be associated with a slightly increased risk. Exertion, fatigue and heat are associated with increased symptoms, probably from the deleterious effects of increased central temperature rather than from active demyelination.

Genetic factors and associated diseases

Multiple sclerosis shows an increased incidence in relatives of affected persons; the risk is about 3% for siblings and 2% for parents. In monozygotic twins there is a 20% chance of concordance for multiple sclerosis but the risk in dizygotic twins is the same as in other siblings. Conjugal partners have no increased risk. The disease is in linkage disequilibrium with HLA-DR2 and -DW2 haplotypes in Europeans. In the UK, HLA-DR2 is present in 19% of controls and 55% of patients with multiple sclerosis. This association is clearly important in relation to the concept that genetic factors confer susceptibility to the disease.

There are no strong associations with other diseases, but myasthenia gravis and systemic lupus erythematosus are rarely associated with multiple sclerosis, and ulcerative colitis is more common in patients with the disease than in controls. These associations suggest that autoimmunity may be important in pathogenesis of the disease.

Investigations

The diagnosis is usually made on clinical criteria (see below) but these may be supplemented by clinical investigations. *Electrophysiological methods*, particularly visual evoked potential (VEP) studies (Fig. 9.1), and, to a lesser extent, brain stem auditory evoked potentials (BAEP) (Fig. 9.2) and somatosensory evoked potentials (SSEP), can be used to delineate lesions in the central visual, auditory

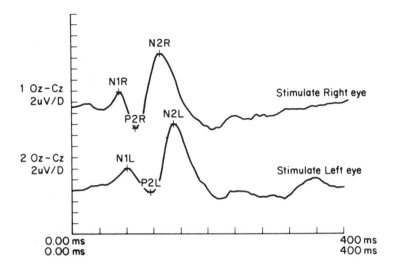

Fig. 9.1 Visual evoked potential recording in multiple sclerosis. On the left there is delay of the P2 (positive deflection); this is associated with demyelination in the left optic nerve.

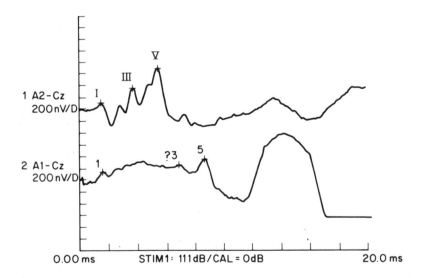

Fig. 9.2 Brain stem (auditory) evoked potential in multiple sclerosis. On the left (lower trace) the first potential (cochlear potential) is of normal latency, but all subsequent potentials are delayed or absent.

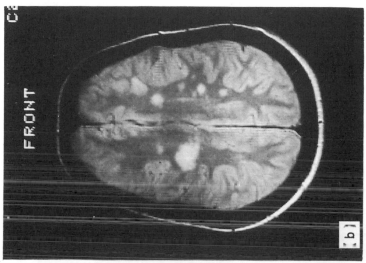

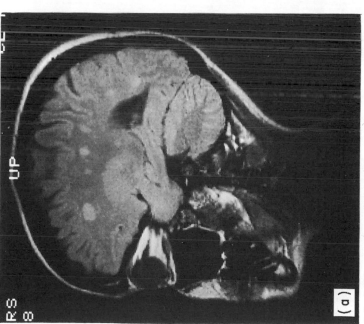

Fig. 9.3 MRI scan in multiple sclerosis. In (a) (sagittal view) a number of lesions shown as white zones, can be seen in the central white matter of the hemisphere. In (b) these lesions are seen situated just superior to the lateral ventricles. These lesions in multiple sclerosis are detected by their proton density, i.e. by their increased water content.

or sensory pathways. Abnormalities of the VEP, consisting of increased latency or increased interocular latency difference of the cortical evoked responses, occur in 89% of patients with optic neuritis, and in 50% of patients with multiple sclerosis *without* clinically evident optic nerve involvement. The yield of abnormality from BAEP and SSEP studies is slightly lower. Generally, the longer the natural history of the disease, the more likely that one of these evoked potential studies will be abnormal. These tests are best regarded as demonstrating additional lesions in the nervous system.

CSF examination has long been used in diagnosis. Thirty per cent of patients have a raised total protein level. The IgG level is raised, when compared with blood IgG levels, in about 75% of patients with the disease, indicating synthesis of IgG within the CNS. Immunoelectrophoresis of this CSF IgG reveals specific oligoclonal bands of IgG protein in more than 90% of patients with typical multiple sclerosis. This is now an important test in diagnosis, since

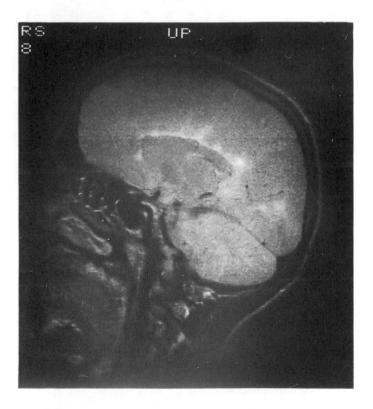

Fig. 9.4 MRI scan in multiple sclerosis showing the typical periventricular location of the demyelination.

it is relatively specific; but similar abnormalities sometimes occur in neurosyphilis, Guillain-Barré syndrome and subacute sclerosing panencephalitis. Sometimes the CSF contains a few monocytes or lymphocytes, but the glucose level is always normal.

CSF examination is relatively invasive and painful. Neuro-imaging, especially *magnetic resonance imaging* (MRI), is capable of demonstrating the plaque-lesions of the disease, and is particularly valuable since it reveals lesions that are not apparent clinically, thus providing evidence of multiple lesions (Figs 9.3 and 9.4). CT scanning, even with contrast enhancement, is much less useful but delayed scanning after high dose contrast increases the yield. In patients with spastic paraparesis, myelography is often considered essential in excluding local, treatable spinal disease, but abnormalities in the visual evoked potential studies, or magnetic resonance imaging, by providing evidence of additional lesions, have made this investigation unnecessary in many patients. The lesions shown by MRI and CT scanning are found particularly in the walls of the lateral ventricles, particularly in the trigone and in the frontal and occipital horns (90% of patients). Brain stem or cerebellar lesions are found in about 50% of patients.

Diagnostic criteria

The lack of a specific diagnostic test for the disease has led to the development of a series of diagnostic criteria based on clinical and investigational data, that classify patients into *definite, probable* and *possible* categories.

Clinically definite multiple sclerosis consists of two attacks, each involving different parts of the CNS, lasting at least 24 hours and separated by at least 1 month. Definite multiple sclerosis may also be diagnosed with laboratory support when there are less certain clinical criteria. In this case one of the two episodes must involve a part of the CNS distinct from that demonstrated on clinical examination or by paraclinical evidence, i.e. electrophysiological, neuro-imaging or CSF examination.

Clinically probable multiple sclerosis is a syndrome of two attacks with clinical evidence of only one lesion, or one attack with clinical or MRI evidence of two lesions, or one attack with clinical evidence of only one lesion but with accompanying paraclinical evidence of another lesion. Laboratory-supported probable multiple sclerosis requires the presence of abnormal CSF.

Possible multiple sclerosis is a common clinical problem in which there is only one lesion, paraclinical evidence is scanty or indefinite, but the clinical symptom is itself strongly suggestive of the disease. For example, trigeminal neuralgia in a patient younger than 40 years, or L'hermitte's phenomenon, are strongly suggestive of multiple sclerosis (see p. 182). The term 'demyelinating disease' is often used to describe such patients.

Epidemiology and pathogenesis

Geographical studies (Fig. 9.5) have shown that the highest incidence of the disease is found in far northern or southern latitudes, and that the disease is uncommon in the tropics. The highest incidence of the disease was found in Iceland, Orkney and Shetland, and the Faroe Islands. In the Faroe Islands there were 24 new cases between 1943 and 1960, but none between 1933 and 1942, and only one between 1961 and 1970. This has been related to occupation of these islands by British troops in the Second World War, and perhaps also to an epidemic of canine distemper at that time. A similar reduction in the incidence of the disease has occurred since 1960 in Orkney and Shetland but the disease remains very common in North East Scotland (140/100 000 prevalence) compared with London (90–100/100 000) (Fig. 9.6). A similar north/south gradient is found in other countries, e.g. in the USA and Canada. In Minnesota the prevalence rate is 196/100 000, whereas in Texas it is 57/100 000. In Australia the prevalence is higher in Tasmania than in more northerly parts of the country.

The global distribution of the disease represents the interaction of genetic and environmental influences. For example, the incidence and prevalence among Afro-Caribbean black people is lower than among white people, even in black people living or born in high

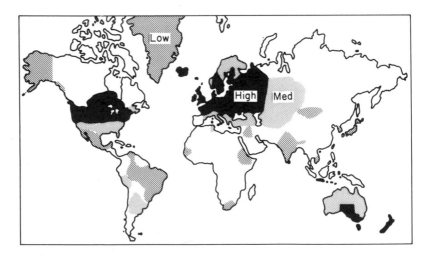

Fig. 9.5 Geographical distribution of multiple sclerosis. There is a higher incidence at latitudes distant from the equator.

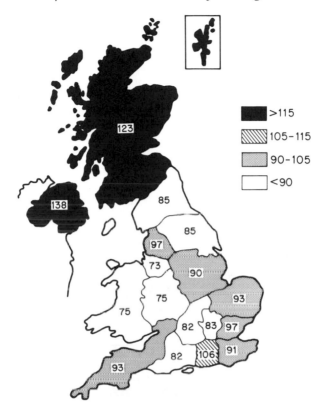

Fig. 9.6 Distribution of multiple sclerosis in the UK, showing the greater incidence of the disease in Scotland and Northern Ireland, compared with England and Wales.

incidence areas. The disease is rare in Japan and in other Oriental peoples, including American Indians and Eskimos, and peoples of the Indian subcontinent. The disease is recognized in Jewish people, and in other Mediterranean and Arab races, including Iranians and the Parsees of India derived from the Zoroastrian migration from ancient Persia.

The effect of migration has been much studied. Generally, individuals migrating from a zone of high risk to low risk take on the risk of their new country provided they migrate before the age of 15 years. Older migrants take their previous risk of the disease with them to their new country. This has been used as evidence that the disease is acquired by susceptible individuals in childhood, but expressed clinically some years later. The nature of this early exposure remains speculative. In support of this general concept, there have been several reports of clustering of the disease in addition to that described above in the Faroe Islands, but there is no evidence of an infective cause. There is no relation to social class, travel or to other socially determined variables. Climate, geology, soil, water and diet have also been studied and excluded as possible factors. Attempts to define the latent period suggest a time of about 4–10 years, but this range is so wide as to defy epidemiological analysis. Many patients with multiple sclerosis show high levels of circulating antibody to measles virus, but the interpretation of this finding is controversial and there is no recognizable association between the disease and measles virus infection.

Pathophysiology

Multiple sclerosis is a multifocal disease (Fig. 9.7). The main feature is demyelination, distributed in 'plaques' (Fig. 9.8). The latter consist of zones of myelin destruction with relative preservation of axons,

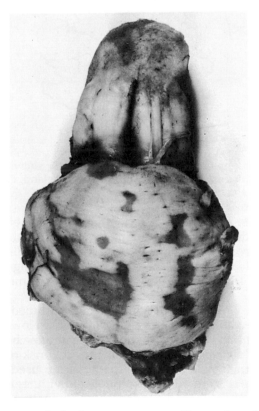

Fig. 9.7   Lesions in the brain stem at autopsy. The patches of demyelination and reactive gliosis are clearly visible on the surface of the pons.

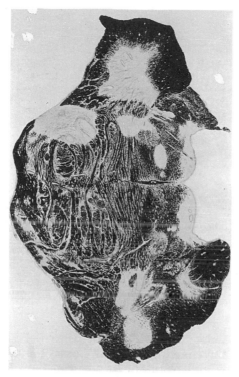

Fig. 9.8 In this myelin-stained section of the pons the circumscribed demyelinated lesions are clearly delineated (from Spielmeyer, *Histopathologie der Nervensystem*, Julius Springer, Berlin 1922)

and an intense astrocytic reactive gliosis (Fig. 9.9). The term plaque is derived from the irregular discoid shape of the lesion in brain sections; the lesions, of course, occupy a volume of tissue. The lesions vary in diameter from 1 mm to about 4 cm. They are mainly located in the periventricular white matter; other sites of predilection include the optic nerves, the cervical spinal cord and the cerebellar hemispheres. They are usually perivenous in distribution and are associated with macrophages, lymphocytes and plasma cells, representing the process of myelin breakdown in its various stages. The early lesions often show partial myelin breakdown. Local oedema is often found in active plaques. The cellular infiltrate in and around the plaque contains immunocompetent T lymphocytes, macrophages and plasma cells, and IgG is demonstrable in relation to these cells, presumably the source of monoclonal IgG in the CSF. There is a marked reduction in the number of oligodendrocytes within the plaque, but there may be increased numbers at the edges, although remyelination is ineffective.

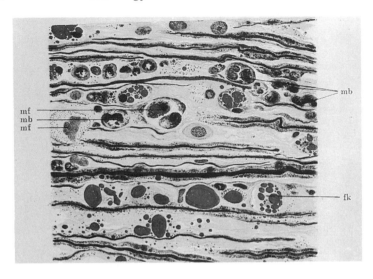

Fig. 9.9 In the lesions of multiple sclerosis, demyelination is patchy, and of variable severity, some axons being spared as in the lower part of this illustration from Spielmeyer's text (see Fig. 9.8).

The symptomatology of multiple sclerosis can be understood in terms of the demyelinating lesions. Loss of myelin results in conduction block with resultant loss of function. When there is partial loss of myelin, or patchy demyelination in a pathway, conduction may be impaired so that there is intermittent conduction block during periods of intense neuronal activity. This may explain the fluctuating symptoms and fatigue that are often noted. In addition, abnormally myelinated fibres are more sensitive to changes in central temperature. Thus, a rise in temperature may lead to failure of conduction, and so to the development, recrudescence or worsening of symptoms (Uhthoff's phenomenon).

Demyelinated or partially myelinated fibres conduct at slower velocities than normal, leading to disturbance of the synchrony and time relation of activity in the affected system, and so to both positive and negative symptoms. In addition, cross-talk (ephaptic transmission) between neighbouring demyelinated fibres may lead to positive derangements of function, such as flashes of light in visual fields during eye movement, seizures, painful paraesthesiae and myokymia. Thus flexion of the neck may cause tingling electric sensations shooting down the spine toward the legs (L'hermitte's sign) when there is demyelination of the posterior columns of the spinal cord. Evoked potential tests in multiple sclerosis often show a striking delay in the latency of the cortical evoked responses, together with a reduction in amplitude. The delay in latency is probably the result of changes associated with delayed conduction, probably due to 'reprocessing time' in the cortex caused by loss of synchrony in the pathway. Reduction in amplitude parallels conduction block, and improves as function in the pathway improves.

Remissions in the disease are not easy to understand. Remyelination is usually scanty, yet functional recovery may sometimes be virtually complete. This may result from recruitment of redundant or alternate pathways, or may be due to resolution of oedema or reconstitution of damaged myelin lamellae. The mechanisms underlying remission and the beneficial effects of steroid treatment are not yet understood, and this problem is complicated by recognition of the surprising extent of clinically silent lesions revealed by autopsy and MRI studies.

Management

The history of multiple sclerosis is peculiarly associated with failed treatments. Virtually every conceivable conventional and unconventional treatment, ranging in recent times from interferon to sunflower seed oil, immunosuppressant drugs to hyperbaric oxygen, and physiotherapy to hypothermia have been tried without success, despite initial enthusiasm. Only short courses of i.m. ACTH or parenteral steroids have been shown to alter the course of acute exacerbations. There is no effective means of altering the course of the slowly progressive form of the disease. The concept of an autoimmune aetiology has led to trials of immunosuppression, including cyclophosphamide, azathioprine, antilymphocytic globulin, thoracic duct drainage, plasma exchange and even total lymphoid irradiation, but these treatments are hazardous and have not been shown to be effective. Oil of evening primrose is believed by many to be effective in preventing relapses, but the evidence from trials is not convincing.

Acute relapses may be treated with ACTH 40–60 I.U. i.m. for 7–10 days, or with methylprednisolone 1.0 g i.v. for 3 consecutive days. This treatment shortens the duration of the relapse but probably does not modify the eventual outcome of the relapse. Drugs such as cyclosporin are currently under investigation. Rest is an important aspect of the treatment of acute relapses and should be continued for 7–21 days, depending on the severity of the deficit. Other treatments are symptomatic. Physiotherapy is important during the recovery phase from motor or sensory deficit, particularly when there is a gait disorder. It should be continued for 3–8 weeks. Catheterization is a useful temporary measure for uncontrollable incontinence or retention. Urinary incontinence results from inappropriate detrusor/sphincter interactions and may be relieved by anticholinergic medications such as terodiline, propantheline or imipramine. Faecal impaction and incontinence are also frequent and may be relieved by manual evacuation and by suitable dietary measures, or by cathartics. Spasticity may be painful and disabling, especially when it is accompanied by flexor spasms. The latter are often indicative of skin or bladder infection, and these require appropriate treatment. Flexor spasms usually respond to diazepam 10–20 mg daily or to baclofen 10–20 mg tds. Spasticity can be improved, although at the cost of dose-related weakness in some patients, by dantrolene 25–75 mg daily or by baclofen 10–20 mg tds. Fatiguability in active patients sometimes responds to amantadine 100 mg bd; the mechanism of action of this drug is unknown.

In patients with chronic or progressive disability the support of a neurologist, with a team of therapists and supporting personnel, is often valuable. The absence of such support implies abandonment, and is a recognition of the non-availability of treatment. Regular surveillance and encouragement, with attention to local causes of pain and discomfort, and appropriate bracing of weak ankles, or advice regarding folding or outdoor wheelchair provision, is invaluable in maintaining independence and confidence in the face of the disability.

Other demyelinating diseases

Although there are other demyelinating diseases of the CNS these are all uncommon (Table 9.1).

Devic's disease (neuromyelitis optica)

This term is used to describe patients in whom a sudden transverse cord lesion develops in close temporal relation with bilateral optic neuritis. This syndrome has been reported during the course of other diseases, e.g. Behçet's disease, systemic lupus erythematosus and in acute disseminated encephalomyelitis, and in some patients it proves to have been the presenting feature of multiple sclerosis itself. As a clinical syndrome it is relatively common in Japanese men; among Japanese people multiple sclerosis itself is relatively uncommon. In most patients, therefore, it probably represents an unusual form of multiple sclerosis.

Acute transverse myelitis (see Chapter 13)

Acute transverse myelitis consists of an acute or subacute complete spinal cord lesion. This may be an isolated event, or may occur as a feature of multiple sclerosis.

Acute disseminated encephalomyelitis

This consists of multifocal inflammatory demyelination associated with viral infection (see Chapter 7).

Central pontine myelinolysis

This disorder presents with the rapid onset of a bulbar palsy, with paralysis of the face, together with involvement of the motor and, to a lesser extent, of the sensory pathways in the pons, causing paralysis of the limbs, especially of the arms ('man in a barrel' syndrome). The pupils are spared and the oculomotor nerves are also unaffected but pontine lateral gaze palsies are a feature. Vision is unaffected when it can be assessed, but deafness is a feature. In most patients the disorder rapidly progresses to coma with rigidity of the limbs and death often occurs. The disorder is due to sudden demyelination in the central and paracentral parts of the pons. Most cases have occurred in the context of malnutrition, liver disease and alcoholism, but cases have also been reported after intractable vomiting or with hypopituitarism, and the common underlying causative factor appears to be hyponatraemia, followed by rapid therapeutic correction of the electrolyte imbalance. It is suggested that the osmotic shift leads to the demyelination and that slow correction of hyponatraemia by fluid restriction may prevent the development of this complication. In survivors recovery may be virtually complete, but is slow during a period of up to 2 years.

Progressive multifocal leuco-encephalopathy

In this syndrome (see Chapter 6) there is patchy, multifocal demyelination in the grey and white matter of the brain stem and cerebral hemispheres, associated with persistent viral infection by a papova virus (SV40 virus). This disease occurs particularly in association with AIDS.

Schilder's disease

There has been confusion as to the nosological position of this disorder. The disease affects children, causing intellectual and visual impairment with progressive spastic weakness, affecting all four limbs. Sensory loss, blindness, incontinence, aphasia, epilepsy and pseudo-bulbar palsy develop. Pathologically there may be multifocal lesions resembling multiple sclerosis, or zones of gelatinous translucent white matter, with sparing of subcortical fibres and relative sparing of axons. The latter lesions may be due to dysmyelination, rather than demyelination, and thus to a leucodystrophy. An indistinguishable X-linked disorder is associated with adrenal atrophy and Addison's disease; this adrenoleuco-dystrophy (sudanophilic leucodystrophy) may involve peripheral nerve myelin also (Addison–Schilder's disease). Diagnosis of these disorders from other leucodystrophies depends on recognition of the pattern of clinical abnormality, and on biochemical studies.

Leucodystrophies

In this group of CNS diseases there is an inherited, usually autosomal recessive, abnormality of myelin metabolism; the clinical manifestations differ according to the biochemical error (Table 9.3). Most begin in childhood. Thus the CNS myelin is abnormal, and undergoes progressive destruction.

Table 9.3 *Leucodystrophies.*

Addison–Schilder's disease (sudanophilic leucodystrophy)
Metachromatic leucodystrophies due to aryl sulphatase A deficiency
  (sulphatide lipidosis)
Krabbe's globoid body leucodystrophy due to galactose cerebrosidase
  deficiency
Canavan's disease
  (spongiform leucodystrophy)
Alexander's leucodystrophy
Pelizaeus-Merzbacher disease

The distinction between *leucodystrophies* and *lipid storage diseases* is to some extent artificial since both involve biochemical errors of metabolism, and both are inherited. In the latter the main abnormality is found in neurons and, in the former, in myelin in the central white matter. Thus leucodystrophies present with progressive neurological disturbances such as spasticity, aphasia, seizures, ataxia and dementia and lipid storage diseases with seizures, myoclonic jerks, dementia and cerebellar signs. Some, such as *metachromatic leucodystrophy*, may also cause peripheral neuropathy, and may present in childhood or adult-onset forms. *Canavan's disease* is associated with spongiform change, lucent zones in white matter in CT scans and megalencephaly. These disorders are all uncommon and tend to occur in isolated populations or in the children of first cousin marriages. No treatment is available, but precise recognition of the various syndromes is important for genetic counselling (see Chapter 17).

10

Dementia

The degenerative disorders of the CNS consist of disorders of neuronal systems and their connections that are recognized by their clinical features and progression and by their pathological features. In some, there are distinct biochemical abnormalities reflecting involvement of particular enzyme systems that lead to the pattern of pathological and clinical abnormality characteristic of the disease. Classification of these disorders thus involves clinical, pathological and biochemical criteria. It is convenient to discuss these disorders in relation to their major clinico-pathological patterns; *dementias, system degenerations* (Chapter 11) and *movement disorders* (Chapter 12).

Definition of dementia

Dementia consists of a global disturbance of higher mental function in an alert patient. In *delirium*, a similar global disturbance of mental function occurs, but there is clouding of consciousness. This distinction is important; delirium may occur in demented patients, causing an abrupt deterioration in mental function. Delirium is sometimes termed an acute confusional state. The current definition of dementia does not imply irreversibility of the mental disorder; thus some dementias are treatable, although most are both irreversible and progressive.

The main features making up the disturbance of mental function in dementia are:
1. reduced ability to register and recall new material
2. impairment of mental grasp, reasoning and learning, with inability to carry out day to day activities
3. disorientation for time, place and person
4. coarsening and blunting of personality
5. deterioration in performance of learned skills, social conduct, personal appearance and self-care
6. aphasia, agnosia and apraxia

These clinical disorders of mental function are found in differing degree in individual patients, and in the different dementia syndromes. They are often exaggerated or obscured by other secondary features, especially depression, clouding of consciousness and concurrent physical disease.

Dementia can be understood by reference to the structural distribution of the causative disease. Thus the disorder may affect the brain as a whole or may be more specifically related to frontal, temporal, parietal or occipito-parietal parts of the brain. *Frontal lobe lesions* cause impairment of judgement, incontinence, loss of social skills, loss of abstractional abilities and impairment of reasoning and decision making. Sequential tasks are particularly affected, causing apraxia in the domain of motor performance. *Temporal lobe lesions* impair processing in relation to time, and result in impairment of short term and recent memory. Data may be recalled inappropriately, causing intrusion errors that are themselves a source of confusion in thought and action. *Left temporo-frontal lesions* cause impairment of language, with relative impairment of executive or receptive language function depending on the location and extent of the lesion. In *parietal lesions* there is spatial impairment that results in geographical disorientation, loss of spatial memory, impairment of tactile, visual or auditory localization and failure of perceptual synthesis, or agnosia. *Occipital lesions* will cause higher-level impairment of visual localization and perception. Thus dementia will have variable clinical features dependent on the extent, severity and distribution of the pathological change. In *sub-cortical dementia* there is particularly severe involvement of basal ganglia, brain stem or other non-cortical structures. Clinically, there is forgetfulness, apathy, slowed thought processes, irritability and focal features, such as corticospinal or cerebellar signs. Thus the dementia of Parkinson's disease, hydrocephalus and progressive supranuclear palsy are subcortical dementias. The clinical features are largely related to interruption of frontal lobe connections, and perceptual disorder is not a feature.

In *delirium* clouding of consciousness is associated with confusion, including disorientation in time, place and person, memory disturbance for the period of the delirium and impairment of perception. The disorder is of abrupt onset and short duration. Fragmentation of speech and thought, and fearfulness with restlessness and inappropriate jocularity are often noted. Delirium is often induced by extraneous factors, superimposed on pre-existing dementia, including pain, sensory deprivation, perceptual isolation, alcohol intoxication, depressive illness or drug intoxication.

Epidemiology of dementia

The prevalence of dementia increases with increasing age. This syndrome is thus particularly a problem of developed countries in which the population is itself ageing. About 10% of people older than 65 years, and 20% of those older than 80 years are demented. The prevalence increases markedly after this age. The majority of these older patients with dementia are women. Dementia has a considerable social cost; about 75% of persons unable to care for themselves in the community are demented. Population increase, and survival of a larger proportion of the population into old age, has meant that the size of the population aged 70 years and over will increase by more than 100% by the year 2000. It is therefore inevitable that the social and medical burden of dementia will increase markedly in the future.

Causes of dementia

Dementia is a syndrome with many different causes (Table 10.1). However, only Alzheimer's disease (60% of cases) and cerebral vascular disease (10–20%) are common, and an undefined, perhaps moderately large proportion of patients suffer both from Alzheimer's disease and cerebral vascular disease. All other causes are relatively rare and only a few of these are amenable to treatment. A distinction between presenile and senile dementia, arbitrarily based on the age of retirement, is of no value in diagnosis or management. However, a treatable cause for dementia (Table 10.1) is more likely to be found in younger people.

Alzheimer's disease

This is the commonest form of progressive dementia in late middle life or senescence. It was first recognized by Alois Alzheimer in 1907, in a woman aged 55 years with progressive dementia. Alzheimer found tangles of abnormal fibrils in neurons in the cerebral cortex (neurofibrillary tangles) and clusters of degenerating nerve endings (neuritic plaques) in the brain of this patient; this pathological change is the characteristic feature of the disease. Similar pathological changes occur, however, although to a less marked degree, in the brains of clinically normal people, and in Down's syndrome a terminal mental deterioration appears to be associated with Alzheimer change in the brain.

In Alzheimer's disease the first clinical abnormality is usually subtle memory impairment, often with insight into this progressive abnormality. Naming difficulty and lack of spontaneous conversation or other intellectual activity may be evident. Later, the features of progressive dementia, with more marked memory disturbance, disorientation, impaired motor abilities (apraxia), lack of initiative,

Table 10.1 *Causes of dementia (after Rossor).*

Common
  Alzheimer's disease
  multi-infarct dementia
  mixed Alzheimer's and multi-infarct dementia

Less common
  Degenerative
    Pick's disease
    Huntington's disease
    Parkinson's disease
    progressive pseudobulbar palsy
    spinocerebellar degeneration

  Infective (Chapter 6)
    syphilis
    Creutzfeldt–Jakob disease
    AIDS
    subacute sclerosing panencephalitis

  Metabolic
    Wilson's disease
    hypothyroidism
    B_{12} deficiency
    lipid storage diseases and leucodystrophies

  Toxic
    drug intoxications
    alcoholic dementia

  Traumatic
    severe head injuries
    boxer's encephalopathy
    subdural haematoma (chronic)

  Neoplastic
    frontal, temporal and parietal tumours

  Others
    occult hydrocephalus
    pseudodementia

dysphasia, naming difficulties and impaired spatial memory and visual perception develop. The normal sleep patterns are often disturbed. There is a striking difficulty carrying out sequential tasks. Later still, loss of personal hygiene, and of social behaviour become disabling problems and incontinence, increased muscle tone and a hesitant apraxic gait result in immobility, followed by emaciation, stupor and death. Extrapyramidal features are sometimes prominent.

In the early stages depression is an important feature, presumed to be a consequence of the patient's recognition of the progressive dementia, and psychotic behaviour may be a problem in management. Seizures occur in about 20% of cases. Generally the disease progresses inexorably but relatively rapid deterioration may develop if the patient is moved from a familiar environment, for example to hospital for investigation; this represents inability to adapt functionally to the new environment. The clinical course is variable, ranging from 2 to 15 years, but most cases are severely disabled 7 years after the disorder has been recognized.

In about 10% of cases the disease appears to be inherited as an autosomal dominant trait but, in view of the late onset of the disease, it is often difficult to ascertain whether or not relatives in a previous generation were affected so that this genetic factor may have been underestimated. Attempts to categorize clinical variants according to age of onset, or rate of progression have not been convincing.

Investigation and diagnosis. The diagnosis is suggested by the clinical features and by the insidiously progressive course. Investigations are designed to show typical features of the disease and to exclude other causes of the dementia syndrome (Table 10.1). Thus, haematological screening tests, with B_{12} and folate levels are useful to exclude B_{12} or folate deficiency, blood calcium and liver function tests, blood electrolytes and blood urea exclude metabolic disorders, and an EEG gives an overall measure of brain electrical activity. The latter is useful in considering metabolic and structural disorders and in excluding epilepsy. In Alzheimer's disease the EEG shows slowing of background rhythms to the theta or even delta range. A serological test for syphilis is important, and HIV-AIDS may cause a dementia syndrome.

Hydrocephalus, cerebral tumours and other focal brain lesions, especially cerebral infarction, can be finally excluded only by CT or MR brain imaging. The CT scan usually shows cortical atrophy with enlargement of the ventricular system, especially the lateral and third ventricles (Fig. 10.1). A CSF examination is unlikely to be of practical benefit, although it can be used to exclude low grade, chronic meningitis, e.g. due to cryptococcal infection. Hypothyroidism can easily be missed and thyroid function tests should always be carried out. Alcoholism is often unrecognized, but may cause a dementia syndrome.

Most of the causes of dementia listed in Table 10.1 are relatively uncommon and show different clinical features or clinical courses from Alzheimer's disease. Nonetheless, some are treatable and therefore justify exclusion by appropriate investigation in people who would otherwise be capable of independent lives. Brain biopsy has been used in the past, but is justified only when genetic factors

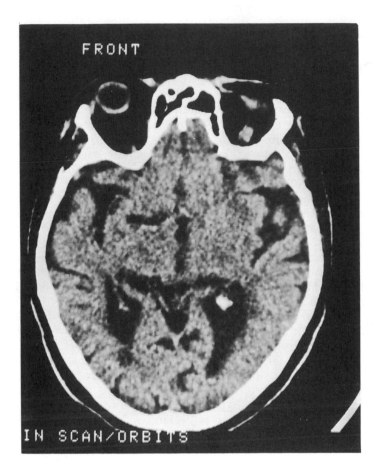

Fig. 10.1 Alzheimer's disease. There is marked atrophy of the brain with increased sulcal markings, and widening of the lateral ventricles in this patient with dementia.

are suspected, and when there are features suggestive of inherited metabolic disorders of the brain, e.g. lipid storage diseases, in which genetic counselling might be important.

Neuropsychological assessment can be useful in the early stages, not only to establish the diagnosis of dementia, but also to help the patient and family adjust to the progressive loss of mental faculties that will occur as the disease progresses. Later, institutional care is often required, with an almost inevitable rapid functional decline in the new environment.

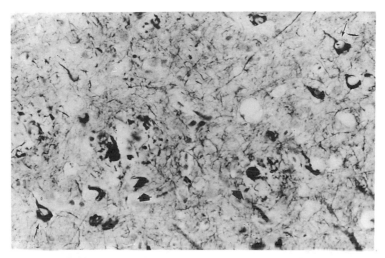

Fig. 10.2 Alzheimer's disease. Silver impregnation of a section of the cerebral cortex, showing neurofibrillary tangles within neurons (arrows) and senile plaques. In the latter the degenerating and regenerating neurites are impregnated with silver (large arrows).

Pathophysiology of Alzheimer's disease. The typical pathology (Fig. 10.2) with neuronal loss, neurofibrillary tangles in neurons, neuritic plaques and granulovacuolar degeneration of neurons is most marked in temporal lobes and in association cortex, but primary motor and sensory cortical areas are spared. Ascending cholinergic fibres arising from the basal nucleus of Meynert, neuronal systems comprising the isodendritic core of the brain, noradrenergic projections from the locus coeruleus, and serotoninergic fibres from the dorsal tegmental nuclei, are strikingly affected. The cholinergic system, important in recent memory function, is particularly severely affected but attempts to improve cholinergic function pharmacologically have not proven useful in the management of the disease, despite preservation of muscarinic receptors in the brain. Neuropeptide levels are relatively normal, apart from somatostatin which is lost in parallel with loss of large neurons in the hippocampus in the disease. The severity of the clinical syndrome correlates fairly well with the numbers of tangle-bearing neurons, and of neuritic plaques in the cortex. There is little correlation, however, with cerebral atrophy, whether of cortical or central white matter, as shown by CT scans. Reaction time measurements are abnormal from an early stage of the disease.

Management. In the early stages depression is often a major feature, with feelings of inadequacy and despondency, and with difficulty sleeping. Treatment with tricyclic drugs may be very effective in managing both these symptoms initially but later the dementia becomes more severe and symptomatic treatment of agitation, wandering and disturbed behaviour with phenothiazines, benzodiazepines and heminevrin may be necessary. Anticonvulsant drugs should be used as appropriate. Specific cholinergic therapy, e.g. tetrahydroaminoacridine has shown promise in experimental trials.

Group therapy, psychological help and psychiatric management, if necessary, in hospital but preferably at home, can be very helpful for the family attempting to cope with this distressing and slowly

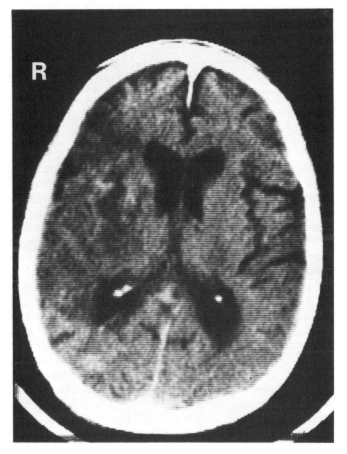

Fig. 10.3 Multi-infarct dementia. There is an infarct in the right fronto-temporal region, with multiple zones of decreased attenuation in the central white matter of both hemispheres, cortical atrophy, and increased ventricular size, especially on the side of the frontal infarct.

progressive disorder. Eventually nursing help and management of incontinence become pressing needs.

Multi-infarct dementia (Fig. 10.3)

The dementia syndrome that may develop in patients with stroke resembles that found in other dementias, especially Alzheimer's disease, but there are a number of differentiating features. In multi-infarct dementia the onset may be abrupt or stepwise. Focal, often transient neurological signs, especially spastic hemiparesis, sensory loss, hemianopia or other visual loss, inco-ordination and prominent early impairment of gait are features that suggest multiple focal and bilateral lesions, rather than a progressive diffuse degenerative dementia. Thus the dementia of multi-infarct disease is typically the result of multiple focal or specific neuropsychological defects, rather than a global disturbance of brain function and information processing, as in Alzheimer's disease. Most patients with multi-infarct dementia are hypertensive, diabetic or have generalized atheroma. Some have valvular heart disease. The infarcts may be small or large.

A problem in the assessment of the cause of dementia in research studies is the coexistence of multiple small cerebral infarcts with dementia of Alzheimer type. Indeed, it has been argued that dementia in patients with multiple cerebral infarcts probably implies the coexistence of these two diseases rather than a dementia due to the multi-infarct state itself. It is worth noting, in this context, that the multiple small infarcts in white matter often thought to cause dementia in 'multi-infarct dementia' may be found without dementia in the CT brain scans of hypertensive patients presenting with multiple small strokes, but without dementia.

Other degenerative diseases (Table 10.1)

Pick's disease

This is an uncommon disorder, occurring with an incidence one-tenth that of Alzheimer's disease, that is difficult to diagnose but recognizable in typical cases by a progressive frontal dementia with restlessness, loss of social inhibitions, volubility and a propensity to make jocular remarks out of context. There is impaired judgement and thinking, with focal symptoms such as aphasia and apraxia. In the latter stages apathy, lethargy and mutism develop. CT scans show atrophy of the frontal and temporal cortex, typically quite circumscribed, an appearance first noted at autopsy.

Pathological studies show that the cortical atrophy spares the posterior two-thirds of the first temporal gyrus. Remaining cortical neurons contain Pick bodies; globular, well defined cytoplasmic inclusions that are well shown in silver impregnations. The aetiology of Pick's disease is not known.

No specific treatment is available.

Huntington's disease

This is a progressive neuronal degeneration, inherited as an autosomal dominant trait that usually presents with a choreiform movement disorder. Dementia is an inevitable feature of the disease that is often evident at presentation but which may precede or follow the development of chorea. In about half the cases the characteristic combination of chorea and dementia is preceded by psychiatric problems, especially failure to conform to the norms of socially acceptable behaviour, e.g. vagrancy, violence, unrest, petty crime and psychosexual difficulties, depression and psychotic behaviour. The disease was first recognized by Huntington in family practice in Long Island, New York, in 1872.

Huntington's chorea usually presents in the fourth decade, although 25% of cases present after age 50 years. Only 5% present before the age of 21 years. Early onset cases are often clinically atypical, with rigidity and akinesia rather than chorea, although dementia, as in other cases, is invariable, leading to a fatal outcome. Cases with paternal transmission have an earlier age of onset than those with maternal transmission. The gene has been located on the short arm of chromosome 4. The life expectancy overall is 17 years but some patients, especially those with onset after age 50 years, may survive as long as 30 years, and early onset cases have a shorter life expectancy. The dominant pattern of inheritance implies a 50% chance of parent to child transmission, but genetic counselling is difficult since most affected people will already have had children before developing overt manifestations of the disease. Although accurate family histories may be difficult to verify because of illegitimacy and late onset of the disease, mutations are very rare, virtually all reported families being traceable to foci of the disease in England, Holland and Scandinavia. Huntington's chorea is rare in Japanese, Chinese and other Asian and African peoples, but there is a high incidence in Venezuela.

In the brain there is severe loss of neurons in the caudate nucleus and in the putamen. Nerve cells are lost, in addition, in the cortex, thalamus and brain stem, and a glial response is found in the striatum. There is a decrease in GABA, choline acetyltransferase and in substance P and enkephalin levels, but other neurotransmitters, e.g. dopamine, TRH and somatostatin, are increased. These findings suggest that the neuronal loss is not limited to cells of any particular functional class.

Clinical features: The onset is insidious. Abrupt, random, non-patterned distal and axial choreiform movements, often prominent in face, tongue and hands, causing a jerky dance-like gait with dysarthria, may be obvious, although the patient and family often deny them. Maintained contraction, as in grasping the examiner's fingers, is interrupted by choreic interruptions of contraction, and whistling or singing a continuous note are also impossible. Eye movements are abnormal, with slowing of lateral and vertical saccades and slowed pursuit movements. The mental disturbance consists of blunting of affect, emotional lability and memory for recent and distant events, so that there are severe difficulties retrieving information both from short term and long term memory. Language is normal and there is no higher-level perceptual defect. Insight is preserved, often even in the terminal stages when anarthria limits communication. These features differ from those found in Alzheimer's disease. Personality disorder, depression and suicide are common in the families of affected persons.

Examination reveals the chorea and the dementia but, except in those cases of early onset with extrapyramidal features (Westphal variant), no other abnormalities occur.

Investigations: The EEG may show a flat pattern that may be a characteristic feature in more advanced cases. Earlier in the disease there is no specific EEG abnormality. CT scan of the brain shows ventricular enlargement with atrophy of the caudate nucleus in most cases, although in some patients the CT image may be normal. Cortical atrophy is not a feature. The CSF and all systemic biochemical tests are normal.

Management: The involuntary movements can be partially suppressed with drugs that interfere with dopamine metabolism, e.g. tetrabenazine, which reduces dopamine release and re-uptake in the striatum, haloperidol and phenothiazines. These medications may lead to drug-induced parkinsonian syndromes that limit their usefulness. Baclofen has also been used. There is no effective therapy available for the dementia. In the late stages the movement disorder is replaced by anarthria and extrapyramidal immobility, with incontinence and difficulty feeding. Dementia is usually profound at this stage but alertness and insight are often relatively preserved.

Genetic counselling: Knowledge of the location of the gene on chromosome 4 suggests that it may be possible to identify the aberrant gene itself and so offer therapeutic abortion. At present, counselling is only possible with large and well-documented pedigrees. Attempts to identify the preclinical phase of the disease by provocative tests with L Dopa and PET scanning tests of glucose metabolism in the corpus striatum are controversial on ethical grounds, and have yielded inconclusive results.

Parkinson's disease (see Chapter 11)

Cognitive impairment develops in about 30% of patients with idiopathic Parkinsonism. There is slowness of thinking, with deficits in language, visuospatial and perceptual/motor functions and a mild disturbance of memory, which amounts to a mild dementia. In these patients this may resemble Alzheimer's disease both clinically and on histological examination of the brain, suggesting that the two disorders coexist more commonly than would be expected from their prevalence rates. Whether there is a specific verbal memory disturbance in Parkinson's disease, representing a form of subcortical dementia, is uncertain. Depression is common in Parkinson's disease and this problem makes assessment of underlying cognitive functions difficult.

Progressive supranuclear palsy

In this neurofibrillary neuronal degeneration, pathological changes are mainly located in brain stem nuclei. There is a mild subcortical dementia that is usually overshadowed by the other neurological manifestations. Treatment does not modify the dementia (see Chapter 11).

Metabolic and toxic dementias

Wilson's disease

Hepato-lenticular degeneration is an autosomal recessive disorder of copper metabolism. There is a hepatic defect in biliary copper excretion, causing copper to accumulate in liver and, later, in extra-hepatic tissues, including the brain. In 40% of cases involvement of the brain is the major clinical problem. In the brain copper is deposited in the basal ganglia, particularly in the putamen. This leads to neuronal loss with characteristic histological changes in remaining neurons in these regions, and in the cortex. Cystic degeneration of the basal ganglia may be found at autopsy, with degeneration of central white matter. The liver shows nodular cirrhosis with high copper levels. In some patients with CNS manifestations, however, liver copper levels are low, although cirrhosis is prominent. Copper is also deposited in other tissues and can be seen as a golden brown ring situated at the margin of the cornea in Descemet's membrane (the Kayser–Fleischer ring). In the blood there is a reduced level of caeruloplasmin, the copper transport protein; 96% of patients with the disease have less than 20 mg/dl. Urinary copper excretion is increased. Measurement of total serum copper levels is not useful in drug users since the combination of a high level of unbound copper and the low level of bound copper may prove misleadingly normal.

Carriers show low serum caeruloplasmin levels and moderately raised hepatic copper content ($<250 \mu g/g$ dry wt: normal $<50 \mu g/g$) but normal liver histology. Homozygotes show higher hepatic copper levels (> 250 μg/g dry wt) and abnormal liver histology. Thus liver biopsy is useful in assessing at risk relatives of patients with Wilson's disease.

Clinical features: The disease is rare; incidence about 30/million. Presentation almost invariably occurs before age 40 years, with involuntary movements consisting of choreiform movements of the face and hands, and a dystonic dysarthria with fixed facial expression. The latter often precedes other manifestations. Progressive difficulty with writing and with learning and intellectual performance is often noted. These early features are often misconstrued as psychiatric in origin. Cerebellar ataxia is prominent in some cases, and may be combined with the dystonia, affecting face and later also limbs, with extrapyramidal tremor and extensor plantar responses. In the terminal stages decorticate and then decerebrate postures develop before death occurs from brain stem failure. The rate of progression is variable. In some patients the course is rapid, very severe disability developing in a few weeks, but in the majority the disease progresses during a period of several months or even a year or more. Other manifestations, due to copper deposition in other organs, include hypersplenism with haemolytic anaemia, Fanconi syndrome, renal calculi, vitamin D resistant rickets, osteomalacia, premature arthritis and skin lesions. Kayser–Fleischer corneal rings are often difficult to detect at the bedside, and slit-lamp examination is a useful technique to demonstrate them.

Investigation and management: Diagnosis depends on recognition of the clinical and biochemical features discussed above. The routine liver function tests are sometimes unusual, despite marked CNS abnormalities. The CT brain scan shows hypodense areas in the basal ganglia, cerebellum and central white matter, with ventricular enlargement, but in 30% of cases the CT scan is normal. Brain stem auditory evoked responses may be abnormal.

Before effective treatment was available death occurred 1 to 6 years after the onset of the disease. Treatment with D-penicillamine 1 g daily in four divided doses is effective in promoting urinary excretion of copper and thus in mobilizing copper from its storage sites in the body. Chelating agents, such as British anti-Lewisite (BAL) and triethylenetetramine are useful in the early stages, and in patients who respond poorly to D-penicillamine. Pyridoxine supplements are necessary. BAL is given as a course of 10–20 i.m. injections daily of 0.3 mg dissolved in oil. The daily administration of elemental zinc (100–200 mg) inhibits absorption of copper from the gut. D-penicillamine should be continued indefinitely. The neurological manifestations improve only slowly, but complete recovery may occur both in brain and liver function. Despite treatment, the more severely affected patients may fail to improve or die.

Lipid storage diseases and other inborn errors of metabolism (Chapter 17)

In this group of disorders there is a disorder of neuronal metabolism often marked by storage of a metabolite. These disorders usually present in infancy or childhood with a combination of progressive dementia, seizures, focal neurological signs and features of involvement of other organs. Most have recognized enzyme defects (see Chapter 17).

Hypothyroidism

Deficiency of thyroid hormone in newborn infants is associated with severe mental retardation and with the systemic features of cretinism. It is usually reversible by treatment with thyroxine. Hypothyroidism developing after the age of 3 years is not associated with retardation but, as in adults, there is placidity, poor memory, slowed thought and behavioural responses and systemic features of hypothyroidism. Paranoid ideation and excitement may occur in adults. The skin is dry and the hair sparse. There may be inco-ordination and cerebellar ataxia. In the elderly, mutism and stupor, with hypothermia, should suggest the diagnosis. Treatment of dementia associated with hypothyroidism in the elderly is only rarely successful, and there is a significant mortality associated with cardiovascular manifestations.

Deficiency of vitamin B₁₂

Dementia sometimes accompanies pernicious anaemia but a variety of mental changes occurs suggesting a non-specific relationship. Mild dementia, confusional states with paranoid ideation and impaired memory may be found. Treatment with vitamin B_{12} results in variable improvement. As in the other neurological manifestations, e.g. myelopathy and peripheral neuropathy, haematological changes may be absent.

Hypercalcaemia and hypocalcaemia

Dementia may accompany hypercalcaemia; the latter is usually of sufficient severity to cause progressive renal failure. Acute hyper-calcaemia, e.g. in metastatic neoplastic invasion of bone, may cause an acute confusional state or even coma. The EEG shows characteristic changes, including bursts of high voltage slow activity. With restoration of normal calcium levels the mental state and the EEG improve. Hypocalcaemia may cause irritability, sleeplessness and seizures.

Table 10.2 *Neurological complications of alcoholism.*

Dementia
Delirium tremens
Wernicke–Korsakoff syndrome
Withdrawal seizures and alcoholic seizures (see Chapter 2)
Alcoholic cerebellar degeneration
Marchiafava–Bignami syndrome
Central pontine myelinolysis (see Chapter 9)
Hepatic encephalopathy
Alcoholic neuropathy and myopathy
Depression and anxiety states
Secondary problems, especially head injuries

Alcoholic dementia and the amnesic syndrome

Alcoholism is associated with a number of neurological complications, but alcoholic dementia has only relatively recently been recognized as common (Table 10.2).

Alcoholic dementia. This dementia is associated with longstanding alcohol abuse and is thought to be due to toxic effects of such abuse on the brain. There is impairment of judgement and affect, with neglect of social skills and self-care. Memory is impaired. The mental syndrome is progressive and involves all aspects of higher cortical function. The CT scan shows cerebral atrophy and ventricular dilatation, and these features may improve with abstinence from alcohol. In some patients clinical evaluation is complicated by a history of other complications of alcoholism, especially head injury, seizures, depression and anxiety, and even delirium tremens. The possibility of multiple causations for the alcoholic dementia syndrome remains. Treatment consists of abstinence from alcohol and vitamin supplements. Improvement occurs, to a varying extent, in 1–2 months.

Alcoholic blackouts. Acute alcoholic debauches are sometimes associated with amnesia for the drinking spree, of up to a day's duration. This syndrome is associated with very high blood alcohol levels, and is indicative of alcohol abuse. It may be associated with delirium tremens during the withdrawal phase.

Delirium tremens

This is an acute toxic psychosis, consisting of excitability bordering on mania, an irregular tremulousness with stimulus-sensitive myoclonus, visual and auditory hallucinosis and tachycardia. The visual hallucinations often consist of formed figures of animals, insects or people, usually reduced in size, moving about the room, bed or walls. They may be frightening. Vestibular disturbances, profuse sweating and hypotension may also be present. Seizures are frequent. The syndrome develops during sudden withdrawal after a long period of progressively more severe alcoholic abuse culminating in an alcoholic debauch. The tachycardia implies alcoholic cardiomyopathy and this may sometimes be fatal. Many patients with delirium tremens have peripheral neuropathy or truncal cerebellar ataxia, additional features of alcoholic brain damage.

Treatment. The patient should be nursed in a quiet room. Sedation is required and heminevrin or diazepam are the drugs of choice. A high fluid intake, but avoidance of hyponatraemia due to alcohol-induced inappropriate ADH secretion, is indicated. Seizures may be controlled by oral or i.v. heminevrin but other anticonvulsants, e.g. phenytoin given parenterally, may be needed. Vitamin supplementation is essential and should be given intravenously; this must include thiamine to prevent thiamine-dependent cardiomyopathy, neuropathy and Wernicke–Korsakoff syndrome. Once recovery has occurred, usually in 2–5 days, arrangements for continued abstinence from alcohol should be recommended to the patient, since this serious complication is often either fatal or subsequently associated with a permanent amnesic syndrome.

Wernicke–Korsakoff syndrome

This syndrome is due to thiamine deficiency. Although most common in alcoholics it is associated with other causes of hypovitaminosis including intractable vomiting and severe dysphagia. In alcoholism it usually develops during recovery from delirium tremens, or in association with intercurrent illness and vomiting. There is a history of inadequate nutrition during several weeks or months prior to the illness. The patient is drowsy or comatose initially and seizures may occur. There is tachycardia. The features of delirium tremens are often present. Ocular palsies, sometimes causing virtually complete ophthalmoplegia, are associated with an acute hallucinatory confusional state, with anxiety, and also with cerebellar ataxia, nystagmus and peripheral neuropathy. The latter is often painful. Examination of the mental state discloses a profound disturbance of short term memory. The patient cannot remember the date, a short string of words or numbers, or the name of the physician or hospital. Despite this, memory for distant personal and public events is intact and recollection of these memories and of other more recent events, even subsequent to the illness, may be inappropriately recalled and presented to the examiner. These intrusions from memory are sometimes termed confabulations, and may be elaborated into complex stories.

Improvement occurs if treatment is instituted early in the illness with thiamine, other vitamins, and restoration of an adequate diet, together with abstinence from alcohol. The ophthalmoplegia usually improves rapidly with intravenous thiamine, but the amnesic syndrome is relatively resistant to treatment and only 20% recover adequately. Few recover fully. The cerebellar syndrome rarely recovers.

The syndrome is associated with necrosis in the medial parts of the thalamus bilaterally, in the central grey matter of the midbrain and upper pons, in the hypothalamic nuclei and especially in the mammillary bodies. It is important to note that the Wernicke–Korsakoff syndrome is quite frequently found unexpectedly at autopsy in patients confused or demented in life, and treatment of confused, drowsy patients with thiamine, especially if malnutrition is evident, is of immense prophylactic value in preventing this potentially disabling amnestic syndrome.

Marchiafava–Bignami disease

This consists of a syndrome of emotional disturbance, seizures, rigidity and paralysis leading to coma and death. It is closely associated with chronic alcoholism. No treatment is available. There is symmetrical degeneration of myelin in the central part of the corpus callosum.

Traumatic dementias (see Figure 10.1)

After *severe closed head injuries* an amnesic syndrome may be prominent, with profound impairment of short term and recent memory, but relative sparing of more distant memories. The patient cannot remember new experiences in verbal, abstract or spatial domains, and there are usually other neuropsychological deficits and associated focal signs of motor and sensory impairment (see Chapter 5). The retrograde amnesia may be very long at first, but this gradually shrinks as recovery occurs during the 12–24 months after the injury.

Subdural haematoma may sometimes present as dementia, particularly when it is bilateral and chronic. Other, more focal features may be present, such as extensor plantar responses, visual field defects and hemiplegia or hemisensory loss. Signs of raised intracranial pressure are not usually present and the diagnosis is made, often unexpectedly, by CT scanning. With treatment by drainage of the haematoma, recovery occurs in a few weeks. In some patients with chronic subdural haematoma, chronic alcoholism is an underlying cause, a head injury having been sustained during a period of alcohol abuse.

Traumatic encephalopathy of boxers. Dementia pugilistica is a syndrome well known amongst professional boxers and their sparring partners, and particularly common in the past in fairground boxers. There is a progressive encephalopathy, developing after some years boxing experience, usually in the context of repeated, stunning blows to the unprotected head, or repeated knockouts. Dysarthria and a change in the tonality of the voice is a prominent early sign. This is followed by unsteadiness of gait, cognitive impairment and spasticity. The disorder often commences some time after retirement from boxing, and progresses for many years. In some cases the combination of psychiatric and extrapyramidal features produces a syndrome resembling Parkinsonism but in most the presence of corticospinal and cerebellar features indicates the underlying relation to the history of boxing-induced head injury. The reason for the progressive nature of the syndrome, after cessation of exposure to repeated head injuries, is not known.

CT scans show cortical atrophy, dilatation of the lateral ventricles and a prominent cavum septum pellucidum. Histologically there is depigmentation of the substantia nigra and neurofibrillary tangles are found in cortical neurons. Treatment is relatively ineffective; L Dopa is sometimes moderately helpful if extrapyramidal Parkinsonian features are prominent.

Most patients show other features of boxing-related injury, especially healed fractures of the metacarpal bones of their dominant hand, arthropathy of the wrists, cauliflower ear on the left, and thickening of facial skin with a broken nose. The facies is often relatively expressionless.

Dementia associated with tumours of the brain. Dementia is not a common presentation of brain tumour. However, very large tumours, especially those located in the frontal or right parietal regions, may cause dementia. This is usually associated with focal signs appropriate to the location of the tumour, for example anosmia and disorders of conduct, socialization and judgement in frontal tumours. Intrinsic CNS tumours usually present with readily recognizable clinical syndromes but large extrinsic tumours, almost invariably meningiomas, may present with much less readily categorizable symptoms and neurological examination is then often normal. The diagnosis is made by CT scanning. Treatment by removal of the tumour, however, is often not followed by rapid or complete recovery, suggesting either that irreversible brain damage has occurred or that another underlying disorder, especially Alzheimer's disease, is present.

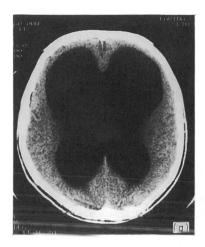 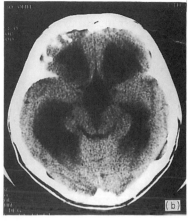

Fig. 10.4 (a and b) 'Occult' hydrocephalus. There is massive dilatation of the lateral and third ventricles, due to aqueductal stenosis. The patient presented aged 35 years.

When patients with dementia are investigated by CT scanning a relatively large number of unsuspected intracranial tumours, especially meningiomas, is discovered. In most cases these are small and clearly insignificant but in some patients larger tumours are found. Unfortunately, removal of these tumours is often not followed by recovery from the dementia. It should be remembered that the one year survival of malignant glioma in patients older than 50 years is only 8%, whatever treatment is given.

Tumours obstructing the ventricular system may lead to dementia by causing obstructive hydrocephalus, and tumours of the third ventricle are particularly likely to cause dementia, not only because they may cause hydrocephalus, but because they may interrupt the ascending non-specific cholinergic fibres of the isodendritic core, arising from the nucleus of Meynert that project to all cortical regions. These fibres are selectively damaged in Alzheimer's disease.

Occult hydrocephalus and dementia. In hydrocephalus there is ventricular enlargement due to obstruction of the flow of CSF out of the ventricular system into the subarachnoid space (obstructive hydrocephalus) or to impaired absorption of CSF at the cerebral convexities (communicating hydrocephalus), but with normal outflow of the CSF from the ventricular system (Fig. 10.4). Increased production of CSF may occur with third ventricle papillomas, but is a very rare syndrome. The causes of hydrocephalus are discussed in Chapter 17.

Communicating hydrocephalus is an ill-understood disorder. It may result from subarachnoid adhesions at the base of the brain, or at the tentorial hiatus, in the Sylvian fissures or at the arachnoid granulations themselves. The arachnoid granulations consist of specialized nodules in the sagittal sinus that are regions of CSF absorption into the venous system, but absorption also occurs into cerebral veins at the cerebral convexities, and fibrosis of the meninges, developing after subarachnoid haemorrhage, head injury or meningitis, may therefore result in the later development of communicating hydrocephalus.

In hydrocephalus the ventricular system, including the temporal horns, is enlarged. This may be associated with raised intraventricular and intracranial CSF pressure, but this is intermittent rather than continuous and attempts to measure pressure are therefore usually unrewarding. However, continuous pressure measurements by intradural transducer placements through twist-drill holes in the skull may reveal increased 'B wave' pressure peaks which, if present for more than 2 hours daily, have been correlated with neurological complications. The typical clinical features of decompensated hydrocephalus consist of progressive dementia, an ataxic/spastic gait with extensor plantar responses and increased tendon reflexes in the legs, often referred to as a gait apraxia. The gait disorder consists of a hesitancy of foot placement with short, rapid steps. In addition, there is incontinence of urine in typical cases. The dementia is of frontal type with disturbances of mood, judgement, serial processing and social skills, but memory and perception are usually unimpaired. There are none of the classical features of raised intracranial pressure.

Much confusion has arisen from attempts to relate mildly increased ventricular size to dementia in the absence of incontinence and gait apraxia. Early optimism about ventriculo-atrial shunt operations to relieve dementia in patients with so-called 'occult' hydrocephalus has not been fulfilled by subsequent experience of this procedure. Further, this procedure is not without complications, including shunt blockage, infection and subdural haematoma. In demented patients with a past history of a possible cause for communicating hydrocephalus the procedure is worth considering nonetheless. In others, however, in whom dementia is associated with ventricular enlargement, but not with cortical atrophy, a cautious approach is relevant.

CT scans of communicating hydrocephalus characteristically reveal periventricular lucencies in the white matter at the frontal and occipital poles, representing leakage of CSF under increased pressure into the adjacent white matter. However, this appearance can be mimicked by lacunar infarction, or by the hypertensive/ischaemic change in the white matter associated with Binswanger's encephalopathy. Attempts to establish the diagnosis by measurement of CSF dynamics after instillation of water soluble contrast by lumbar puncture, using serial CT scanning of the brain, have proved unreliable, and other tests, such as clearance of TC^{99m} labelled, micro-aggregated human serum albumin, pressure monitoring and CSF perfusion studies, have also yielded conflicting results. Further, obstructive hydrocephalus, although usually of more abrupt or rapid onset than communicating hydrocephalus, is rarely accompanied by dementia (see Chapter 17).

Pseudodementia. This consists of apparent intellectual impairment in a patient with a primary psychiatric disorder, resembling organic brain disease. Depression alone may present in this way, but many patients with true dementia become depressed and improvement results after appropriate treatment. In a few patients the pseudodementia is a manifestation of a hysterical conversion syndrome and the underlying personality disorder can then usually be recognized during the clinical assessment.

Pseudodementia usually has a relatively rapid or abrupt onset and shows a phasic but variable course. The patient usually appears withdrawn or depressed and sleep disorder is evident. There may be a history of affective disorder. Psychological testing reveals disparity in the results of sub-tests and clinical assessment usually shows no consistent features of agnosia, apraxia or aphasia. There are thus well-marked inconsistencies in the clinical syndrome. The patient often complains bitterly of memory disorder, but testing does not confirm this. Investigation is normal and treatment with antidepressant drugs results in marked improvement.

Recognition of *depression* in patients with dementia, in some respects the converse of pseudodementia, is also important since antidepressant drug therapy will result in substantial improvement in mental performance, allowing the underlying dementia to be adequately assessed.

11

Parkinson's Disease, Tremor and other Extrapyramidal Disorders

The term *involuntary movement disorders* is often used to describe the diseases listed in Table 11.1, in which the major features are a disturbance of posture and the presence of involuntary movements or spasms, often with a superimposed disturbance of voluntary movement. Parkinson's disease and essential tremor are the commonest of these disorders. All are the result of diseases of the basal ganglia or their connections.

Clinical features of basal ganglia (extrapyramidal) diseases

The classification used in Table 11.1 implies that extrapyramidal disorders may cause either *akinetic/rigid syndromes* or *dyskinesias*. The former are predominantly associated with rigidity and relative absence of spontaneous or automatic movement, termed poverty of movement by Parkinson. The latter are disorders in which there is an excess of spontaneous movement, consisting of involuntary movements that are superimposed on resting posture or voluntary movement patterns. In practice, many of the disorders listed in Table 11.1 show a predominance of rigidity/akinesia or of dyskinesia, while exhibiting features of both.

Tremor, chorea, myoclonus, torsion dystonia (athetosis) and *tics* are well-defined involuntary movement syndromes. *Tremor* consists of involuntary periodic oscillation of a body part which is rhythmic and continuous when present. It may be *resting* or *static*, i.e. present when the affected part is supported or, as in *action* tremor, present only when the body part is moved. *Chorea* consists of brief, jerking, unpredictable, simple or complex movements that may affect any body part but are often marked in fingers and face. *Myoclonus* consists of sudden jerks, which are involuntary, irregular and brief, affecting individual muscles or muscle groups. *Torsion dystonia* consists of involuntary, prolonged tonic contractions of muscles or muscle groups. *Tics* are purposeless, stereotyped jerking movements

Table 11.1 *Involuntary movement disorders (after Marsden, 1982).*

Akinetic/rigid syndromes	Dyskinesias
Parkinson's disease	Tremor
Post-encephalitic parkinsonism	essential tremor
Drug-induced parkinsonism	cerebellar tremor
Multiple system atrophy	Chorea
Shy–Drager syndrome	Huntington's disease
striato-nigral degeneration	rheumatic (Sydenham's) chorea
olivopontocerebellar atrophy	chorea gravidarum
Progressive supranuclear palsy	systemic lupus erythematosus and
Wilson's disease	other causes
Hallervorden–Spatz disease	Myoclonus
Rigidity in other diseases	myoclonic epilepsy
multi-infarct dementia	essential myoclonus
Alzheimer's disease	symptomatic myoclonus
traumatic encephalopathy	post-anoxic
post-anoxic rigidity	with cerebellar degeneration
spastic dystonia	Torsion dystonia
	hereditary (dystonia musculorum
	deformans)
	symptomatic
	paroxysmal
	focal dystonia, e.g. spasmodic
	torticollis, writer's cramp,
	blepharospasm, hemifacial
	spasm, Meige's syndrome
	Tics
	organic and functional

mainly affecting facial and head and neck muscles. They may be simple or complex patterned acts or fragments of motor acts. *Rigidity* is found on clinical examination and consists of resistance to passive movement of the body part.

Akinetic/rigid syndromes

Parkinson's disease

This disease was described by James Parkinson in 1817 from his observations made in Hoxton, London. He summarized the clinical features as:

> Shaking palsy (paralysis agitans). Involuntary tremulous motion, with lessened muscular power, in parts not in action and even when supported; with a propensity to bend the trunk forward, and to pass from a walking to a running pace: the senses and intellects being uninjured.

Epidemiology and pathogenesis. Parkinson's disease is a common disorder, affecting about 1% of people older than 50 years in the UK. Its incidence increases with advancing age. It is less common in Black people than in caucasians. There is no evidence of a genetic factor. Men are affected slightly more commonly than women (1.4 : 1.0). The disease is rare before age 40 years.

The cause of the disease is unknown. Since the experience of the development of post-encephalitis parkinsonism following the pandemic of influenza and encephalitic lethargica in 1916–1926 a viral cause was suspected, but no evidence in support of this hypothesis has been discovered. Dietary factors appear irrelevant. The most recent clue to the aetiology of the disease has come from the observation that self-administration of MPTP, a derivative of pethidine, by drug addicts in California, is followed by the rapid development of typical parkinsonism. This substance is a highly selective toxin for the pars compacta dopaminergic neurons of the substantia nigra and seems to produce an experimental model of idiopathic Parkinson's disease. However, the disease has been known at least from the time of Parkinson and probably from Galen and thus if an environmental toxin is responsible for the idiopathic disease, it must be a naturally-occurring substance. A parkinsonian syndrome also occurs in miners and steel workers exposed to manganese ore.

Clinical features. Two-thirds of patients present with tremor. This is usually asymmetrical, commonly affecting upper limbs. The tremor is distal, coarse, variable in amplitude, and has a typical 'pill-rolling' rotary element at 4–5 Hz. It is most marked at rest and usually disappears during movement and in sleep. The tremor has often been present for many months or longer before presentation, since the disease has an insidiously progressive course. It is worsened by anxiety. In many patients there is a prodromal personality type, consisting of depression, lethargy and obsessionality traits, with fatigue, aches and pains and cramps. These may represent the earliest phase of the disease. Presentation with gait disorder, especially progressive slowing of gait, a shuffling gait, stiffness and difficulty on rough ground or stairs accounts for most of the remaining third of the patients, but some present with dysarthria or with speech or writing problems. Undue quietness of the voice, a festinant dysarthria and micrographia (tiny handwriting) may lead to medical consultation. Axial postural reflexes are defective, causing difficulty swimming, turning over in bed and getting in and out of a bath.

On examination the main features are *akinesia* and *rigidity* (Fig. 11.1). There is a poverty of spontaneous movement with a tendency to maintain unusual postures. This immobility may be

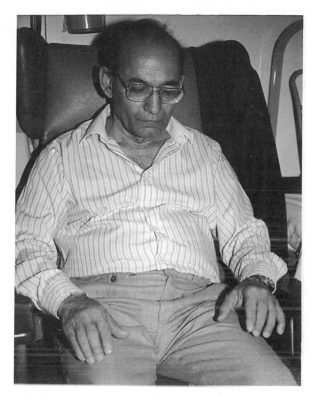

Fig. 11.1 Parkinson's disease. There is resting flexion of the upper limbs with an immobile posture. Note that the hands are not resting on the knees

particularly evident in the face, with reduced blink frequency, lack of emotional expression and of gestural language, and by oedema of the dependent affected hand. Rigidity of a peculiarly characteristic cogwheel type is found in the limbs, especially on rotation of the passive wrist or elbow. *Tremor* is present at rest or on maintenance of a posture. The tongue may be affected and drooling of saliva is often prominent (sialorrhoea). The complexion may be greasy, with seborrhoeic dermatitis. The posture is unusually flexed both at rest and standing. The gait shows this flexed posture, with absence of arm swing, short steps and a tendency to accelerate the gait cycle as though falling foward (*festination*) after marked initial hesitation. *Retropulsion*, consisting of a tendency to walk backwards if gently pushed in that direction, is often a feature in more advanced cases. Postural reflex loss can be demonstrated by observing difficulty moving about on a bed and a tendency to fall if displaced suddenly laterally. The tendon reflexes are normal and the plantar reflexes are flexor. Eye movements are affected, with impaired convergence, and with jerky interruption of smooth pursuit movements, and slowed saccadic movements. Repetitive tapping on the glabella causes an exaggerated, non-fatiguing blink reflex response, a paradoxical sign in the virtual absence of spontaneous blinking.

In the later stages of the disease about 30% of patients develop a mild dementia (Chapter 10), perhaps related to Alzheimer change in a proportion of cases. The disease progresses at variable speed; some patients seem not to progress at all during many years. Autonomic neuropathy resembling that of multiple system atrophy with postural hypotension, dysphagia, constipation, urinary incontinence and impaired sweating develops in some cases. These late complications indicate that the degenerative process has extended beyond the nigro-striatal pathway.

The disease tends to be less severe in young people and is often rather worse in women than in men.

Pathology and pathogenesis. Parkinson's disease is a neuronal degeneration (Fig. 11.2). There is selective loss of dopaminergic neurons, especially in the substantia nigra pars compacta. Remaining neurons in the substantia nigra show reduced neuromelanin content, and many contain eosinophilic cytoplasmic inclusions (Lewy bodies) (Fig. 11.2). These contain ubiquitin, a highly-conserved heat shock protein involved in degradation of intermediate filament proteins. This loss of neurons is accompanied by reduction in nigral and striatal dopamine content. As much as 80% of dopamine content and neuronal number in the substantia nigra must be lost before the features of Parkinson's disease appear. Dopaminergic receptors in the striatum, especially in the putamen, may be increased, representing a compensatory process for reduced dopaminergic activity in the nigro-striatal pathway, or decreased as in the later stages of the disease. There is also a mild reduction in dopamine levels in other dopaminergic pathways, especially in the hypothalamus and in cortical and limbic areas. Noradrenaline levels in the hypothalamus and locus coeruleus are slightly decreased. Choline acetyltransferase levels, reflecting acetylcholine metabolism, may be slightly reduced in frontal cortex, perhaps associated with the Alzheimer-type dementia of the later phase of the disease. However, the motor defects are explained by the dopaminergic deficit in the nigro-striatal pathway.

Treatment with L-Dopa. The akinesia and rigidity respond well to dopaminergic therapy, but tremor is relatively less well relieved by this treatment. Since dopamine crosses the blood–brain barrier only poorly the drug is administered as its precursor L-Dopa, which is metabolized in the body and brain to the active neurotransmitter

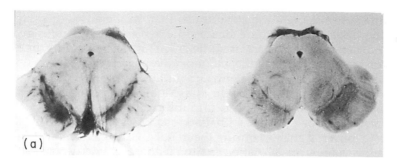

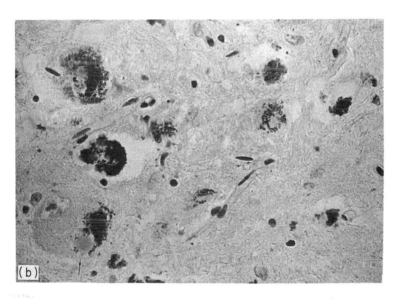

Fig. 11.2 Parkinson's disease. (a) The substantia nigra in the mid brain slice from the patient with Parkinson's disease (right) is depigmented, indicating loss of melanin-containing neurons. The slice on the left is from a patient without Parkinson's disease, but matched for age. (b) Lewy bodies (arrow) in the remaining pigmented neurons in the substantia nigra in a patient with Parkinson's disease.

dopamine. High circulating dopamine levels cause tachycardia, hypotension and gastrointestinal hyperactivity and L-Dopa is therefore usually administered together with a peripheral decarboxylase inhibitor which itself will not cross the blood–brain barrier. Systemic breakdown of L-Dopa is thus inhibited and more of the drug is available to brain neurons for metabolism. The clinical response to L-Dopa treatment is dependent on the ability of remaining nigral neurons to synthesize dopamine for neurotransmission in the striatum so that, in the advanced stages of the disease, when there has been extensive loss or damage of nigral neurons, there are insufficient neurons remaining in the nigrostriatal system for sufficient dopaminergic activity to be induced by dietary L-Dopa supplementation and the clinical features prove unresponsive to treatment. In these patients striatal dopamine receptors are usually reduced in number.

About 75% of patients with Parkinson's disease regain nearly normal physical abilities during the initial phase of treatment. There is improvement in all patients and, if there is no response, the diagnosis should be questioned. However, after 6 years of treatment half the patients fail to maintain benefit or develop intolerable side effects necessitating a change in the regimen.

L-Dopa should be started in low dose, in a preparation containing a peripheral decarboxylase inhibitor; the dose is slowly increased, using frequent doses rather than large intermittent doses until a satisfactory response is achieved. The best possible response should not be sought since this is likely to be followed by the rapid development of dyskinetic and psychiatric unwanted effects which may limit subsequent treatment. Improvement sufficient to restore normal activity of daily living is the ideal (see Table 11.2). Because of these side effects low dose regimes of L-Dopa have been advocated, despite the incomplete clinical response that is then inevitable.

Table 11.2 *Drug management of Parkinson's disease.*

Disease severity	Management
Mild disability, e.g. tremor	Anticholinergic drugs Amantadine
Moderate disability with tremor and hypokinesia	Amantadine L-Dopa; in small doses 3 or 4 times daily
Severe disability	L-Dopa; in *frequent* dosage, avoiding dyskinesias and confusion Add dopamine agonist in small initial dosage
Decreasing response to L-Dopa or on/off phenomena etc.	Reduce dose of L-Dopa, but give medication 3–4 hourly Add Selegiline or dopamine agonist

Unwanted effects of L-Dopa: These relate to changing blood and brain levels of L-Dopa and dopamine, and to striatal receptor hypersensitivity to dopamine. *Peak-dose dyskinesias* are repeated orofacial, axial and limb movements, often of a contortional or grimacing nature, that occur at times of high brain dopamine levels, usually 30–60 minutes after oral L-Dopa dosage. They may suddenly cease, giving way to sudden immobility and speechlessness at the height of the dopamine release in the brain (*peak-dose akinesia*, or *freezing*). In patients with marked receptor hypersensitivity dyskinesias may occur throughout the 2–3 hour active period after dosage. End-of-dose deterioration may also develop abruptly, with immobility, salivation, tremor and rigidity. These effects result in swings of responsiveness and immobility, which can be very distressing. As the disease progresses these problems become more prominent, necessitating frequent, smaller doses of drug. Visual hallucinations and toxic confusional states indicate overdosage and should be avoided. '*Off periods*' denote periods, usually toward the end of a day, when the patient is unresponsive to treatment. The treatment of longstanding Parkinson's disease thus becomes increasingly difficult once the patient is established on L-Dopa therapy.

Other treatment. Dopaminergic drugs are also used, but these carry the same risk of unwanted effects as L-Dopa itself. *Bromocryptine* is the most frequently used, and slowly incrementing dosages are usually tried, often in combination with L-Dopa treatment. It seems to have no significant clinical benefit over L-Dopa, although it may be a useful adjuvant when L-Dopa therapy has been associated with fluctuating responses. Other dopaminergic drugs, such as lergotrile, lisuride and pergolide, are little used. *Selegiline* (Éldepryl) is an inhibitor of MAO B receptors in the brain, causing a selective stimulant action at dopaminergic receptors. The drug is used in a dose of 5–20 mg daily with L-Dopa therapy and tends to improve the clinical response to this treatment. It is advisable to decrease L-Dopa dosage by about 20% when adding selegiline to an established regimen. Subcutaneous apomorphine with an antiemetic (Maxolan) may be useful when on/off effects are pronounced.

Amantadine, an antiviral agent, also has weak dopaminergic actions and few unwanted effects. It has been used in patients with mild Parkinson's disease and has a place in delaying the necessity for L-Dopa treatment. Similarly, *tricyclic antidepressants* have weak anti-Parkinsonian effects. *Anticholinergic drugs,* such as benzhexol, orphenadrine procyclidine and methixene, are moderately effective for tremor and sialorrhoea in Parkinson's disease, but do not relieve bradykinesia. In addition, they cause anticholinergic unwanted effects, e.g. glaucoma, urinary retention, constipation and confusion, and their use is restricted either to mild Parkinson's disease or as an adjuvant to L-Dopa therapy when tremor is severe (Table 11.2).

Stereotaxic thalamotomy, in which a small (2–3 mm diameter) lesion is induced in the ventromedial thalamus by cryoprobe under mathematical and physiological control, is useful in a few selected patients to control severe tremor; it does not modify the other features. Transplants of adrenal medullary cells, or of foetal substantia nigra have recently been tried; these procedures are of uncertain benefit.

Other measures. Physiotherapy, occupational therapy and the provision of help at home for patient and family are important in long term management. Incontinence may be a problem requiring nursing help or even catheterization. The development of dementia may require nursing home management rather than home care but, in other circumstances, hospitalization should usually be avoided, since it provokes confusion and immobility, with difficulty in rehabilitation.

Drug-induced parkinsonism. Drugs that deplete nigro-striatal neurons of dopamine such as tetrabenazine or reserpine, or that block dopamine receptors such as phenothiazines, may cause parkinsonian syndromes. Initially this effect is dose related. Withdrawal of dopamine-depleting drugs results in rapid improvement of the parkinsonian symptoms, especially of rigidity, akinesia and tremor, but withdrawal of neuroleptic drugs may not be followed by rapid resolution of symptoms. In the latter case, improvement occurs during the following 6 months but many patients remain parkinsonian. In addition, oro-facial dyskinesias may develop representing the direct effects of the antipsychotic drug on dopaminergic striatal receptors. These are often refractory to treatment with sedatives, anticholinergics and other drugs (see below). L-Dopa can be used to manage drug-induced parkinsonism but, usually, anticholinergic drugs are moderately effective in managing this side effect. In some patients there is a clinical suspicion that these antipsychotic drugs may damage the striatal receptors enough to precipitate the features of idiopathic Parkinson's disease, implying that there was pre-existent subclinical loss of neurons in the substantia nigra. MPTP toxicity (see above) is a specific toxin for substantia nigra pars compacta neurons.

Post-encephalitic parkinsonism

Encephalitis lethargica occurred in epidemic proportions in Europe and later in other countries between 1915 and 1930. It was an acute illness, usually accompanied by fever, with somnolence, ophthalmoplegia and other focal disturbances such as hemiplegia and aphasia. In a second form hyperkinesis, chorea, myoclonus and sleep disturbances occurred and, in a third type, an acute parkinsonian syndrome, sometimes with a catatonia-like stupor, was observed. Half of the survivors developed parkinsonism in the

5 years after the infection; the mortality in the acute illness was 40%. The disease still occurs sporadically but is uncommon.

Post-encephalitic parkinsonism differs from idiopathic Parkinson's disease in the relatively non-progressive course once the syndrome is established, and in the occurrence of oculo-gyric crises. The latter consist of maintained deviation of the eyes laterally and usually upwards with akinesia and relative unresponsiveness occurring suddenly and lasting seconds or minutes. The physiological basis of this feature is unknown. Post-encephalitic parkinsonism is accompanied by rigidity and tremor, with dysarthria and there are sometimes pupillary abnormalities, focal neurological signs and abnormalities of the ventilatory rhythm. Corticospinal involvement is relatively frequent.

Pathologically there is damage to the substantia nigra and to the locus coeruleus, but the remaining neurons, unlike those in idiopathic Parkinson's disease, contain neurofibrillary tangles. Lewy bodies are absent. There is some cortical involvement, representing a sequel to the encephalitis.

Treatment resembles that of the idiopathic disease, but the response to L-Dopa is less dramatic. Since the disorder is non-progressive the long term prognosis of L-Dopa treatment is rather better.

Progressive supranuclear palsy

This is a progressive, sporadic disorder beginning in middle life or in the senium, of unknown causation. There is a supranuclear ophthalmoplegia with inability to look downwards. Axial dystonic rigidity is present with severe pseudobulbar dysarthria, pseudobulbar palsy and mild dementia. Cerebellar, corticospinal or parkinsonian features may also be present. The disorder begins insidiously and progresses to death from hypostatic pneumonia about 6 years after the onset. Pathological examination has shown neurofibrillary neuronal degeneration with gliosis in the red nucleus, pontine tegmentum, oculomotor nuclei and superior cerebellar peduncles. In its early stages the disorder may be mistaken for idiopathic Parkinson's disease but the absence of resting tremor, symmetrical onset, early gait disturbance, extensor rigidity and poor response to L-Dopa therapy should suggest the diagnosis. The head is held in extension, despite the impaired downward gaze. CT scanning shows enlargement of the third ventricle and interpeduncular cistern. Treatment with various drugs, including anticholinergics, amitryptoline and L-Dopa has proved only moderately useful, the results varying from case to case. The dementia, which is of subcortical type, is unresponsive to treatment.

Multiple system atrophy

This disorder, striato-nigral degeneration and olivo-ponto-cerebellar atrophy are system degenerations that are described in Chapter 12. Striato-nigral degeneration is difficult to diagnose on clinical grounds since it closely resembles idiopathic Parkinson's disease, but there is only a poor response to L-Dopa or other anti-parkinsonian drugs.

Rigidity in other diseases

Extrapyramidal rigidity occurs in conditions other than Parkinsonian syndromes (Table 11.1). In multi-infarct dementia, Alzheimer's disease, traumatic encephalopathy, anoxic encephalopathy and spastic dystonia, rigidity is common, consisting of a resistance to passive manipulation of the joints when the patient is relaxed. The increased tone is often more marked when the rate of displacement is varied, but tends to affect extensors and flexors equally. When tremor is superimposed a cogwheel effect results. The rigidity of these non-specific and diffuse lesions is sometimes termed paratonic rigidity (Gegenhalten: go/stop) to describe the tendency of the patient's limb to oppose any interposed displacement. The rigidity of chronic spasticity, e.g. in cerebral palsy, termed spastic dystonia, differs in that there is flexor predominance in the upper limb and extensor predominance in the lower limb, and in that there is spasticity on dynamic stretching of the limb. Decerebrate and decorticate rigidity and posturing shows features of spasticity and does not represent an extrapyramidal disorder.

Dyskinesias

Tremor

The periodic rhythmic oscillation that is the characteristic feature of tremor may be an asymptomatic normal phenomenon (physiological tremor), represent an exaggeration of normal tremor (anxiety tremor), or be due to disease of the nervous system. Tremor can be classified according to its presence at rest, during maintained posture, or with action or the intention to action (Table 11.3). Classification by frequency is imprecise in clinical practice but measurement of tremor frequency has been used in research. The amplitude of tremor has little diagnostic value, but rhythmicity is important. For example, parkinsonian tremor is rhythmic, but cerebellar action tremor is irregular.

In *resting tremor*, the tremor is present only when the affected body part is supported or relaxed. Parkinson's disease is the typical

Table 11.3 *Causes of tremor and tremor frequencies.*

Resting tremor	
Parkinson's disease	4–5 Hz tremor
parkinsonian syndromes	
Postural tremor	
physiological tremor	7–11 Hz tremor
exaggerated physiological tremors	
thyrotoxicosis	
anxiety	
alcohol withdrawal	
drugs, e.g. lithium	
mercury salts	
β_2 receptor agonists, e.g. ventolin	
cimetidine	
neuroleptics	
benign familial (essential) tremor	5–8 Hz tremor
peripheral neuropathy	
Intention tremor	
cerebellar disease	4–6 Hz tremor
(essential tremor)	
(Parkinson's disease)	

example of resting tremor, in which there is a distal, alternating contraction of agonist and antagonist muscles, e.g. flexors and extensors, or supination and pronation movements. The tongue and face may also be affected. *Postural tremor* is a tremor that appears when the body part is actively maintained against gravity. It often persists or is increased during voluntary movement of the part. Physiological tremor and benign essential tremor are the commonest examples; other causes are listed in Table 11.3. *Lower frequency tremors*, at 2–4 Hz, also occur, merging in nomenclature with involuntary movements. These often affect proximal muscles and the head and neck and are principally associated with multiple sclerosis or in survivors of severe closed head injury. In *peripheral neuropathy* a coarse distal tremor, due to fasciculation of enlarged motor units, may develop; the tremor involves fingers and is strikingly irregular.

Essential tremor. This form of tremor is commoner than Parkinsonian tremor. It is a postural tremor and is absent at rest. It occurs at a frequency of 5–8 Hz with a dominant frequency of about 6.5 Hz and particularly involves the arms. It is not made strikingly worse by movement and is not associated with signs of Parkinson's disease or cerebellar disease, although it is worse in the outstretched than in the flexed arm. It is more marked distally than proximally and is worsened by emotional stress and sympathomimetic drugs. During a period of many years it gradually worsens, involving both upper limbs, the head and neck, and even the voice. In half the cases there is a family history of tremor, suggesting dominant inheritance. Essential tremor differs from physiological tremor by its slower frequency, progressive course and asymmetry but it is often difficult to distinguish these two forms of tremor. Essential tremor characteristically improves with alcohol, even with small doses such as a glass of sherry. Most patients notice improvement with β adrenergic blocking drugs, especially propranolol 30–120 mg daily. Propranolol blocks both peripheral β_2 receptors and central β_1 receptors and both these actions are important. Primidone may be useful but at the cost of sedation and other side effects at the relatively high doses needed. The drug should be commenced with low doses, e.g. 62.5 mg daily, and increased gradually to a maximum of 250 mg tds. Propranolol and primidone therapy may be given in combination. The pathophysiology of essential tremor is uncertain, but these drugs are thought to be effective by their CNS actions. Parkinson's disease has been reported to be associated with essential tremor, and a trial of anti-parkinsonian drugs, e.g. benzhexol, may be worthwhile.

Drug-induced and physiological tremor. Many drugs (Table 11.3) may exaggerate physiological tremor and essential tremor. These drugs, including caffeine, isoprenaline, lithium, steroids and L-Dopa, may stimulate tremorogenic peripheral receptors. The increased tremor of anxiety and alcohol withdrawal probably have central origins. *Physiological tremor* is a normal phenomenon; its pathophysiology is not understood but probably involves a combination of central and peripheral mechanisms. It is exaggerated by posture, as in the outstretched hand with abducted fingers, but is always relatively fast (7–11 Hz) and of small amplitude. It does not require treatment, but its exacerbation by stress can be suppressed by propranolol, an effect that has been utilized by professional musicians and snooker players to enhance performance.

Intention (action) tremor. Cerebellar tremor is absent at rest, and induced by movement. When severe, it may also be induced by posture, as in alcoholic cerebellar degeneration, Wilson's disease or multiple sclerosis. It is usually tested by the heel-shin or finger-nose tests, which demonstrate that the tremor is at right angles to the intended direction of movement and not in the direction of movement itself, and that it is most marked in the middle range of movement. Cerebellar tremor results from lesions in the cerebellar peduncles and the brain stem connections of the dentate, fastigial and interpositus nuclei of the cerebellar hemispheres. Mid-line cerebellar lesions, e.g. of the vermis, result in mid-line, truncal ataxia, and more laterally placed lesions cause limb ataxia. Nystagmus occurs with lesions in the cerebellar hemispheres, cerebellar roof nuclei, peduncles and brain stem connections.

Drug therapy for cerebellar ataxia is ineffective. Damping the oscillations of ataxic limbs with weights may be of slight benefit to some patients. The output of the cerebellum is inhibitory and neurosurgical attempts to alleviate the tremor by lesioning the thalamic nuclei have also proved ineffective, although electrostimulation of the cerebellum has shown mild benefit in a few patients.

Hysterical tremor. Tremor is a relatively common manifestation of hysteria. The involuntary movement is present at rest or in action, is relieved by suggestion, and increased by observation and by inducing emotional distress. It can often be relieved by gently stroking the limb. It does not interfere with motor control when attention is directed away from the tremor. It is usually at about 4–5 Hz, the natural resonant frequency of the limb, and almost always affects an arm or the head and neck. The legs are rarely affected. The symptom is a conversion reaction, and is accompanied by features of hysterical personality disorder. The underlying cause is usually related to emotional, financial and especially sexual problems and improvement results when this disturbance is relieved. The prognosis, as in other forms of hysteria, is rather poor. In some patients there may be an underlying organic neurological disorder that becomes recognizable when the conversion symptom has resolved.

Chorea

Chorea consists of brief jerking movements affecting tongue, head, face, respiratory and limb muscles, both at rest and during voluntary movement. The involuntary movements may be subtle or coarse, and are irregular, unpredictable and non-repetitive. They thus differ from tremor. They may be sufficiently severe to interfere with voluntary movement, e.g. with gait, posture, speech, swallowing and respirations.

The most common cause of chorea (Table 11.4) is Huntington's chorea, a dominantly inherited disorder (Chapter 10). All the forms of chorea listed in Table 11.4 are generalized except hemiballismus, which usually involves only one side of the body. Hemiballismus follows a lesion in or near the sub-thalamic nucleus, usually vascular or neoplastic.

Inherited chorea. Most patients with inherited chorea have Huntington's disease. In some families a benign form of chorea

Table 11.4 *Causes of chorea.*

Inherited chorea
  Huntington's disease
  chorea/acanthocytosis syndrome
Acquired chorea
  hemichorea (hemiballismus)
  Sydenham's chorea
  systemic lupus erythematosus
  thyrotoxicosis
  pregnancy
  hypoparathyroidism
  drug-induced
    L-Dopa and dopamine agonists
    phenothiazine
    anticonvulsants, especially phenytoin overdose
  polycythaemia rubra vera

occurs without dementia, usually developing after the sixth decade. This has been termed benign hereditary chorea or senile chorea, but in many if not most instances this is a late-onset form of Huntington's disease. Sporadic senile chorea is likely to be due to Alzheimer's disease or to cerebrovascular disease.

Chorea/acanthocytosis syndrome (neuroacanthocytosis). This syndrome consists of chorea, myoclonic jerks and tics, with a severe bulbar dystonia causing dysphagia. There may be mutilation of the lips. There is an associated axonal peripheral neuropathy with a raised blood creatine kinase level, and spiky erythrocytes (acanthocytes) are found in peripheral blood films. These syndromes are inherited as autosomal recessive or sex-linked traits. They develop in childhood or in adult life, and represent a heterogenous group of conditions.

Acquired chorea. The acquired choreiform involuntary movement disorders do not have a uniform underlying pathophysiological cause, but may be due to focal or diffuse brain disease (Table 11.4).

Hemichorea. This is the most dramatic form of chorea. Its alternative name, hemiballismus, indicates the rapid, throwing movements of the limbs and body that occur. The limb alternates from a position of extension and elevation to any intervening posture, and there is an impression of continuous flinging motion that is both tiring and distressing to the patient, and a cause of injury against furniture. It has been suggested that hemiballismus represents an unstable alternation of the postures of decerebration and decortication, and this aptly describes the extent of the involuntary movement.

However, during recovery the choreiform movement gradually subsides through a stage of typical chorea to normality, chorea being induced only by fatigue and stress. The commonest cause of hemichorea is infarction of the contralateral sub-thalamic nucleus, or of the white matter close to this nucleus in the field of Forel. Occasionally, encephalitis or a metastatic tumour in this region may cause hemichorea and, rarely, the syndrome may be bilateral.

In hemichorea due to infarction there is usually an associated hemiparesis. Recovery occurs gradually in a period of days or weeks. The involuntary movements can be suppressed to a useful degree with fentazin 15 mg tds or tetrabenazine 12.5 to 25 mg tds. This therapy is useful in reducing the risk of self-harm from the movement, but may cause depression and dose-related parkinsonism as unwanted effects. The hemichorea disappears in sleep and is activated by anxiety and emotional distress, and sedation is often useful in management of the acute phase.

Sydenham's chorea (St Vitus' dance). Rheumatic chorea (chorea minor) is often preceded by features of rheumatic fever following streptococcal infection. The chorea is accompanied by non-specific mental complaints, especially lassitude and irritability, with lack of concentration. Rarely there may be an acute psychosis. There is generalized chorea, usually consisting of small-amplitude fidgety movements. The latter may not be noticed at first, but may be exaggerated by anxiety and by attempts to sustain unusual postures. Facial twitchiness is rather characteristic, but the arm movements are often quasi-purposeful, being absorbed into coincidental voluntary movements. Most cases occur in children between the ages of 5 and 15 years. In contemporary practice in developed countries Sydenham's chorea is rare, due either to a change in virulence of the organism, to host resistance, or to the use of antibiotics. Recovery is usually complete in 6 months, but in 30% of cases there are residual symptoms, consisting of anxiety, mild chorea and tics.

Treatment: Bed rest and antibiotic treatment have been recommended in the acute stage because of the association with rheumatic carditis. Prophylaxis of streptococcal throat infections with penicillin for several months has also been recommended. The chorea can be treated with haloperidol, tetrabenazine or diazepam.

Chorea gravidarum. Chorea of generalized type, closely resembling Sydenham's chorea, may complicate pregnancy. It nearly always develops in the second trimester of the first pregnancy, and may recur in subsequent pregnancies, but rarely occurs for the first time in multipara. A similar form of chorea occurs occasionally during treatment with oral contraceptives. This form of chorea may sometimes be unilateral. Chorea gravidarum, and contraceptive induced chorea, is probably hormonal in origin, but its pathogenesis is unknown. Chorea associated with oral contraceptive treatment resolves in a few days when these drugs are stopped. Chorea gravidarum resolves after delivery.

Other forms of chorea. In *thyrotoxicosis*, and less commonly in *hypoparathyroidism*, choreic involuntary movements may be evident. These subside when the endocrine disorder resolves with treatment. Generalized chorea also occurs in *systemic lupus erythematosus*, unassociated with other CNS manifestations of this disorder but indicating lupus encephalopathy. In *polycythaemia rubra vera*, chorea may be one of the neurological manifestations, together with seizures, confusion and drowsiness or stroke, but as in systemic lupus erythematosus, chorea can develop without other CNS abnormalities. In both polycythaemia rubra vera and systemic lupus erythematosus chorea resolves when the underlying cause is relieved. *Drug-induced chorea* is relatively common, occurring with L-Dopa therapy of Parkinson's disease, as an unwanted effect of phenothiazine therapy and as part of anticonvulsant toxicity, especially with phenytoin overdosage, with blood levels greater than about 30 mg/litre. *Electrolyte imbalance*, especially hypernatraemia, may induce chorea.

Pathogenesis and treatment of chorea. The cause of chorea in generalized or metabolic disorders is unknown. Although hemichorea can be due to a lesion in the contralateral subthalamic nucleus (corpus Luysii), diffuse cortical abnormality, perhaps due to vasculitis in Sydenham's chorea and systemic lupus erythematosus, and to changes in blood flow in polycythaemia rubra vera, may be important in the encephalopathies associated with chorea. In Huntington's chorea striatal abnormality, associated with glutamate depletion, may be important but in L-Dopa toxicity changes in striatal dopamine receptors are clearly causative. Thus, chorea is probably a symptom of disordered motor control associated with relative hyperexcitability of motor systems, but due to several possible mechanisms. Whatever its cause, chorea improves with management of the underlying cause and can be suppressed by haloperidol or tetrabenazine therapy, or by phenothiazines and, to a lesser extent, by diazepam or other sedatives. Chorea is always relieved by sleep.

Myoclonus

The sudden jerks of myoclonus are involuntary, brief and irregular, affecting individual muscles or muscle groups. Myoclonic movements may be repetitive and localized (segmental myoclonus) or generalized. The term myoclonus is used to describe a number of different phenomena all arising in the CNS (Table 11.5).

While myoclonus may occur in many different disorders, classified in Table 11.5 as symptomatic myoclonus, several different physiological disturbances underlie the production of myoclonic jerks. These have been classified as *cortical myoclonus, reticular myoclonus* and *segmental myoclonus* from brain stem or spinal cord disease. Focal and segmental myoclonus presents a different clinical problem from generalized myoclonus in that the clinical phenomenon is strikingly limited to one part of the body. *Palatal myoclonus* is the best known example of focal myoclonus; other examples include persistent hiccough following brain stem infarction or viral encephalitis, and rhythmic segmental (spinal) myoclonus associated with viral infection, e.g. Herpes zoster myelitis, tumours of the spinal cord, multiple sclerosis and spinal infarction.

Cortical myoclonus. The characteristic feature of cortical myoclonus is that the muscle jerk is generated by a discharge arising in the cerebral cortex. This discharge may occur spontaneously, as in *spontaneous cortical myoclonus*, or in response to an external stimulus, as in *cortical reflex myoclonus*. If it occurs repetitively the syndrome of *epilepsia partialis continua* results. These cortical events are related to epilepsy in that local spread of a cortical myoclonic discharge can lead to a Jacksonian seizure, and generalization of the discharge might produce a major generalized convulsion. Thus, cortical myoclonus is often associated with epilepsy. The myoclonic jerk can be correlated with electrical discharges recorded in cortex by EEG, or located by back-averaging from the jerk. In *cortical reflex myoclonus* giant responses can be recorded from the cortex after cutaneous or peripheral nerve stimulation. These responses have been associated with cerebellar disorders, e.g. Ramsay–Hunt syndrome, perhaps indicating loss of the inhibitory cerebellar cortical output. Similarly, EEG studies of the time relationships of *spontaneous cortical myoclonus* to electrical discharges in the cortex suggest a sub-cortical origin, perhaps in basal ganglia or brain stem, for this type of myoclonus. Epilepsia partialis continua, also, may arise subcortically, rather than from the motor cortex itself. In Alzheimer's disease and Creutzfeldt–Jakob disease myoclonus of cortical type are prominent features.

Reticular myoclonus. In reticular myoclonus the EEG discharge, if present, is not directly temporally related to the myoclonus. The myoclonus is generalized, triggered by external stimuli such as touch, stretch or movement, and is accompanied by a generalized EEG discharge indicating a central reticular origin for the generalized myoclonic jerk. *Post-anoxic myoclonus* is a form of reticular myoclonus that is both triggered, i.e. reflex, or spontaneous in origin. Other

Table 11.5   *Causes of myoclonus.*

Physiological myoclonus
  arousal and startle responses
  sleep jerks
  hiccough
Essential myoclonus
Epileptic myoclonus (see Chapter 2)
  isolated epileptic myoclonic jerks
  epilepsia partialis continua
  photosensitive myoclonus
  petit mal
  childhood myoclonic epilepsy
Symptomatic myoclonus
  storage diseases
    Lafora body disease
    lipidoses (e.g. Tay–Sachs' GM2 gangliosidosis)
    ceroid-lipofuscinosis (Batten's disease)
    sialidosis
  Ramsay–Hunt syndrome
  basal ganglia degenerations, e.g. Wilson's disease
  dementias
    Alzheimer's disease
    Creutzfeldt–Jakob disease
  viral encephalopathies
    subacute sclerosing panencephalitis
    Herpes simplex encephalitis
  metabolic encephalopathies
    renal, hepatic, electrolyte imbalance
    non-ketotic hyperglycaemic encephalopathy
  other diffuse encephalopathies
    post-anoxic encephalopathy
    carbon monoxide poisoning
    heat stroke
    post-traumatic
  drugs

disorders, such as myoclonic epilepsy, petit mal epilepsy, subacute sclerosing panencephalitis and essential myoclonus are probably also reticular in origin. *Essential myoclonus* is a familial syndrome in which myoclonus is associated with dystonia. The myoclonus is absent at rest but induced by action, consisting of chaotic irregular jerks of all muscle groups. It is not associated with other abnormalities, and is improved temporarily by alcohol.

Startle syndromes, such as startle myoclonus, consisting of a sudden bodily jerk in response to startle, or startle epilepsy, are probably also reticular in origin. *Hypnic jerks,* sudden bodily jerks when drowsy, are normal reticular responses that are experienced by almost everyone. Noctural myoclonus consists of sudden jerks of the legs, often asymmetric, occurring during non-REM sleep.

Ramsay–Hunt syndrome and progressive myoclonic dementia syndromes. The term Ramsay–Hunt syndrome represents a clinical description of patients with myoclonus and cerebellar ataxia, associated with a mild seizure disorder. This syndrome has many causes, including spinocerebellar degenerations, and various metabolic disorders. The *progressive myoclonic dementias* consist of a group of disorders characterized by the early onset of myoclonic jerks, dementia and seizures, with ataxia and other manifestations in some cases. This clinical syndrome may occur with Lafora body disease, with neuronal storage disorders and with mitochondrial encephalomyopathies.

Dystonic syndromes (athetosis)

Dystonia implies a tendency to maintain a relatively fixed, abnormal posture. Thus dystonia is a feature of hemiplegic stroke (posthemiplegic dystonia) and of decerebration or decortication. The term torsion dystonia has come to be used in recent years to describe involuntary and prolonged tonic contraction of muscles or muscle groups. *Dystonias are characterized by simultaneous contraction (cocontraction) of agonist and antagonist muscles.*

Focal dystonias involve a single part of the body. Involvement of two or more contiguous parts, e.g. hand and forearm, is termed *segmental dystonia. Generalized dystonias* usually commence as focal dystonias. Generalized dystonia begins before the age of 20 years, but *focal dystonias* begin later, usually after the age of 30 years.

There are many different syndromes of dystonia, but in most the dystonia is only an additional manifestation of the underlying disorder, rather than a primary or major manifestation. The focal dystonias listed in Table 11.6 are all relatively common, acquired

Table 11.6 *Focal and segmental dystonias.*

Spasmodic torticollis: rotation, extension and tilting of head due to tonic contraction of sternomastoid, trapezius and other nuchal muscles; associated with tremor and jerking of head
Blepharospasm: dystonia of facial and periorbital muscles
Oromandibular dystonia: dystonic jaw, face and tongue movements with forced opening and closing of mouth
Meige's syndrome: blepharospasm and oromandibular dystonia
Dystonic dysphagia: pharyngeal muscle dystonia
Dystonic dysphasia: adductor spasm of the larynx
Writer's cramp: dystonic spasms and jerks of hand, forearm and arm
Lower limb dystonias: variable localized patterns of leg and pelvic dystonia
Occupational cramps: in musicians and others

forms of dystonia. There are areas of overlap between the different syndromes; for example blepharospasm and oropharyngeal dystonia may occur separately, or together (Meige's syndrome) and some patients presenting with the latter syndrome also show features of torticollis or of writer's cramp.

Writer's cramp is of particular interest since, like torticollis, it has often been considered an hysterical disorder. Characteristically it develops in people dependent on writing for their livelihood, consisting of an increasing tendency to grip a pen fiercely, to develop spasmodic and jerky co-contraction of agonist and antagonist muscles acting at elbow, wrist and fingers and so to prevent writing *without* affecting mobility and facility of these muscles in relation to other activities. Work then becomes impossible. This disorder is now generally regarded as an organic, acquired focal dystonia, representing an acquired physiological disturbance of motor control in relation to writing. A similar focal dystonic syndrome occurs in musicians, darts players and other performing artists, perhaps

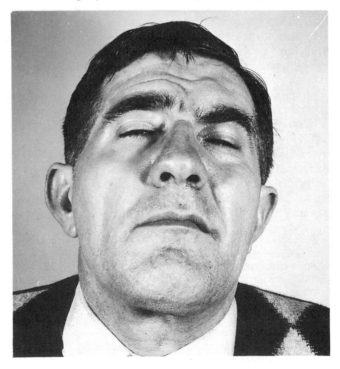

Fig. 11.3 Blepharospasm. There is forced, chronic eye closure with facial muscle spasms and abnormal positions of the head and neck. This was a progressive disability associated with dystonia of one upper limb. No structural or metabolic cause was found despite extensive investigation.

representing an overuse syndrome. Most focal dystonias are worsened by anxiety and emotional distress, and show fluctuating disability during clinical observation over several weeks or months. They are absent during sleep and are often not markedly evident at rest, but are worsened by attention, or by attempts to perform certain tests, e.g. writing, speaking, swallowing etc. as is appropriate for the particular syndrome. Examination reveals spasm or dystonia of muscles in the affected region of the body without abnormality of power, reflexes or sensation. *Torticollis*, similarly, is not associated with specific abnormalities on examination, although the affected sternomastoid, trapezius and nuchal muscles, as in other forms of dystonia, may be hypertrophied. *Blepharospasm* (Fig. 11.3) may be so severe as to cause loss of vision because of permanent closure of the eyes. A similar blepharospasm may occur with L-Dopa induced dyskinesias and, occasionally, in post-encephalitic parkinsonism.

Treatment. A number of drugs have been tried in the treatment of focal dystonias but none is consistently effective. The principal drugs are anticholinergic drugs, such as artane or trihexyphenidyl (40–100 mg/day), baclofen, tetrabenazine, carbamazepine and benzodiazepines. Focal dystonias can also be relieved by local injections of botulinum toxin into the affected areas; this causes conduction block at neuromuscular junctions and weakness of the affected muscles with a beneficial response until recovery occurs in up to 3 months. The treatment can then be repeated. This treatment is also useful in writer's cramp, torticollis and blepharospasm. In torticollis, section of the spinal accessory nerve may be successful.

Generalized dystonia may be idiopathic or symptomatic (Table 11.7).

Idiopathic torsion dystonia. The disorder usually commences in childhood before the age of 11 years, involving one part of the body, usually a foot but sometimes an arm. Later onset cases, beginning in the third decade, begin in an arm. Progression to generalized dystonia occurs in about 85% of cases of early onset but is rare in later onset cases and never occurs in those beginning in the fifth decade. The disorder is disabling and may be fatal. Initially dystonic movements are intermittent and often particularly induced by certain movements or tasks but later they become continuous, although of variable severity. They are always abolished by sleep or drowsiness and are usually attenuated by sensory stimulation, especially by bodily contact, for example by leaning back against a wall or by lying in a bed or chair. Similarly, focal dystonias can be relieved by cutaneous contact; for example torticollis is often modified by lightly

Table 11.7 *Generalized dystonia, classified by aetiology.*

Idiopathic dystonia (torsion dystonia; dystonia musculorum deformans)
  Hereditary: autosomal recessive torsion dystonia (severe)
                autosomal dominant form (mild)
  Sporadic

Symptomatic dystonia
  Hereditary:
    degenerative, e.g. Huntington's disease
    metabolic: Wilson's disease
                aminoacidurias, e.g. homocystinuria
                storage diseases, e.g. Batten's disease
                hyperuricaemia, e.g. Lesch–Nyhan syndrome
  Acquired:
    perinatal brain injury or haemorrhage
    kernicterus
    encephalitis
    post-traumatic
    multiple sclerosis
    following cerebral infarction
    drug-induced, e.g. L-Dopa, phenytoin toxicity, phenothiazines
    associated with Parkinson's disease
    poisoning with manganese or carbon monoxide
    psychogenic dystonia

touching the chin with the hand and blepharospasm by contact of a finger on the periorbital skin.

Idiopathic torsion dystonia is not associated with other neurological abnormalities. For example, intelligence and mental development are normal and there are no other motor, sensory or reflex abnormalities on examination, apart from released grasping and avoiding reactions in the hand. In contrast, patients with symptomatic dystonia show neurological features consistent with the underlying neurological disease including mental retardation, seizures, cerebellar features and striking corticospinal and other systemic abnormalities. Dystonia at rest is also more likely in symptomatic than in idiopathic hereditary dystonia. Patients with idiopathic torsion dystonia tend to show a progressive course with periods of relatively rapid progression and sometimes with periods of remission. Hereditary torsion dystonia has been recognized especially amongst Jewish peoples, but occurs in all races. It is inherited as an autosomal dominant trait with incomplete penetrance.

Treatment: Idiopathic torsion dystonia can be extremely disabling with the development of fixed, contorted postures, and life expectancy in such cases is diminished. Treatment is difficult. Surgical treatment by thalamotomy helps some patients, particularly those with limb dystonia rather than axial dystonia, and those requiring only a unilateral surgical procedure. Drug treatment has been disappointing. Rarely, particularly in those with fluctuating dystonia, there may be a response to low dose L-Dopa therapy. Anticholinergics, especially benzhexol or trihexyphenidyl, beginning at 2.5 mg bd and increasing until an effect is obtained or tolerance is exceeded, are also useful. As in the treatment of focal dystonias, baclofen, diazepam and carbamazepine and tetrabenazine may also be helpful. Physiotherapy has an important role in modifying muscular tone and in preventing joint contractures; it is particularly useful when used in brief, intensive courses of treatment.

Symptomatic dystonias. These disorders can be recognized on the basis of the features of the underlying disease. Presentation with lateralized dystonia, with other neurological signs, with features of systemic disease and with mental retardation, dementia or seizures particularly suggest an underlying cause. Intensive investigation may be required to define the cause. This should include thorough clinical evaluation, including family history, EEG and CT scan, biochemical investigation including full blood count, ESR, liver function tests and uric acid and blood calcium estimations. Wilson's disease must be excluded by serum caeruloplasmin measurement and slit lamp examination of the cornea, and blood lysosomal enzyme measurements are useful. In appropriate cases urine amino acid screening tests and blood pH measurements are indicated. Mitochondrial cytopathy can be excluded by muscle biopsy and EMG, including nerve conduction studies. Other tests, including fibroblast or white blood cell culture for exclusion of lipid storage disorders may be necessary in doubtful cases.

Dystonia occurring with antipsychotic medication, or with metoclopramide treatment for nausea and vomiting may occur acutely. It is reversed by diphenhydramine injection or by anticholinergic drugs and its occurrence does not imply any propensity to the development of torsion dystonia or other dyskinesias.

Tics and mannerisms

This term has an imprecise definition, overlapping in some respects with certain forms of chorea, and myoclonus. The synonym 'habit spasms' gives a clear idea of the jerky, repetitive movements, involving discrete muscle groups, which mimic normal co-ordinated movement and which can temporarily be suppressed by an effort of will. Tics are often patterned, seeming to consist of a fragment of voluntary movement, and are relatively easy to imitate. Patients often complain of an irresistible urge to move, and that voluntary suppression of the involuntary movement is accompanied by increasing inner tension that can be relieved only by movement. Tics are worsened by anxiety, anger or embarrassment, and partially relieved by concentration, drowsiness and sexual arousal. They disappear in sleep.

Tics can be distinguished from myoclonus since the latter cannot be controlled at will, and myoclonus is not associated with a conscious urge to move. Chorea, like tic, may consist of complex movements, but it is not repetitive and stereotyped, and is not accompanied by the inner tension and urge to move characteristic of tic. A problem in the recognition and definition of tics is that tic-like movements have been described in relation to other involuntary movement disorders, for example Huntington's chorea and focal dystonias. This observation serves to strengthen the notion that tics are a manifestation of neurological disease, rather than a psychologically determined phenomenon.

Mannerisms represent acquired tic-like movements consisting of a stereotyped movement or fragment of a movement that becomes a necessary preliminary or component of a complex motor act or task. In this sense mannerisms represent characteristic but exaggerated movement patterns that come to form part of the expression of an individual's personality or eccentricity. They occur in context, rather than without purpose and thus differ from tics.

Tics occur in various disorders (Table 11.8). Tics are common in childhood, occurring in up to 15% of normal children. They consist of head twitching, blinking and limb movement or rocking motions, usually developing between the ages of 5 and 8 years. The tic resolves and is rare after adolescence. They are often associated with periods of personal or emotional stress, sometimes sufficient to require psychiatric help. About 20% of affected children show features consistent with minimal neurological abnormality, e.g. reading difficulty, clumsiness, stammering, enuresis or hyperactivity

Table 11.8 *Diseases in which tics occur.*

Primary tic of childhood
Hereditary tics
　Gilles de la Tourette syndrome
　Huntington's disease
　torsion dystonia
Secondary tics
　infections, e.g. viral encephalitis
　post-traumatic
　multi-infarct states
　dementia and other degenerative disorders
　schizophrenia
　drug-induced akathisia, e.g. phenothiazines, L-Dopa
　senile tic
　restless legs syndrome
　mental retardation

---

syndrome. Reassurance and attention to underlying social or emotional problems is usually associated with a favourable outcome. Medication, such as benzodiazepine drugs, should be avoided.

Gilles de la Tourette syndrome

This is the major tic syndrome, occurring with a prevalence of 5/million. It consists of multiple tics, with involuntary vocalizations consisting of sudden loud grunts and sounds, coprolalia (obscene utterances), echolalia (repetitions of the speech of others) and repeated motor actions copied from recently observed movements. For example, the patient will repeat conversation or the mannerisms of those around him, or will imitate others. The tics are often complex and repetitive. Intelligence and orientation is normal, but educational abilities are limited by a short attention span. The illness begins in early childhood; before the age of 10 years. The sex ratio is 3 : 1 male to female, and Jews seem more susceptible than others. Life expectancy is normal but affected people are poorly adapted to society, or even outcasts, unable to hold down a job and often severely socially disadvantaged. Many show compulsive/obsessive traits. In Tourette's syndrome sleep is disturbed with somnambulism and arousals; tics may occur during these episodes. There is a family history of tics in approximately a third of cases, but usually not amounting to the full Tourette syndrome. The pathophysiology or biochemistry is unknown.

Treatment: No specific treatment is available. Severe chronic tics may respond to benzodiazepines, or to clonidine (0.25–0.9 mg/day). Behavioural therapy and psychotherapy are not effective. Haloperidol, a dopamine receptor antagonist drug, is the most effective drug beginning in a dose of 0.25–0.5 mg daily. Children usually respond to doses of 5 mg/day or less but much larger doses, up to 100 mg/day, may be required in adults. The severity of the syndrome varies from month to month and treatment should vary with this factor.

Symptomatic tics

These should be managed according to the underlying cause. Tics are particularly prominent in the mentally retarded and in schizophrenia, but do not usually require specific treatment. In encephalitis and post-traumatic encephalopathies the tic syndrome usually slowly improves with time, except in survivors of encephalitis lethargica in whom tics sometimes persisted for many years. In *restless legs syndrome* there is a peculiar compulsion to move the legs; this syndrome has been associated with subclinical peripheral neuropathy and occasionally with Parkinson's disease. Tics also occur in dementia syndromes, and in non-demented elderly people, and haloperidol can be useful in their management.

12

System Degenerations: Hereditary Ataxias, Spastic Paraplegias and Anterior Horn Cell Diseases

Degenerations of functionally related neuronal systems and their connecting tracts form a group of genetically-determined diseases called system degenerations. These include the hereditary ataxias and hereditary spastic paraplegias. Genetically-determined degeneration of anterior horn cells and of the lower motor neuron, called spinal muscular atrophies, can be classified within this general category of inherited neuronal and system degenerations. Motor neuron disease, although only rarely an inherited disorder, consists of degeneration of upper and lower motor neuron pathways and can thus be related to this group of diseases. Classification of the hereditary ataxias is complex, but can be simplified by separation of those disorders with recognized metabolic cause, and of early and late onset types in the case of those without known metabolic cause. Other disorders such as Parkinson's disease, in which there is a specific neuronal degeneration, are not classified as system degenerations since there is associated degeneration of other or of diffuse neuronal networks (Table 12.1).

Table 12.1 *System degenerations.*

Hereditary ataxias with metabolic cause
Hereditary ataxias of unknown cause
early onset, e.g. Friedreich's ataxia
late onset, e.g. autosomal dominant ataxias
Multiple system atrophy
Hereditary spastic paraplegia
Anterior horn cell disorders
spinal muscular atrophies
Motor neuron disease

Hereditary ataxias of metabolic cause

The hereditary ataxias with known metabolic cause (Tables 12.1 and 12.2) all commence in childhood, most before the age of 5 years, and are inherited as autosomal recessive or, rarely, sex-linked recessive traits. Most are serious problems and many are associated with other systemic or cerebral manifestations that are potentially fatal. These disorders are rare. In some, for example the neuronal lipid storage disorders, cerebellar ataxia is a minor feature in relation to the severe encephalopathy. Similarly, in the hyperammonaemias, encephalopathy and mental retardation are severe problems in survivors.

Several of these metabolic disorders can be managed by dietary regimes and sometimes by dietary supplementation, e.g. arginine supplements are useful in arginosuccinate synthetase deficiency. Some of the mitochondrial cytopathies have responded to dietary supplementation of the electron transport chain with coenzyme Q. In abetalipoproteinaemia the neurological abnormalities appear to be secondary to impaired absorption of vitamin E, due to absence of short chain fatty acids; improvement follows dietary supplementation with large doses of vitamin E. Cerebro-tendinous xanthomatosis is associated with deposition of cholestanol in the tissues and improvement occurs when cholestanol is mobilized and broken down by chenodeoxycholic acid, which can be given orally. The disorders of DNA repair are associated with cerebellar ataxia, but this is a relatively unimportant feature in relation to the other clinical manifestations, for example, in xeroderma pigmentosum there is

Table 12.2 *Hereditary ataxias with metabolic cause.*

Intermittent ataxic syndromes
  with hyperammonaemia,
    e.g. ornithine transcarbamylase deficiency
  aminoacidurias (without hyperammonaemia),
    e.g. Hartnup's disease
  disorders of pyruvate and lactate metabolism,
    e.g. mitochondrial cytopathy
Progressive ataxic syndromes
  abetalipoproteinaemia (Bassen–Kornzweig disease)
  hexosaminidase deficiency
  cerebrotendinous xanthomatosis (cholestanolosis)
  neuronal storage disorders
    e.g. sphingomyelin storage disease
      ceroid lipofuscinosis (Batten's disease)
  disorders of DNA repair,
    e.g. xeroderma pigmentosum
      ataxia telangiectasia

dermal sensitivity to sunlight with recurrent cutaneous cancers, and CNS tumours may also develop. In the neuronal storage disorders cerebellar ataxia is a minor feature.

Hereditary ataxias of unknown cause

These disorders are conveniently grouped into early onset and late onset types; the clinical manifestations of these two types differ strikingly. In addition, the late onset types are all dominantly inherited, and the early onset types are autosomal recessive traits, e.g. Friedreich's ataxia (Table 12.3).

Friedreich's ataxia (Table 12.3)

This is the commonest form of hereditary ataxia. It begins before the age of 20 years, at a mean age of 10 years. The prevalence is 1/50 000. The disorder is inherited as an autosomal recessive disease; the genetic locus is on the short arm of chromosome 9. It begins with unsteadiness of gait, dysarthria, spasticity and weakness of the legs, with impaired joint position sense in the feet leading to difficulty walking in the dark (with a positive Romberg sign). The ankle jerks are absent, there is pes cavus and the plantar responses are extensor. Nystagmus is present in half the cases and most have reduced visual acuity due to pigmentary retinal degeneration with primary optic atrophy. Scoliosis is almost invariable and most patients have a cardiomyopathy. The latter may lead to cardiac failure, arrhythmia and death. Deafness occurs in some patients and distal muscular atrophy, probably resulting from the peripheral neuropathy, is frequent. Diabetes mellitus occurs in about 10% of cases. Ophthalmoplegia and pupillary abnormalities may also develop and some patients become mildly demented in the late stages. Incontinence may develop.

The CSF shows a raised protein level and nerve conduction studies show slightly slowed motor and sensory nerve conduction velocities,

Table 12.3 *Hereditary ataxias of unknown cause.*

Early onset ataxias
  Friedreich's ataxia
  ataxias with other associated features,
    e.g. deafness, myoclonus, mental retardation
Late onset ataxias
  olivopontocerebellar atrophy syndromes
  cerebellar ataxia without other features (Holmes type)
  with deafness, or with essential tremor

consistent with axonal degeneration. However, evoked potential studies show marked abnormalities. Brain stem evoked potentials are usually absent, visual evoked responses are greatly delayed and dispersed, or absent, and somatosensory responses are delayed. These studies reflect the abnormalities in the auditory, visual and somatosensory afferent pathways. The ECG shows T wave inversion and the heart is enlarged, with septal hypertrophy on echocardiography. CT brain scans are usually normal but some atrophy of the cerebral hemispheres and of the vermis may be seen.

Management. No treatment is available for this condition. Symptomatic management of immobility, heart failure, diabetes and incontinence are important in relieving suffering. A wheelchair is necessary from a relatively early age and scoliosis and pes cavus can be alleviated by appropriate physiotherapy, postural advice and surgical treatment. Genetic counselling is important. Death occurs within about 20 years from the onset.

Ataxias with other associated features (Table 12.3)

There have been many reports of families with hereditary ataxias accompanied by certain associated features, relatively specific to the family reported. These include hypogonadism, deafness, myoclonus, dystonia, mental retardation or dementia. These disorders differ from Friedreich's ataxia in their clinical features, which lack the constant association of retinal, cerebellar, corticospinal, posterior column and peripheral nerve manifestations, together with pes cavus, scoliosis and cardiomyopathy, that is so constant in Friedreich's ataxia. The prognosis in these disorders, despite the early onset, tends to be better than in Friedreich's ataxia.

Pathology. In Freidreich's ataxia there is loss of Purkinje cells, with degeneration of the posterior columns, corticospinal tracts and posterior spinocerebellar tracts in the spinal cord; the cells of Clarke's nucleus, and of the gracile and cuneate nuclei degenerate. Reactive gliosis is prominent in the degenerating spinal pathways. Cells in the posterior root ganglia degenerate and there may be loss of anterior horn cells. There is loss of large and intermediate sized myelinated axons in peripheral nerves, especially in distal parts of long nerves, such as the sural nerve. The heart shows fibrosis, fatty degeneration and loss of myocardial cells. The optic nerve shows gliosis and loss of fibres and there is degeneration of cochlear and vestibular neurons in the brain stem.

The pathological features of the early onset hereditary ataxias are less well defined, but may involve loss of Purkinje cells, cerebellar atrophy and olivo-dentate atrophy.

Olivopontocerebellar atrophy syndromes (Table 12.3)

This syndrome is defined by its pathological features but the designation *olivopontocerebellar atrophy* (OPCA) has come to be applied to a clinical syndrome characterized by cerebellar ataxia, extrapyramidal features and features of involvement of corticospinal tracts, and of the peripheral and autonomic nervous systems. These clinical features are variable and are not associated with uniform pathological features so that the clinical syndrome of OPCA is not equivalent to any pathological definition of this term. Nonetheless the diagnosis is in common clinical use.

OPCA is a progressive syndrome beginning in middle age. When genetic transmission is evident in the family history autosomal dominant inheritance is usual but autosomal recessive forms have been recognized. The disorder begins with a gait disturbance; this is either bradykinetic with rigidity, i.e. an extrapyramidal gait disorder; or unsteady, i.e. cerebellar in type. Speech is dysarthric and cerebellar tremor of the upper limbs is usually present, but nystagmus is not a feature. The ankle jerks are often absent. Later, dementia, spasticity and extensor plantar responses become prominent and a supranuclear ophthalmoplegia may develop. Parkinsonian tremor is found in some cases. Autonomic dysfunction is also a frequent late feature, including urinary incontinence and constipation, postural hypotension, impotence and anhydrosis.

Investigation. CT scans and MR images show atrophy of the pons, medulla and cerebellum. There is no specific biochemical defect, since the clinical syndrome of OPCA is heterogeneous but some cases show glutamate dehydrogenase deficiency in fibroblasts, platelets or leucocytes. Excess amounts of glutamate, an excitatory transmitter, may accumulate in toxic concentrations in the CNS causing the progressive deterioration.

Multiple system atrophy

This consists of progressive autonomic failure (Table 12.4), with other features suggesting involvement of other systems, particularly olivopontocerebellar atrophy (OPCA) and striatonigral degeneration. The latter disorder consists of an akinetic and rigid form of Parkinson's syndrome, without other parkinsonian features such as tremor, and without cerebellar degeneration, as found in OPCA. The term Shy–Drager syndrome is often used to describe the syndrome of primary orthostatic hypotension with other features of autonomic failure, and with cerebellar and extrapyramidal abnormalities. In addition muscular atrophy and fasciculation are present.

Table 12.4 *Autonomic disorders.*

CNS diseases
  progressive autonomic failure
  progressive autonomic failure with parkinsonism
  progressive autonomic failure with multiple system atrophy:
  (Shy–Drager syndrome)
  Parkinson's disease
  Holmes–Adie syndrome

Peripheral nervous system disease (see Chapter 13)
  acute and subacute autonomic neuropathy
  autonomic dysfunction associated with peripheral neuropathy
  e.g. diabetic neuropathy, Guillain–Barré syndrome

This syndrome is now more usually called multiple system atrophy, since this term allows variability of clinical expression in the different phases of the disease, and between OPCA and striato-nigral degeneration with autonomic failure (Table 12.4). In Parkinson's disease (Chapter 11), autonomic failure may be a late complication.

Progressive autonomic failure

This is a disorder, occurring in isolation or as part of a more complex multiple system atrophy, in which there is degeneration of the central and, to a lesser extent, of the peripheral parts of the autonomic nervous system.

The autonomic nervous system consists of sympathetic and parasympathetic components which, although mutually antagonistic, function in concert in the control of visceral, skin, cardiovascular, sphincteric and sexual functions. The central pathways descend from the hypothalamus. Sympathetic fibres synapse with cells of the intermediolateral column in the spinal grey matter from T1 to L2 levels. Parasympathetic fibres arise in the craniosacral nuclei, i.e. in third, seventh, ninth and tenth cranial nerves, and in sacral S2–4 roots, and synapse in ganglia located in the periphery close to their target organs, e.g. salivary ganglia, ciliary ganglia, enteric plexus and ganglia, and vesical ganglia. This parasympathetic outflow is subject to central hypothalamic modulation. The hypothalamus itself has central connections with orbito-frontal and cingulate cortex, and with reticular neurons, related to higher functions such as emotional and sexual responses. Preganglionic sympathetic fibres are cholinergic and post-ganglionic sympathetic fibres, except sudomotor fibres and some vasodilator fibres in muscle, are noradrenergic. The parasympathetic system is entirely cholinergic. The myenteric plexus of the gut is neither catecholaminergic nor cholinergic but uses purinergic, glutamatergic, and complex molecules such as vasoactive intestinal peptide (VIP), bombesin and somatostatin for neurotransmission and neuromodulation. The enteric nervous system is thus largely independent of other parts of the autonomic nervous system.

In progressive autonomic failure there is degeneration of all parts of the autonomic nervous system. In the early stages the peripheral components of the sympathetic nervous system are particularly involved, leading to orthostatic (postural) hypotension, absence of heart rate responses to changes in posture and cardiac output, and impairment of sweating responses. Horner's syndrome is often present. Involvement of other components of the autonomic nervous system leads to urinary and faecal incontinence, intractable constipation with megacolon, and impotence with failure of erection and ejaculation. Hoarseness of the voice from denervation of the abductor muscle of the larynx also occurs in this syndrome, often in temporal relation to degeneration of sacral motoneurons controlling bladder sphincters, and with urinary incontinence. Sleep apnoea, from damage to the CO_2 responsiveness of the brain stem centres, is a potentially fatal feature. The other features of multiple system atrophy depend on involvement of other, non-autonomic pathways in the CNS.

Clinical tests of autonomic function. The principal non-invasive tests used in the clinical assessment of progressive autonomic failure, or of other disorders of autonomic function, depend on cardiovascular abnormalities. These tests define the clinical abnormality but do not localize the site of the autonomic defect. Sweating tests, and quantitative tests of pupil responsiveness (pupillometry) are also useful, and video cystometrograms provide a useful assessment of both sympathetic and parasympathetic function. There are five main tests of cardiovascular function (Table 12.5).

The heart rate responses to breathing and changes in posture reflect vagal parasympathetic function. Changes in blood pressure on standing and with isometric exercise and sweat tests are largely related to sympathetic afferent and efferent function. Plasma noradrenaline levels also evaluate sympathetic function. Other invasive tests, for example the baroreceptor response to an infusion of pressor drugs such as phenylephrine or angiotensin, can be used for research purposes in the assessment of afferent sympathetic function.

Management: Orthostatic hypotension is the major life-threatening problem, since it may be severe enough to cause syncope with cerebral ischaemia and infarction. A tight-fitting elastic garment around the abdomen and elastic stockings are often useful in preventing postural hypotension. The patient should sleep with the head of the bed raised 20°, a posture that maintains blood volume.

Table 12.5 *Tests of autonomic function.*

1. Cardiovascular responses
   (a) Blood pressure response to standing (from lying)
       —a fall > 30/15 mm Hg (systolic/diastolic) is abnormal
   (b) Heart rate response to standing (from lying)
       —R : R response at 30th beat, and 15th beat (30 : 15 ratio)
       < 1.04 is abnormal
   (c) Heart rate variation during deep breathing
       —maximum : minimum heart rate < 10 beats/minute is abnormal
   (d) Blood pressure response to sustained handgrip (isometric exercise)
       —30% maximum grip for 5 minutes; increase in diastolic BP
       < 10 mm Hg is abnormal
   (e) Heart rate response to Valsalva manoeuvre
       —expiratory pressure > 40 mm Hg for 15 seconds (using sphygmo-
       manometer : longest : shortest R : R interval ratio < 1.1 is abnormal
2. Sweating responses to body heating
3. Pupillary responses: to light
                        to methacholine drops
                        parasympathetic lesion: pupillary constriction
                        to hydroxyamphetamine
                        sympathetic lesion: lack of pupillary dilatation
4. Bladder responses by cystometrography
5. Gut motility and transit studies

The most effective drug therapy is fludrocortisone (9αfluorohydro-
cortisone). This promotes an increase in blood volume by its salt
retaining properies, induces noradrenaline release from post ganglionic
sympathetic nerve endings and sensitizes vascular receptors to
circulating pressor amines. Treatment with 0.1–1.0 mg daily is
necessary. Indomethacin, clonidine, ephedrine and dihydroergot-
amine may also be useful. Incontinence can be managed only by
catheterization, although bethanechol can be tried. Catheterization
should be used as an intermittent twice daily procedure to prevent
infection and calculus formation. Failure of penile erection can be
managed, if indicated, by penile implantation with a rigid or inflatable
device, but injection of 5 mg phenoxybenzamine, or 40 mg papaverine
into the cavernous part of the penis will cause erection for up to
4 hours. Retrograde ejaculation can be treated by desipramine, which
promotes contraction of the α-adrenergically innervated bladder neck.
This condition is usually fatal within several years of the onset from
a combination of respiratory, cardiovascular and thermoregulatory
problems, despite optimal treatment.

Holmes–Adie syndrome

There are two major components to this benign syndrome. The Adie
pupil is characterized by absent or delayed pupillary constriction

to light or to accommodation. Once constricted the pupil dilates only slowly, whether in response to darkness or to far gaze. The pupil may thus appear small or large initially and this may lead to confusion with Horner's syndrome, or with the Argyll Robertson pupil of neurosyphilis. The Adie pupil is frequently unilateral, causing unequal pupils (anisocoria). It is often suddenly noticed, usually in the second or third decade of life, and may cause some blurring of vision on near gaze from loss of the accommodation response. It is due to parasympathetic denervation from a lesion in the ciliary ganglion of unknown cause. Gordon Holmes noted the association of unilateral or bilateral areflexia with the Adie pupil. The site of the lesion responsible for areflexia is not known, but is probably at the synapse of afferents from muscle spindles with the anterior horn cells, since the reflexes may return if a corticospinal lesion, for example due to stroke, develops coincidentally. In some patients with Holmes–Adie syndrome autonomic dysfunction with sweating disorder and postural hypotension develop.

Horner's syndrome

This syndrome (Fig. 1.2), consisting of narrowing of the palpebral fissure, constriction of the pupil, absence of sweating on the corresponding forehead, side of face and neck, absence of the ciliospinal reflex (dilatation of the pupil on pinching the skin of the ipsilateral side of the neck, and absence of dilatation of the pupil on shading the eye) is due to a lesion of the cervical sympathetic, or of the sympathetic pathways in the cervical spinal cord, brain stem or hypothalamus. The syndrome may also occur with lesions in the sympathetic fibres in the wall of the carotid artery *en route* to the eye. The commonest site for the lesion, however, is at the level of the first rib close to the vertebral column where lymphatic enlargement, trauma, infection and neoplastic invasion, e.g. from Pancoast tumour of the lung, selectively damage the sympathetic outflow or the stellate ganglion.

Hereditary spastic paraplegia

This is a rare disorder characterized by slowly increasing spasticity and weakness in the legs. Pure and complicated forms have been described. In the latter involvement of other systems may include optic atrophy, extrapyramidal features, dementia, mild amyotrophy and cerebellar ataxia. In pure hereditary spastic paraplegia spasticity is far more prominent than weakness, the disorder presents before the age of 35 years with dominant inheritance, and there may be a history of developmental delay in achieving motor milestones.

A rare recessive form with distal sensory loss and urinary incontinence is recognized, of later onset but more rapid progression.

Pathologically there is degeneration of corticospinal tracts in the spinal cord below the level of the decussation of the pyramids, with some degeneration of posterior columns. Life expectancy is normal. Treatment is symptomatic. Antispasticity drugs such as baclofen and dantrolene may provide useful relief of spasticity without increase in weakness if the dose is carefully titrated.

Anterior horn cell disorders

Diseases affecting anterior horn cells may present at any age. In children the disorder is usually limited to anterior horn cells but in adults involvement of the upper motor neuron is common. The former are usually autosomal recessive disorders, termed spinal muscular atrophies (although bulbar muscles are often affected), and the latter are usually sporadic disorders of unknown origin, termed motor neuron disease (Table 12.6).

Table 12.6 *Anterior horn cell disorders*

Spinal muscular atrophies (SMA)
Type I (Werdnig–Hoffmann disease)
Type II (intermediate SMA)
Type III (Kugelberg–Welander disease)
Type IV (adult-onset SMA)
other clinical syndromes of SMA
Motor neuron disease

Spinal muscular atrophies (SMA). These disorders are classified (Table 12.6) according to age of onset, clinical features and pattern of inheritance; the underlying biochemical disturbances leading to these disorders are unknown. They usually present with proximal weakness but rare varieties of SMA may present with distal, asymmetrical, scapulo-peroneal or bulbospinal weakness. Within individual families there is a high degree of consistency in the clinical syndrome. Autosomal recessive inheritance is invariable in all except a few rare clinical syndromes.

In this group of disorders there is degeneration of anterior horn cells, and of the lower motor neuron, including motor end-plates and muscles. There is no involvement of any other neuronal system of the brain, and sensory pathways are intact. The upper motor neuron is not affected.

Type I SMA: Werdnig–Hoffmann disease is a fatal disorder, death occurring in most cases before the age of 18 months. It occurs in 1 : 25 000 live births. In about a third of cases the disease begins *in utero*, with feeble fetal movements. All are affected by the age of 5 months.

The child is usually hypotonic with weak limb and trunk movements. Head control is poor and the child cannot roll over or sit unsupported. Swallowing and sucking movements are weak, and respirations are shallow. External ocular movements are normal. Facial involvement and fasciculation of the tongue develop, but fasciculation of other muscles may be difficult to recognize. On palpation the limb muscles are atrophic. Joint deformities are uncommon. Death occurs from respiratory failure and pneumonia.

Type II SMA: The intermediate form of SMA presents after the age of 6 months, usually before the first birthday, with delayed motor milestones. The child is able to sit but independent standing and walking are not achieved normally. The disease may sometimes begin relatively suddenly. Weakness is generalized with a proximal emphasis, but bulbar and external ocular muscles are spared. There is often only slow deterioration and 30% of affected children can still walk, but only with assistance, at the age of 10 years. Fasciculation of atrophic muscles is usually evident. Weakness of truncal and axial muscles is usually severe, leading to the development of scoliosis that can be partially prevented by appropriate management. Type II SMA is less common than Types I and III SMA.

Type III SMA (Kugelberg–Welander disease): Kugelberg–Welander disease presents between the ages of 2 and 15 years. The first symptoms are due to weakness of proximal muscles of the legs, leading to difficulty climbing stairs, and getting up from low chairs or the floor. The gait is waddling, due to pelvic girdle muscle weakness. Hypertrophy of the calves develops in a quarter of cases. Weakness of the arms, pectoral girdle and periscapular muscles develops later. Affected muscles are wasted but fasciculations are rarely clinically evident. External ocular muscles are spared and bulbar muscles are less severely affected. The tendon reflexes are diminished or absent. Joint contractures and scoliosis are uncommon.

The clinical presentation of Type III SMA resembles that of limb girdle muscular dystrophy, and many cases have been mistakenly classified. Since the prognosis of Type III SMA is relatively benign, with a relatively normal life expectancy despite disability of increasing severity in the third to sixth decades, full investigation, including electromyography (EMG) and muscle biopsy is important.

Type IV SMA: The adult-onset form of SMA is benign, but rare. Unlike the other forms, dominant inheritance has been noted in about a third of cases.

Other forms of SMA: These are classified according to the distribution of muscular weakness and wasting. They include an

X-linked recessive bulbo-spinal form in which gynaecomastia and dysphagia develop, distal SMA, asymmetrical SMA, and scapulo-peroneal SMA with severe weakness of periscapular and anterior tibial muscles.

Investigations and management: The creatine kinase is moderately increased in chronic, slowly progressive forms of SMA, especially Type III SMA, reflecting the development of work-induced hypertrophy and secondary myopathic change from wear and tear effects in weakened muscles. The EMG shows features of a neurogenic disorder, especially fibrillation potentials, fasciculations and complex motor unit action potentials of increased amplitude and duration, indicating a combination of denervation and compensatory reinnervation of motor units. Motor and sensory nerve conduction velocity studies are normal. The muscle biopsy shows features of denervation (Fig. 12.1), reinnervation with fibre type grouping, fibre hypertrophy and some foci of fibre degeneration and regeneration (secondary myopathic change). The CSF is normal.

No specific therapy is available. The most important factor is prevention of scoliosis in the Type II and Type III forms of SMA, since long survival is possible and scoliosis can be a severe deformity, even compromising respiration when there is weakness of respiratory muscles. Splinting of weakened joints may help when weakness is very severe but, in most cases, regular exercise and physiotherapy

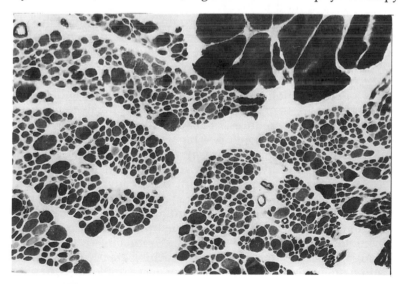

Fig. 12.1 Spinal muscular atrophy (Type 2 of infancy). There is marked atrophy of fascicles of muscle fibres. These fibres are rounded and of variable staining reaction in this adenosine triphosphatase (ATPase) preparation. In one fascicle the muscle fibres are of normal size.

to maintain muscle tone and fitness, even in weakened muscles, is crucial in maintaining independence. A period of bedrest may lead to marked weakness. Calipers may be helpful in Type II SMA.

Motor neuron disease. This progressive disorder of the motor system is a disease of late middle life. Age-specific incidence increases with increasing age until the eighth decade. It is uncommon before the age of 40 years. The male/female ratio is 1.5 to 1.0, and about 10% of cases are familial. It acounts for 1 in every 1000 adult deaths.

The first symptom is weakness or undue fatiguability. Weakness is frequently focal, presenting as a foot drop, or with weakness of a hand, but some cases present with paraparesis or with bulbar symptoms, especially dysphagia and dysarthria. As in the other anterior horn cell disorders atrophy accompanies weakness. The external ocular muscles and sphincter muscles are characteristically spared. Fasciculations, consisting of random contractions of groups of muscle fibres producing a twitch-like contraction of part of a muscle, visible through the skin and most easily seen in the tongue, are a common and almost pathognomonic feature of the disease. They are found in a widespread distribution unrelated to fatigue or recent muscular activity. Benign fasciculations, not indicative of neurogenic disease, are particularly related to exertion, occur at a faster rate, and tend to involve the same part of a muscle.

Muscle cramps and stiffness are common early features that, like fasciculations, may precede weakness and atrophy. Sooner or later, despite the focal onset, the disease becomes generalized. At this stage the characteristic combination of upper and lower motor neuron signs is found. Atrophy, weakness and fasciculation are found in combination with hyperreflexia, spasticity and extensor plantar responses. In other diseases causing wasting the tendon jerks are almost invariably reduced or absent. This combination, together with fasciculation of the tongue, is highly characteristic of the disease and has led to the term *amyotrophic lateral sclerosis* to describe the combination of atrophy and corticospinal abnormalities. *Progressive bulbar palsy* consists of predominant bulbar involvement, and in *primary lateral sclerosis* the disability is limited to corticospinal tract involvement. Both these latter syndromes are rare in isolation but represent clinical variants of motor neuron disease.

In motor neuron disease sensory abnormalities do not occur, although patients often complain of aching pain, presumably of postural origin, and paraesthesiae from nerve or plexus entrapment are not infrequent. Incontinence does not occur. Dementia is very rare and should lead to suspicion of other diseases, especially Creutzfeldt–Jakob disease, in which progressive dementia with myoclonus and fasciculation may occur.

Prognosis: Motor neuron disease is a progressive disorder. Disability develops relatively rapidly and depends on the relative distribution of neurological abnormality. Patients with bulbar symptoms become disabled from dysarthria and dysphagia, with cachexia and pneumonia, relatively quickly. In most patients severe weakness of limb and trunk muscles develops, inexorably leading to dependence on others for tasks of daily living, and life expectancy is then short. The mean survival from diagnosis is about 3 years, only 20% of cases surviving longer than 5 years, and 10% more than 10 years. Familial cases have a similar prognosis.

Diagnosis: The EMG shows similar neurogenic changes to those found in spinal muscular atrophy. Some muscles are more affected than others, and giant motor units are recorded in very atrophic muscles, indicating prominent reinnervation in surviving motor units. The CSF protein is slightly raised or may be normal. The CK level is slightly raised or normal. There is no systemic abnormality, and no clue to the cause of the disease is revealed by investigation. CT scans of the brain, myelography and muscle biopsy are often used to exclude other possible diagnoses such as spinal cord compression.

Differential diagnosis: The main problems are lumbocervical spondylosis with cord compression and multiple root lesions, in which the combination of upper and lower motor neuron lesions, so characteristic of motor neuron disease, may occur. Hyperthyroidism may also cause fasciculation and proximal muscle weakness. Motor neuropathies can be recognized by absence of distal reflexes, by the relative absence of fasciculation, and by the more symmetrical weakness and atrophy. EMG and CSF examination may be helpful in these cases.

Management: No specific therapy is available. Fatigue, when prominent, may be helped by anticholinesterase drugs such as neostigmine or pyridostigmine. Spasticity is rarely severe enough to warrant treatment with drugs such as baclofen or dantrolene. Cramp is often troublesome and responds to quinine sulphate in some cases. Dysphagia may be improved by cricopharyngeal myotomy. Physiotherapy has little place. Arrangements for terminal care at home or in a hospice are important and home care with daily visits from a nurse is often a great relief to both patient and family. A wheelchair will be required. Artificial ventilation is rarely used since the prognosis is hopeless.

Causation: The 10% incidence of familial cases suggests the possibility of a genetic background but this factor is not yet understood. Many extraneous factors have been considered, including latent poliovirus infection, other virus infection, heavy metal intoxication, autoimmune destruction of the motor system, dietary deficiencies and toxins derived from the natural environment, e.g. cycad nuts, or from industrial waste. Although these factors may lead to damage to anterior horn cells they do not cause classical motor neuron disease.

Patients infected with poliomyelitis in youth may develop progressive weakness in the weakened muscles many decades later. This post poliomyelitis syndrome represents additional weakness developing in weakened muscles from a combination of age-induced anterior horn cell loss and secondary myopathic change in the weakened muscles. There is no increased incidence of motor neuron disease in survivors of poliomyelitis.

An association of motor neuron disease and plasma cell dyscrasia with monoclonal gammopathy has been noted in about 5% of patients with the disease. In a few of these plasma exchange has resulted in some temporary improvement. Three foci of higher incidence of motor neuron disease are known. These are in Guam, the Kii peninsula of Japan and western New Guinea. In the latter country motor neuron disease syndromes are 100 times as common as in Western countries. However, the disease differs clinically and pathologically by its association with parkinsonism and dementia and by the occurrence of neurofibrillary tangles in damaged neurons. These foci therefore seem to represent a different form of anterior horn cell disease.

13

Peripheral Neuropathies and Plexus Syndromes

Diseases of the peripheral nervous system may affect the peripheral nerves at any site from the nerve roots, through the nerve plexus close to the spine, to the peripheral nerves themselves as they extend through the body and limbs to innervate skin, muscle and internal organs. Thus motor, sensory and autonomic components of the peripheral nervous system may be involved.

In *mononeuropathies* individual nerves are affected. This is usually due to compression or entrapment as the nerve traverses a narrow space between bones or ligaments, to trauma or to infarction. Rarely tumours arising in peripheral nerves, e.g. Schwannomas, may cause a mononeuropathy. *Peripheral neuropathies* consist of symmetrical motor, sensory and autonomic disturbances, usually commencing distally, due to disease of peripheral nerve axons or of the Schwann cells that myelinate the peripheral nervous system. *Plexus* lesions cause problems in a distribution involving root and peripheral nerve patterns.

Clinical features of mononeuropathies and polyneuropathies

The clinical features of mononeuropathies depend on the nerve involved, consisting of weakness, sensory features or a mixture of these two groups of symptoms and signs. Pain may be a feature in acute mononeuropathies. Polyneuropathies are usually slowly progressive. Distal sensory disturbances, consisting of diminished sensory acuity or numbness are characteristic and these may be associated with tingling, pins and needles sensations (paraesthesiae) or spontaneous painful sensations (dysaesthesiae). Sometimes the affected skin feels painful to touch (hyperpathia). Motor problems may also occur, particularly distal weakness and atrophy with an abnormal 'high-stepping' gait as a compensatory mechanism for foot drop. The features of lower motor neuron lesion, with areflexia, are

Table 13.1 *Causes of mononeuropathies.*

Entrapment:	constriction of a nerve by fibrous bands, or in a fibro-osseous tunnel, e.g. carpal tunnel syndrome
Compression:	sustained pressure on a nerve, e.g. Saturday night radial palsy
Nerve injury:	blunt or sharp trauma
Stretch of nerves:	usually associated with trauma; may be a factor in entrapment or occupational palsies
Infarction:	may affect multiple nerves, e.g. polyarteritis nodosa
Predisposition to mononeuropathies:	susceptibility to compression or entrapment, e.g. diabetes mellitus
Tumours of nerves:	Schwannomas in neurofibromatosis, and malignant invasion from lymph nodes
Infections:	leprosy, Herpes zoster

thus present. Polyneuropathies are typically always symmetrical. Autonomic disturbances are usually localized to the affected distal portion of the limbs but, in the autonomic neuropathies themselves, pronounced and disabling symptoms result from autonomic denervation involving the cardiovascular, gastro-intestinal and urogenital systems.

Mononeuropathy syndromes

Mononeuropathies have several different causes and these tend to affect some nerves more than others (Table 13.1). Entrapment, compressive and stretch-induced neuropathies result from disruption of myelin lamellae at a site of predilection, leading to motor and sensory deficits distal to the nerve lesion. There may be local and referred pain and discomfort. Tapping the nerve at the site of damage elicits 'electric' dysaesthesiae in the sensory distribution of the nerve (Tinel's sign). These neuropathies recover relatively quickly when the cause is removed, provided that irreparable deformity of the nerve and axon loss have not occurred. These are the most common forms of mononeuropathy.

Carpal tunnel syndrome

This is the commonest of the entrapment neuropathies. The median nerve is compressed and trapped beneath the flexor retinaculum at the wrist because the fibro-osseous tunnel is constricted by ligamentous thickening, or by the effects of an old wrist fracture. Women are affected three times more commonly than men, and the syndrome characteristically occurs during pregnancy and at the menopause. In 40% of cases the syndrome is bilateral but the dominant hand is nearly always more severely affected.

The most prominent symptoms are numbness in the median innervated skin of the hand, with pain in the wrist and flexor aspect of the forearm. These sensory symptoms are especially prominent at night, on waking in the morning and after repetitive movements of digits and wrist as in sewing, knitting, typing etc. In some patients pain may extend more proximally. Difficulty recognizing objects or manipulating coins between thumb and forefinger may be noted. Weakness of the thumb is a less common complaint, but may become evident doing buttons and tying shoelaces, or in unscrewing bottle caps.

Examination reveals impaired sensation on the palmar surface of the hand on its radial side, extending into the thumb, index and middle fingers, and involving half of the fourth finger, but sparing the little finger. The sensory disturbance extends proximally to the wrist crease, or a few centimetres onto the forearm but it does not involve the dorsal surface of the hand, apart from the skin of the distal parts of the radial fingers, near the nail beds. This sensory distribution is of major importance in diagnosis; in C6 root lesions the sensory disturbance involves dorsal and palmar aspects of the hand and extends onto the forearm as far as the elbow. In early cases of carpal tunnel syndrome sensory abnormalities may be subtle, perhaps only recognizable as impairment of two point discrimination on the pulps of the thumb, index and middle digits, or may be absent altogether. Subtle wasting of the abductor pollicis brevis muscle, with weakness of this muscle is often found and there is also weakness of opponens pollicis and of the lumbricals of the index and middle digits. These latter features are not easy to recognize. Sometimes Tinel's sign may be positive on tapping the flexor surface of the wrist, or forced flexion of the wrist may reproduce the sensory symptoms (Phalen's sign). Wrist deformity may be evident when there has been previous trauma. There are usually no other features of peripheral nerve disease but in some patients an underlying mild polyneuropathy may be present which has led to undue susceptibility to the nerve entrapment, perhaps only manifest by absent ankle jerks.

Management. In mild cases a wrist splint, with the wrist in a neutral or slightly extended posture, worn at night, prevents nocturnal symptoms. This treatment is useful in pregnancy but is less effective in other cases. An injection of hydrocortisone into the carpal tunnel is often used and this produces temporary benefit. Patients with sensory signs or weakness of the abductor pollicis brevis are best managed by surgical decompression of the nerve at the wrist. Recovery from sensory symptoms is relatively rapid, but weakness recovers more slowly. In bilateral cases the more severely affected side should be treated first.

Ulnar nerve palsy

The ulnar nerve is vulnerable to compressive or traumatic injury in the olecranon groove at the elbow. This produces tingling paraesthesiae on the medial border of the hand in the little and ring fingers, both on the palmar and dorsal aspects, extending just above the wrist. In severe cases weakness and atrophy of the hypothenar muscles and of all the interossei develops. This may lead to a characteristic deformity involving the ring and little fingers with flexion of the interphalangeal joints and extension of the metacarpophalangeal joints.

Management. Rest and prevention of injury to the elbow by avoiding leaning the point of the elbow on hard or upholstered surfaces is important. Surgical exploration and transposition of the nerve is useful if there is severe arthropathy at the elbow, but although this may prevent progression it is not often followed by improvement.

Radial nerve palsy

The radial nerve is vulnerable as it winds round the medial surface of the humerus in the spiral groove. This lesion typically occurs during sleep when the arm hangs over a chair (Saturday night palsy). There is weakness or dorsiflexion of the wrist and fingers, producing wrist and finger drop, with only a small area of sensory loss in the web between the thumb and index finger. Tinel's sign is positive at the humerus in the spiral groove. Recovery occurs spontaneously in a few days or weeks.

The *posterior interosseous branch* of the radial nerve arises at the elbow, innervating the extensors of the thumb and fingers, but not the wrist extensor. This nerve has no sensory innervation. The nerve is usually injured from compression by lipoma, or in a fibro-osseous tunnel through the extensor compartment of the forearm and surgical exploration can be effective in promoting recovery.

Common peroneal nerve

This nerve winds round the neck of the fibula, where it can be palpated, to enter the fibular tunnel. It may be injured by recurrent compression, e.g. due to a posture of sitting with the legs crossed, or against a mattress or the side of a bed. There is foot drop (Fig. 13.1), with weakness of tibialis anterior, peroneal muscles and extensor hallucis longus, and there is sensory loss on the lateral

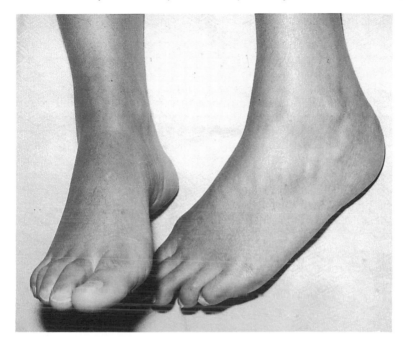

Fig. 13.1 Left foot drop. The left foot is unable to dorsiflex or evert, and so takes up an inverted position on the bed; the characteristic posture of common peroneal palsy.

aspect of the lower leg and foot resembling that of an L5 root lesion. However, inversion at the ankle is normal, the ankle jerk is present, and Tinel's sign may be positive at the head of the fibula. Recovery occurs spontaneously if recurrent injury is prevented. An ankle splint can be useful in alleviating the foot drop. The lesion can be prevented by careful attention to preventing compression of the nerve during extended periods of bed rest.

Meralgia paresthetica

This common syndrome is due to compression of the lateral femoral cutaneous nerve of the thigh beneath the inguinal ligament. It is common in obese persons. There is an oval zone of dysaesthetic sensory impairment on the lateral aspect of the thigh. The nerve has no motor component.

Management. In most cases the symptom resolves. Weight loss is important. The nerve can be decompressed at the inguinal ligament, or sectioned at this site. Local steroid injection may also be of value.

Sciatic nerve syndromes

The sciatic nerve may be damaged by direct trauma, hip surgery, fracture-dislocation of the hip and by accidental iatrogenic injections misplaced into the nerve in the buttock. It may be compressed by a Baker's synovial cyst in the popliteal fossa, and sciatic nerve injuries may also follow traumatic forceps delivery. The common peroneal component is usually more severely affected than the tibial component. There is weakness of hamstrings, and of all the muscles below the knee, with extensive sensory loss below the knee and on the skin of the back of the thigh. The ankle jerk is usually absent.

Management. Treatment is nearly always conservative, but exploration may be indicated when the nerve is compressed in the popliteal fossa, or in traumatic injuries in assocation with fractures of the hip and pelvis.

Tarsal tunnel syndrome

There is intermittent burning pain and numbness of the palmar surface of the foot, aggravated by standing and walking, including the heel.

Femoral nerve

This nerve is rarely vulnerable to injury, but is involved in some patients with diabetic neuropathy.

Cranial mononeuropathies

The facial, oculomotor and abducens nerves are relatively frequently damaged in isolation but mononeuropathies of other cranial nerves are rare.

Bell's palsy (facial nerve)

There is sudden paralysis of one side of the face, due to a lower motor neuron lesion, affecting the nerve in the stylomastoid canal. The weakness is accompanied by pain in the mastoid region, and develops over a period of a few hours. It is often preceded by upper respiratory tract infection a week or so previously. Taste on the anterior two-thirds of the tongue may be lost and hyperacusis from weakness of the stapedius may be a feature in more proximal lesions. The whole side of the face, including eyelid, forehead and perioral muscles, is affected. There is rarely sensory loss but a small area in the tragus of the ear may be hypoesthetic. Rarely the disorder is bilateral or recurrent.

Herpes zoster infection can cause facial paralysis associated with herpetic vesicles in the external auditory canal. There is a higher incidence of Bell's palsy in diabetics, and facial palsy may be a feature of sarcoidosis, and of Guillain–Barré syndrome.

Management. Spontaneous recovery is complete in more than half the cases, especially in young people. Recovery continues for up to 6 months after onset. In the first few days after the onset of the palsy, treatment with prednisolone 40–60 mg daily for 5 days is often recommended in the hope that it might improve the prognosis in severe cases. Fewer than 5% of patients are so disabled that surgical reconstruction of the paralysed face is indicated. The prognosis of H. zoster infection is poor, and steroids are contraindicated.

During recovery there may be aberrant regeneration within the branches of the nerve, leading to co-contraction of the eyelid and mouth on movement either of the eyelid or mouth, and even to cosmetically distressing spasm of the face. This develops gradually during 3–12 months after the onset. Lateral tarsorrhaphy may be necessary to narrow the palpebral fissure and protect the cornea from abrasion. Protective spectacles are also useful.

Hemifacial spasm

This is a rare disorder, in which writhing, involuntary, tonic and clonic activity occurs in the facial muscle of one side of the face. It is thought to be due to vascular compression of the nerve in the posterior fossa at its exit from the brain stem. Two-thirds of cases are women. Treatment by mobilization of the nerve in the posterior fossa, or by the paralytic effect of botulinum toxin injected into the affected part of the facial muscle is often effective.

Oculomotor nerve palsy

There is ptosis, dilatation of the pupil with loss of the reactions to light and to accommodation, and paralysis of all the external ocular muscles except the superior oblique (fourth nerve) and lateral rectus (sixth nerve) muscles (Fig. 13.2). The eye is deviated laterally and some depression and intorsion is possible. If the nerve is only partially damaged the syndrome is incomplete. Thus, in lesions in the superior orbital fissure the pupil, medial and elevator muscles are affected but the other muscles are spared.

The third nerve may be damaged by inflammation in the orbit, tumours in the orbit, or with lesions behind the orbit, e.g. aneurysms of the posterior communicating artery, meningioma, pituitary tumour and metastatic tumour or chronic meningitis (tuberculosis

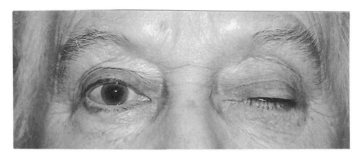

Fig. 13.2 Third nerve palsy in a patient with diabetes mellitus. There is ptosis on the left, with impaired adduction, elevation and depression, but with normal abduction, and a normal pupil. Recovery occurred in 12 weeks.

or sarcoidosis). One of the commonest causes of third nerve palsy is infarction of the nerve in diabetes mellitus. In this syndrome there is sudden painful paralysis of the third nerve, but the pupillomotor fibres are spared so that the pupillary reactions are normal. A similar, pupil-sparing third nerve palsy may occur as part of the mononeuritis multiplex of polyarteritis nodosa. Recovery is often incomplete. Orbital trauma may also cause third nerve dysfunction particularly when the fracture involves the superior or inferior orbital fissure. In 'blow-out' orbital trauma and fracture the fourth nerve is characteristically involved causing vertical diplopia and a compensatory head tilt.

Abducens palsy

This is a relatively common, non-specific cranial nerve palsy. It occurs as a feature of raised intracranial pressure, after trauma, lumbar puncture and meningitis, and in orbital disease. It frequently recovers.

Other cranial nerve palsies

Involvement of the *trigeminal nerve* is relatively common in basal skull disease, especially metastatic carcinoma or lymphoma. There is sensory loss, especially in the inferior mental branch of the third division (numb chin syndrome) and weakness of the mandibular musculature. The *eighth nerve* is frequently affected by acoustic neuroma, and by metastatic carcinoma of the meninges. The lower cranial nerves are involved unilaterally with lesions near the hypoglossal foramen or jugular foramen, as in tumours of the glomus jugulare.

Table 13.2 *Features of peripheral neuropathies.*

Axonopathy	Myelinopathy
Ascending distal sensory impairment	Mild distal sensory loss
Distal dysaesthesiae	
Absent distal reflexes	All reflexes absent
Distal weakness	Proximal or distal weakness
Distal atrophy	Atrophy in long-standing cases (tremor). Nerves may be slightly thickened.
CSF normal	CSF protein raised
Mild slowing motor nerve conduction velocity	Markedly slowed motor nerve conduction velocity (<30 m/s in arms)
Slow recovery possible	Rapid recovery possible

Polyneuropathies

Peripheral neuropathies may be symmetrical and generalized, focal or multifocal. Symmetrical generalized polyneuropathies result from disease affecting myelin, i.e. Schwann cells (myelinopathy), or the nerve axons (axonopathy). This syndrome can also result from diffuse infiltration of the peripheral nerves, e.g. by lymphoma, but this is rare. Polyneuropathies usually present with distal sensory impairment and distal weakness and wasting (see Table 13.2).

In axonopathies there is a toxic or metabolic disturbance in the nerve cell and/or in the nerve axon itself (proximal/distal axonopathy).

Table 13.3 *Causes of peripheral neuropathies.*

Axonopathies	Myelinopathies
Metabolic	Immunological
diabetes mellitus	Guillain–Barré syndrome
uraemia	Toxic
endocrine disorders	diphtheria
porphyria	Genetic
nutritional deficiencies	Refsum's disease
Toxic	sulphatide lipidosis
drugs, e.g. isoniazid, alcohol	Type I Charcot–Marie–Tooth
industrial toxins, e.g.	syndrome
triorthocresylphosphate	
n-hexane	
Malignant disease	
Myeloma	
Genetic	
Type II Charcot–Marie–Tooth syndrome	

Virtually all drug-induced neuropathies are axonal in type, and most metabolic neuropathies are also due to axonal or nerve cell (anterior horn cell and dorsal root ganglion cell) disease. There are fewer causes of myelinopathy. It should be remembered that peripheral nerve myelin is different immunologically, biochemically and structurally from CNS myelin, and that the two forms of myelin are manufactured by different cells, the Schwann cells in the peripheral nervous system and the oligodendroglia in the central nervous system. Demyelination in the CNS is therefore *not* associated with demyelination in the peripheral nervous system. The common causes of axonopathies and myelinopathies are shown in Table 13.3.

Diabetic neuropathy

Diabetes mellitus is associated with several different clinical patterns of neuropathy (Table 13.4). Virtually all patients with Type 1 or Type 2 diabetes have evidence of peripheral neuropathy if sophisticated clinical tests of sensation, or electrophysiological methods are used in assessment, but this is only important when it is symptomatic and disabling.

Diabetic neuropathy may present abruptly, especially proximal motor neuropathy, or insidiously. In adult-onset Type 2 diabetes neuropathy may be the presenting feature, but in childhood-onset Type 1 diabetes neuropathy is a complication of glucose intolerance that develops months or years after onset of the diabetes. Diabetic neuropathy may commence, or worsen, during periods of poor control of diabetes and it can be related to poor control of hyperglycaemia. Diabetic neuropathies of all types are associated with increased CSF protein, but this does not correlate with the severity of the neuropathy.

Sensorimotor neuropathy. This symmetrical mixed sensory, motor and autonomic neuropathy is the commonest clinical type of neuropathy in diabetes. It is often mild with varying degrees of the three principal clinical components. Tingling in the feet and toes is

Table 13.4 *Diabetic neuropathies.*

Distal symmetrical polyneuropathy
   sensorimotor, usually with autonomic involvement
   predominantly sensory
Focal and multifocal neuropathies
   asymmetrical proximal motor neuropathy (diabetic amyotrophy)
   cranial neuropathy
   multiple mononeuropathies
   entrapment neuropathies

---

common, but weakness is often slight. Autonomic disturbances such as postural hypotension, impotence, incontinence and diarrhoea may be present. The skin appears red and shiny in the extremities.

Sensory neuropathy. Ascending, distal, symmetrical, stocking-and-glove sensory impairment without weakness or other features develops in association with autonomic problems. The sensory disturbance may be mild or severe, with ulceration at pressure points and incoordination due to sensory deprivation (sensory ataxia). Spontaneous shooting pains resembling the lightning pains of tabes dorsalis may be present.

In *small fibre sensory neuropathy* there is decreased pain and temperature sensation, with spontaneous pain, but with relatively preserved position and vibration sense, and reflexes. In *large fibre sensory neuropathy* there is a predominance of position sense disturbance with sensory ataxia, and with absent reflexes.

Asymmetrical proximal motor neuropathy. In diabetic amyotrophy, asymmetrical weakness and atrophy develops relatively abruptly in proximal muscles of the thighs and hips. There is often pain in the anterior compartment of the thigh, and weakness of hip flexion and of knee extension is the main feature. This syndrome nearly always affects the pelvic girdle muscles but involvement of upper limb muscles has been described. There is always some associated diabetic distal polyneuropathy of sensorimotor type. Diabetic amyotrophy often begins at a time of rapid weight loss during a period of poor control of diabetes, or as the presentation of Type 2 diabetes in adults.

Cranial neuropathy. Acute painful ophthalmoplegia in a complete or partial third nerve distribution, but with sparing of pupillary reactions to light and accommodation, is characteristic of diabetes mellitus. A similar syndrome may occur rarely in polyarteritis nodosa. Less commonly other cranial neuropathies, affecting fourth and seventh nerves, may develop acutely in diabetes mellitus, and nearly 10% of Bell's palsies are associated with diabetes mellitus. These acute cranial neuropathies improve, or even resolve completely during a period of 3–6 months.

Entrapment neuropathies. Diabetic patients are particularly susceptible to develop entrapment neuropathies at the usual sites of predilection, e.g. carpal tunnel syndrome. In most patients these mononeuropathies improve with better diabetic control, but decompression is indicated if there is marked sensory loss or muscular atrophy.

Management of diabetic neuropathies. In some patients the diagnosis of diabetes will not have been made, and tests of glucose tolerance are indicated in patients with polyneuropathies of unknown origin. The key to successful management is strict control of diabetes by dietary control or by oral hypoglycaemic drugs. Insulin therapy is indicated only if these measures fail to control diabetes. In brittle diabetics with severe neuropathy insulin pump therapy may produce good results. Attention to the skin at pressure points, and on the feet is important and when there is anaesthesia of the feet this is mandatory in order to prevent painless injuries. Footwear should be carefully chosen. Patients with position sense loss may develop painless traumatic arthropathies (Charcot joints). Pain in diabetic neuropathy is difficult to manage; treatment with carbamazepine, imipramine, phenothiazines, phenytoin and diflunisal are all useful in some patients.

Other metabolic axonopathies

There are many metabolic neuropathies but most, e.g. uraemic and hypothyroid neuropathies, are usually mild. The neuropathy responds to treatment of the underlying cause.

Uraemic neuropathy. Neuropathy occurs in about 30% of patients treated with haemodialysis as a gradually progressive and disabling sensorimotor neuropathy. Renal transplantation is the most effective treatment, but recovery is slow.

Porphyria. Porphyria is a disorder of haem biosynthesis. Neuropathy is particularly characteristic of *acute intermittent porphyria*, but it also occurs in *variegate porphyria* and in *hereditary coproporphyria*. Acute intermittent porphyria is an autosomal dominant disorder that is latent until adolescence. The disorder is characterized by episodes of abdominal pain, often combined with constipation, vomiting and fever. These episodes are associated with agitation and irritability or even delirium. An acute motor neuropathy may follow such an episode either acutely or subacutely. Weakness may be proximal or distal, symmetrical or asymmetrical, but it usually involves proximal arm muscles more than other muscles and in severe cases there may be quadriplegia with paralysis of respiratory muscles. Pain may be a feature but sensory abnormalities are much less striking than the weakness, involving pain and temperature sensibility, but sparing joint position sense. The ankle jerks are usually present, although other reflexes are absent. Tachycardia is prominent and may suggest the diagnosis. Attacks of acute porphyria may occur spontaneously, but many are precipitated by drugs, especially barbiturates, sulphonamides, antibiotics and anticonvulsants.

The neuropathy progresses in severity during several weeks and death may result from cardiorespiratory problems. Recovery is slow but is usually complete during a period of several months or years. The diagnosis is suggested by brown-coloured urine, a colour that develops when the urine is allowed to stand. Delta aminolaevulinic acid and porphobilinogen are found in the urine.

Alcoholic/nutritional neuropathy. Neuropathy in the alcoholic is due to thiamine deficiency. Other B group vitamins may also be deficient but thiamine deficiency occurring without other nutritional deficiencies can also produce neuropathy (dry beri-beri neuropathy). Alcohol itself is toxic to peripheral nerves. The initial symptoms are aching and discomfort in soles and calves with distal sensory loss in the feet and absent ankle jerks. Intense burning feelings and tenderness in the feet are strongly suggestive of the diagnosis. Foot and wrist drop may be present.

The neuropathy is frequently associated with other complications of alcoholism, especially Wernicke–Korsakoff syndrome, ataxia and seizures. Treatment with thiamine and other B vitamin supplements, dietary improvement and alcohol abstinence results in improvement in the neuropathy.

Neuropathy also results from pyridoxine deficiency or excess and is a feature of the neurological manifestation of vitamin B$_{12}$ deficiency.

Vitamin B$_{12}$ deficiency. The peripheral neuropathy of vitamin B$_{12}$ deficiency is less prominent than the manifestations of the spinal cord disorder. The ankle jerks are diminished and there is distal sensory impairment. In addition, there is striking loss of position and vibration sense, with impaired two point discrimination in the feet, ankles and even knees. The upper limbs are less involved. Loss of joint position sense is accompanied by sensory ataxia and Rombergism. There are also associated corticospinal signs, with increased knee jerks, despite the diminished ankle jerks, and extensor plantar responses.

There is usually a macrocytic anaemia with undifferentiated white cell precursors in the blood, and with a megaloblastic bone marrow. The blood B$_{12}$ level is low. The tongue may appear atrophic in advanced cases and mild jaundice may be evident. Treatment with hydroxocobalamin 1 mg i.m. weekly for a month, followed by monthly or two-monthly maintenance doses is effective.

Toxic neuropathies

A large number of drugs and industrial chemicals can produce neuropathy. This is a typical painful mixed sensorimotor neuropathy of axonal type. It is of varying severity depending on dose, duration and neurotoxicity of the causative agent. Some substances cause

Table 13.5   *Neuropathies of malignant disease.*

Subacute sensory polyneuropathy
Sensorimotor polyneuropathy
Neuropathies associated with paraproteinaemia

systemic effects. Treatment of all these syndromes depends on cessation of exposure. In some instances the biochemical mechanism is understood and in these the neuropathy seems to be due to disturbed axonal transport mechanisms. Isoniazid neuropathy is readily prevented by coincidental pyridoxine therapy (10 mg tds) since it is due to an interfering effect of isoniazid on pyridoxine metabolism.

Neuropathy of malignant disease

Polyneuropathy occurs commonly in patients with malignant disease but this remote manifestation of the malignancy is only rarely a serious problem and is often barely detectable. In many cases, in contemporary practice, it is not possible to distinguish the polyneuropathy of malignant disease from polyneuropathy caused by cytotoxic chemotherapy, e.g. vincristine (Table 13.5).

Subacute sensory neuropathy

In this rare syndrome there is a relatively rapid onset, during several days or weeks, of sensory polyneuropathy. There is marked sensory loss particularly involving position sense, vibration sense and light touch (discriminatory sensation) but with less involvement of pain and temperature sensibility. There is a marked sensory ataxia, with pseudo-athetoid involuntary movements affecting distal extremities, and the reflexes are absent. Autonomic involvement with postural hypotension and pupillary areflexia may be found. In most cases there is an underlying small cell carcinoma of the lung but the sensory neuropathy may precede discovery of the cancer by many months. Treatment of the neoplasm does not modify the neuropathy.

Mixed sensorimotor neuropathy

This is the commonest peripheral neuropathy associated with neoplasia, particularly with carcinoma of lung, breast and stomach, but also found with lymphomas. It may be acute, insidious or relapsing, but is only rarely severe.

Neuropathies associated with paraproteinaemias

A mixed sensorimotor neuropathy, with predominant motor features, may occur in patients with myeloma or lymphoma, in association with monoclonal paraproteinaemia. Treatment of the underlying disease, especially when there is solitary plasmacytoma and paraproteinaemia, may improve the neuropathy. Plasma exchange is not often useful. Patients with benign paraproteinaemia may also develop polyneuropathy, often with relatively low levels of circulating paraprotein, and treatment in these cases usually has little or no beneficial effect on the neuropathy. In some patients with myeloma, neuropathy is due to amyloid deposition in the peripheral nervous system; no treatment is available for this complication.

Genetic polyneuropathies

The common form of the genetically determined neuropathies is a slowly progressive, symmetrical disorder in which peripheral neuropathy, predominantly motor in type, is associated with deformities of the foot, especially pes cavus. Pes cavus itself, however, can occur without peripheral neuropathy. These genetic neuropathies are classified according to their metabolic basis, if this is known, or by their clinical features, if it is not (Tables 13.6 and 13.7). The metabolically-determined polyneuropathies are all rare. The *familial amyloid polyneuropathies* are dominantly inherited and tend to occur in relatively closed communities, e.g. in Northern Finland, Portugal and in the USA. In some families the peripheral nerves are enlarged. Some are painful and presentation with carpal tunnel syndrome is a well-known feature.

Refsum's disease is an autosomal recessive disorder which may pursue a remittent course with periods of relatively abrupt deterioration. The main features are hypertrophic polyneuropathy with dry flaking skin (ichthyosis), night blindness, sensorineural deafness, optic atrophy, cerebellar ataxia and pes cavus. There is often a cardiomyopathy, which may prove fatal. The disease is due to storage of a vegetable lipid, phytanic acid, in the nervous system.

Table 13.6 *Some metabolically-determined genetic polyneuropathies.*

Familial amyloid polyneuropathies
Refsum's disease (phytanic acid storage)
Lipid storage polyneuropathies, e.g. metachromatic leucodystrophy

Table 13.7 *Genetically-determined neuropathies without known metabolic cause.*

Hereditary motor and sensory neuropathy (HMSN)
Hereditary sensory and autonomic neuropathies (HSAN)
Friedreich's ataxia
Other rare hereditary neuropathies

Improvement occurs, but only slowly, when all vegetables and vegetable products except potatoes, and proteins derived from vegetable-eating animals, e.g. beef and lamb, are excluded from the diet. Vitamin supplementation is necessary since this diet is extremely limited.

The typical example of genetically-determined polyneuropathy without known metabolic cause is Charcot–Marie–Tooth syndrome (hereditary motor and sensory neuropathy: HMSN), of which several distinct types exist. The older term 'peroneal muscular atrophy' is still often used.

Hereditary motor and sensory neuropathy. This is the most common of this group of diseases. Dominant and recessive forms have been described. Most patients present with distal muscle weakness, foot drop and atrophy of the anterior tibial muscles. There is pes cavus, consisting of a high arched foot due to muscular imbalance of small intrinsic foot muscles and the long flexors and extensors acting across the foot. The distal atrophy gives way proximally to relatively normal muscles. Atrophy of small hand muscles may be present. There is mild distal sensory loss. In 25% of cases the peripheral nerves are enlarged distally and tremor may be present. The disease commences before the age of 20 years.

In the Type II form, which is usually recessively inherited, the motor conduction velocity is only slightly slowed, but in the Type I, dominantly inherited form, it is markedly slowed, usually < 20 m/s in the legs. In the latter form the tendon reflexes are all absent, the peripheral nerves are enlarged and the CSF protein may be strikingly raised, features that suggest a predominantly demyelinating process. This Type I form of the disease is the commonest form and is generally more severe than the Type II variant. An infantile-onset, recessive type of the disease (Déjerine–Sottas disease) is also associated with very slow conduction velocity, severe weakness, sensory ataxia and areflexia.

Management: Care of the hypoesthetic feet is essential. Unperceived skin and bony injuries cause infection and deformity, including Charcot joints and loss of toes, and these secondary features lead to disability. Shortening of the Achilles tendon is common, causing toe walking and instability. Careful attention to footwear and intermittent physiotherapy are important. Bracing the foot can be useful provided the braces are light and comfortable. Fixation of the forefoot by surgical fusion is often used to maintain a plantigrade posture. Life expectancy is normal but many patients progress to wheelchair dependency after 20–30 years.

Hereditary sensory and autonomic neuropathies. This is a rare group of disorders in which there is a slowly ascending sensory neuropathy with pain, trophic distal ulcers and autonomic disturbances of variable severity. *Familial dysautonomia* (Riley–Day syndrome) is the best known type, characterized by vomiting episodes, feeding problems in infancy, recurrent pneumonia, gastric distention and urinary retention, distal impairment of pain and temperature sensation and absence of the fungiform papillae of the tongue with absent taste sensation. The disorder is usually fatal in the second decade.

Hereditary susceptibility to pressure palsies. Families with susceptibility to pressure mononeuropathies, and to brachial plexus palsies, have been described, in which there is an inherited abnormality in myelin structure. These disorders are autosomal dominant traits.

Guillain–Barré syndrome (post-infectious polyradiculoneuritis)

This syndrome is important because it is acute and recovery is usually complete, but there is a risk of death from ventilatory failure. The disorder usually follows an infection of viral type, often involving the upper respiratory tract some 2–3 weeks earlier. The neuropathy is predominantly a motor disorder, with symmetrical weakness that involves the trunk and proximal limb muscles, usually mainly involving the lower limbs. Bulbar muscles may also be involved. Sensory features may be insignificant, but distal pain and paraesthesiae are sometimes troublesome. The respiratory muscles are involved in some patients, particularly those with bulbar weakness, and difficulty in breathing may occur at a time when the limbs are relatively strong. In 80% of cases the clinical disability reaches a peak within 2 weeks of the onset. The tendon reflexes are reduced or absent. External ocular muscles are almost always unaffected. Autonomic disturbances, including incontinence, hypotension, hypertension or tachyarrhythmias may be prominent, or even life-threatening.

Investigations. The CSF protein is raised after an interval of several days, and reaches a peak 2–4 weeks after the onset of the disease. Motor nerve conduction velocity may be slowed especially in proximal segments of the nerves. There are no specific diagnostic tests.

Management. Most patients will recover completely within a few months, but the prognosis is less good in the elderly and in very severe cases. Ventilatory muscle weakness is life-threatening and may not be recognized in the face of apparently reasonable limb strength. Tests of vital capacity and forced expiratory volume (FEV) are therefore an essential part of the management, and should be repeated, e.g. with peak flow measurements, hourly at the bedside until it is established that this is not a problem. A vital capacity < 1.5 litres is an indication for considering the necessity for ventilatory assistance. These measurements are not always reliable when there is facial weakness leading to leakage of air around the mouthpiece. About 10% of cases require ventilation.

The patient will require full nursing care, with attention to pressure sores. Catheterization may be necessary. Nutrition is important. Although no specific treatment is available plasma exchange, especially when used in the first 10 days of the illness, may be followed by relatively rapid recovery. The role of steroids is doubtful. Any secondary infection should be treated immediately with appropriate antibiotics. Physiotherapy and simple analgesics are important in the early stages to relieve postural discomfort. Later, physiotherapy is helpful in restoring strength, mobility and confidence.

Chronic relapsing polyradiculopathy. A chronic relapsing course develops in about 5% of otherwise typical cases of Guillain–Barré syndrome. These patients are usually steroid-responsive. High dose steroids are needed to induce remission, and smaller maintenance doses given on alternate days may be necessary to maintain normality. This form of the disease has been linked with HLA DRW2.

Miller–Fisher syndrome. This is a rare variant of Guillain–Barré syndrome, consisting of the acute onset of ophthalmoplegia, ataxia and areflexia, with pupillary paralysis. The prognosis for recovery in a few days is excellent and few patients with this syndrome develop more typical features of Guillain–Barré syndrome.

Mononeuritis mulitplex

This term is used to describe a multifocal disorder of peripheral nerves. The essential feature of mononeuritis multiplex is therefore

Table 13.8 *Causes of mononeuritis multiplex.*

Vascular
diabetic microangiopathy
polyarteritis nodosa and other autoimmune vasculitides
rheumatoid arthritis and vasculitis
Infections
leprosy
Neoplastic
invasion of peripheral nerves and roots

the finding of clinical features suggesting involvement of two or more separate nerves. The clinical features are usually asymmetrical. Proximal mononeuropathies, e.g. femoral or radial neuropathies, tend to produce mainly motor effects, and distal neuropathies, e.g. median or common peroneal nerve lesions, produce a mixed sensorimotor disturbance. Most patients with mononeuritis multiplex describe a relatively acute onset. There are several causes of this clinical syndrome (Table 13.8).

Treatment of mononeuritis multiplex is that of the underlying cause. The importance of the syndrome is that it is frequently the presenting feature of an underlying systemic disorder (Table 13.8).

Nerve plexus lesions

The brachial and lumbosacral plexuses are susceptible to damage from trauma, infiltration with cancer or inflammatory processes, and from localized immunological damage, as in brachial neuritis. The brachial plexus is more commonly involved by these processes than the lumbar plexus.

Brachial plexus

The brachial plexus is the site of formation of the sensorimotor nerves innervating the arm and shoulder; it is made up of C3–T1 nerve roots. The brachial plexus is rarely involved in its entirety in any disease process. The clinical features depend on the distribution of abnormality with respect to the upper, middle and lower portions of the plexus, involvement of the cervical sympathetic chain, especially the stellate ganglion at C8, and the rate of progression of the process. Thus Horner's syndrome is an important feature of lower brachial plexus lesions.

Lesions of the upper trunk usually affect biceps, deltoid and spinatus muscles, with C5/6 sensory disturbance. In lower plexus lesions there is weakness of the hand and triceps, with sensory disturbance in C8/T1, and with Horner's syndrome. Although there are many causes of brachial plexus lesions only brachial neuritis

Table 13.9 *Causes of brachial plexus lesions.*

Post-infectious brachial neuritis
Trauma, e.g. traction on an arm in motor cycle accidents during childbirth
Malignant infiltration, e.g. carcinoma of breast carcinoma of lung (Pancoast syndrome) lymphoma
Delayed effects of radiation therapy

(neuralgic amyotrophy), trauma and neoplastic invasion are common (Table 13.9).

Neoplastic vs radiation plexopathy

The distinction between these two processes is not always easy. Neoplastic invasion, e.g. in Pancoast's syndrome, usually causes damage to the lower trunk of the plexus, with weakness of the hand, Horner's syndrome and severe root pain in C8–T1. Radiation plexopathy, on the other hand, usually affects the upper trunk, with weakness of deltoid and biceps; pain is not such a major feature.

Traumatic brachial plexopathy

This injury occurs when an arm is tethered or is the site of a sudden traction force as in motor cycle injuries and in certain industrial accidents. This injury can also occur to an infant during childbirth. The injury may affect the whole plexus but more commonly affects upper or lower trunks of the plexus. The limb is atrophied, with sensory impairment, and spontaneous persistent burning pain may be a major feature. This neuralgic pain is difficult to relieve. Recovery from injuries such as these can occur provided the nerve roots and trunks are not severed, and that the vascular perfusion of the arm is maintained. In some cases surgical exploration is justified in order to suture divided nerves. The lesion may be preganglionic, i.e. proximal to the posterior root ganglion, in which case the histamine flare triple response is preserved in anaesthetic skin, and the sensory nerve action potential is also retained. Myelography with CT scanning is useful since damaged nerve roots can usually be readily recognized (Fig. 13.3). Pain may require opiates but these are often unsuccessful and carbamazepine (up to 800 mg daily) and diflunisal (20 mg b.d.) may be useful. If some sensation is preserved useful function can be learned even when there is severe weakness and atrophy, but an anaesthetic, flail and atrophied limb is not only useless but may be a potential source of infection and injury.

Brachial neuritis (neuralgic amyotrophy)

This is probably the commonest form of brachial plexopathy. The syndrome often follows immunization or a viral infection but may occur spontaneously. Up to 2 weeks after the antecedent event there is acute severe pain in the shoulder, arm and neck. Within a few days weakness of the deltoid, shoulder girdle and biceps muscles (upper trunk syndrome) develops without objective sensory loss except for patchy disturbance in the circumflex territory on the outer aspect of the shoulder. About 25% of cases are bilateral, although asymmetrical.

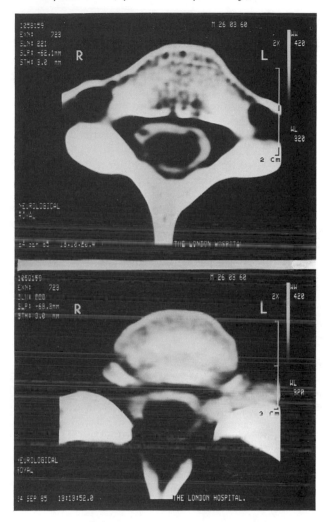

Fig. 13.3 Brachial plexus traction injury. This injury is often associated with rupture of the brachial roots as shown in this CT scan of the C6 level, made during myelography. In the upper picture the normal right sided nerve root can be seen outlined against the central cord shadow. In the lower picture contrast is seen leaking into the soft tissues of the neck through the avulsed root on the left side.

Recovery begins within a few weeks and is virtually complete in most cases 3 years after the onset. Management is symptomatic since there is no specific treatment and the prognosis is good. The syndrome is sometimes recurrent, and a rare hereditary form is recognized in which palsy of the ipsilateral recurrent laryngeal nerve is a feature.

Lumbosacral plexus

The lumbosacral plexus is less vulnerable to trauma than the brachial plexus, being deeply situated within the pelvis. The commonest cause of lumbosacral plexopathy is diabetic proximal neuropathy, a disorder that only rarely affects the brachial plexus. Conversely lumbar neuritis, unlike brachial neuritis, is uncommon. Retroperitoneal disease, especially neoplasm, haemorrhage, and inadvertent injury during orthopaedic and gynaecological operations and, rarely, in difficult forceps delivery, may also lead to lumbar plexus lesions. The clinical features depend on the distribution of the lesion in the plexus; the L2 and L4 components of the lumbar plexus are more frequently affected than other components. The clinical differentiation of lumbar plexus lesions from lumbar root disease is not easy. Cauda equina disease is usually bilateral but diabetic lumbar plexopathy is also frequently bilateral and the recognition of an associated distal polyneuropathy is important in the latter diagnosis.

14

Myopathies, Myositis and Myasthenia

Diseases of muscle are characterized by muscular weakness which is usually proximal and symmetrical; this weakness is usually painless and slowly progressive, except in inflammatory myopathies. Muscular wasting is frequently a feature and the tendon reflexes are usually present. Diagnosis of the cause of the muscular syndrome depends on variations in these features, especially age of onset, family history, sex, associated clinical features of disease in other systems, fatiguability and pseudohypertrophy of muscles.

The commonest muscular disease is polymyositis but clinically unimportant muscular weakness is frequent in endocrine disorders, especially thyroid disease. Many of the well-known myopathies, e.g. Duchenne dystrophy, are relatively uncommon. *Myopathy* is a term used to describe muscular disease; *myositis* implies inflammation as in the inflammatory myopathies (polymyositis); *muscular dystrophies* are inherited, progressive myopathies in which severe structural changes occur in muscle without abnormalities in the motor innervation; *myasthenia* is muscular weakness occurring on effort, i.e. undue fatiguability, due to impaired neuromuscular transmission.

Muscular dystrophies

The muscular dystrophies are classified according to their clinical and genetic characteristics (Table 14.1); the causation of these disorders is only incompletely understood.

Duchenne muscular dystrophy

This severe, progressive muscular dystrophy is inherited as an X-linked trait so that it is expressed in boys and transmitted in female carriers. It affects 1 in 3500 live male births. It can usually be recognized by the age of 3 years by difficulty walking and climbing

Table 14.1 *Muscular dystrophies.*

X-linked muscular dystrophies
   Duchenne muscular dystrophy
   Becker muscular dystrophy
Limb-girdle muscular dystrophy
Facio-scapulo-humeral muscular dystrophy
Scapuloperoneal muscular dystrophy
Myotonic dystrophy

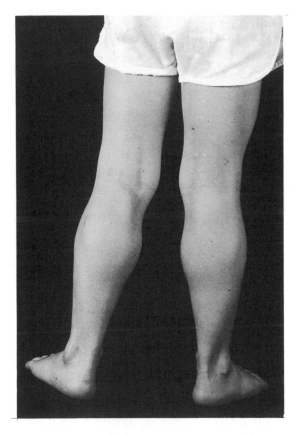

Fig. 14.1 Duchenne muscular dystrophy. There is pseudo-hypertrophy of the calf muscles with shortening of the Achilles tendons in this 8 year old boy.

stairs. Affected boys never run normally and cannot hop. Weakness is first evident in pelvic girdle muscles, and difficulty rising from the floor is a characteristic feature. This is often recognized by a peculiar method of getting up in which the child seems to climb up his legs after straightening the knees while in the 'all fours' position. The gait is waddling and there is a pronounced lumbar lordosis. The muscular weakness progresses rapidly after the age of 8 years so that a wheelchair is necessary by the age of 12 years, and in the majority of cases death occurs by the age of 20 years. Pseudohypertrophy of muscles (Fig. 14.1), especially of calves, deltoids and serratus anterior, is an important diagnostic feature. These enlarged muscles are weak. Joint contractures and scoliosis with respiratory difficulty develop, but ocular, facial and distal hand muscles are relatively spared, even in the late stages of the disease. There is mild intellectual impairment in many cases, and ECG evidence of cardiomyopathy.

Becker muscular dystrophy

This is a slowly progressive muscular dystrophy that resembles Duchenne muscular dystrophy, but with a later age of onset (15–18 years), slower progression and longer life expectancy. Survival into the fifth decade is usual, and most can still walk in the third decade.

Investigation of X-linked muscular dystrophy

The diagnosis is usually evident after clinical assessment. In Duchenne dystrophy the blood creatine kinase (CK) level is greatly raised, reaching very high levels (30–300 times normal) in infancy and becoming lower later in the course of the disease as muscular atrophy progresses. In Becker dystrophy the CK level is somewhat lower. Creatine kinase is an intracellular enzyme important in oxidative muscular metabolism that leaks out of muscle cells into the circulation during muscle fibre necrosis, or when the muscle cell membrane is 'leaky'.

The *EMG* shows myopathic motor unit potentials; the motor and sensory nerve conduction velocities are normal. The *muscle biopsy* (Fig. 14.2) shows rounding of muscle fibres, marked variation in fibre size with hypertrophy, atrophy, degeneration and regeneration of muscle fibres, and marked endomysial and interfascicular fibrosis. Pink, hyaline fibres in haematoxylin and eosin stained section are characteristic of both these X-linked dystrophies.

Pulmonary function tests show restrictive defects from kyphoscoliosis and respiratory muscle weakness.

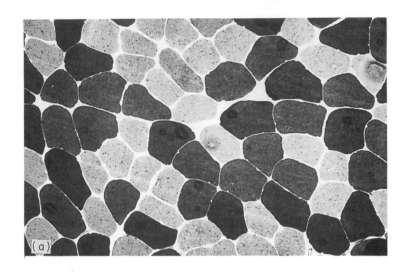

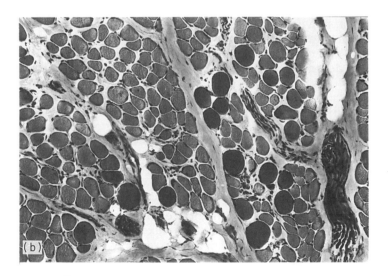

Fig. 14.2 (a) Normal muscle biopsy, ATPase pH 9.4. The dark fibres are Type 2 (phasic contracting) and the pale fibres Type 1 (tonic contracting). These two fibre types are arranged in a pseudo-random mosaic 'checkerboard' pattern. (b) Duchenne muscular dystrophy, haematoxylin and eosin. There is interstitial fibrosis and fat replacement, rounding of muscle fibres, and scattered hypertrophied, dark fibres. A normal nerve fibre bundle is present to the right.

Genetics and carrier detection. Half the sons of a carrier female will be affected and half the daughters will be carriers. It is generally thought that about 30% of cases are the result of spontaneous mutations of the gene site on the short arm of the X chromosome at Xp21. The genetic locus has been identified as that coding for dystrophin, a protein important in maintaining the integrity of the muscle cell membrane. Dystrophin, a membrane protein, is absent in muscle cells in Duchenne dystrophy, and abnormal in Becker dystrophy. These abnormalities can be applied as a test *in utero* to babies at risk of inheriting the disease.

Carrier detection may also be possible by genetic investigation in the future. Conventional assessment relies on the presence of minimal features of the genetic disorder (manifesting carrier status) such as slight hypertrophy of calf muscles, mild elevation of the serum CK or even muscular weakness. Definite (obligate) carriers are women who have two affected sons (ruling out mutation as a cause) or one affected son and another, closely-related, affected male relative.

Management. Attention to physiotherapy to prevent joint contractures is important in maintaining ambulation and independence. Provision of seating with adequate back support partially prevents scoliosis. Infections should be treated immediately. Provision for education and occupation at home are important. Suitable shoes and calipers, and mechanical aids for those seriously disabled, e.g. page-turning equipment, computers etc. are valuable. No effective treatment is available to delay the progression of Duchenne or Becker disease.

Limb-girdle muscular dystrophy

This clinical syndrome is probably heterogeneous. The term limb-girdle muscular dystrophy is used to describe patients with progressive proximal muscular weakness beginning in the second or third decades, due to a myopathic process. The weakness is often asymmetrical and may particularly affect certain muscle groups, e.g. quadriceps muscles. Disability becomes severe about 20 years after the onset. Most cases are inherited as an autosomal recessive trait. Enlargement of calf muscles is an unusual feature.

The blood CK is moderately raised (up to 10 times normal). The main differential diagnosis is from Type III spinal muscular atrophy. Clinical, CT scanning of muscles (Fig. 14.3), and EMG and biopsy assessment are necessary to assess these patients, since the prognosis of the two disorders is rather different.

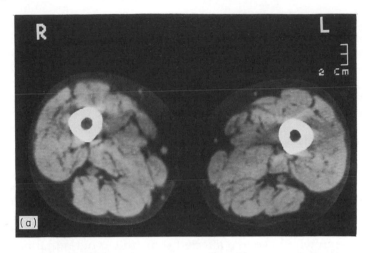

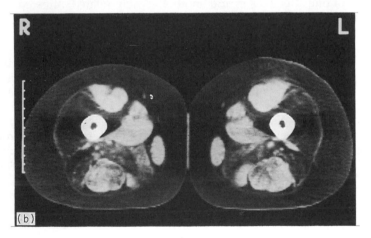

Fig. 14.3 (a) CT scan of normal thigh muscles in an adult. (b) CT scan of thigh muscles in limb-girdle muscular dystrophy. Some muscles, especially vastus lateralis and the lateral hamstring muscles show markedly reduced attenuation but others, e.g. gracilis and rectus femoris, are normal.

Other muscular dystrophies

These are classified according to their clinical features, particularly the distribution of muscular weakness and atrophy. The best known of these rare disorders are facio-scapulo-humeral muscular dystrophy and scapuloperoneal muscular dystrophy (Fig. 14.4). The former is an autosomal dominant trait, but the inheritance of the latter is variable.

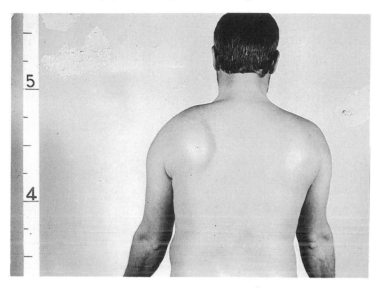

Fig. 14.4 Facio-scapulo-humeral muscular dystrophy. Scapular winging is evident as the patient begins to elevate the left arm.

Myotonic dystrophy and other myotonic syndromes

This is the commonest of the adult-onset muscular dystrophies (about 5/100 000). It is inherited as an autosomal dominant disorder, but the children of affected mothers tend to develop a more severe form of the disease, earlier in life, than the children of affected fathers, an observation suggesting that a cytoplasmic factor may be relevant. The gene is located on chromosome 19. Penetrance is variable so that incomplete forms of the disease are common.

The clinical features are characteristic (Fig. 14.5). There is ptosis, weakness and wasting of distal muscles in the limbs, and of the sternomastoids and facial muscles. There is hollowing of the temporal fossae and cheeks and the face is long, with the lips slightly parted. Systemic involvement is almost invariable with cataract, mental abnormalities, testicular atrophy and infertility, glucose intolerance, dysphagia from involvement of oesophageal muscle and cardiomyopathy, e.g. heart block. Sleep apnoea, associated with alveolar hypoventilation, is a serious and sometimes fatal aspect of severe cases of the disease.

The most characteristic feature of this disease is myotonia, consisting of persistent contraction of a muscle or of a group of fibres in a muscle following cessation of voluntary contraction of the muscle or in response to a mechanical stimulus, e.g. a blow from a tendon

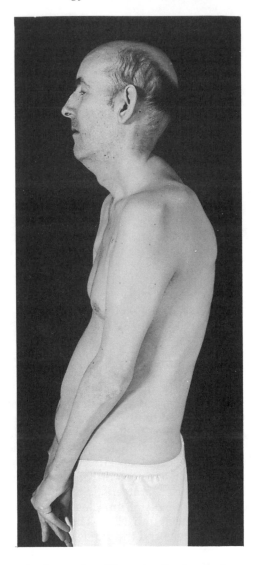

Fig. 14.5 Myotonic dystrophy. There is distal muscle atrophy, frontal baldness, a myopathic facies, and a swan-neck posture, with wasting of the sterno-mastoid muscles.

hammer onto the belly of the muscle. The patient is unable to release objects and the combination of facial weakness and myotonia leads to a slurring dysarthria. Myotonia is always worse after rest or in cold weather, and may itself be a cause of disability in myotonic dystrophy. Myotonia can almost always be detected clinically but

EMG assessment is useful in recognizing the characteristic 'dive-bomber' sound of myotonic discharges.

Neonatal myotonic dystrophy is a severe form presenting in the neonatal period in children of myotonic mothers, even in mildly affected mothers. Hypotonia, poor sucking and swallowing and respiratory distress with facio-bulbar weakness are evident but myotonia develops in survivors only a year or so later. Many affected neonates are severely mentally retarded.

Management. Treatment of myotonia is sometimes helpful; phenytoin, quinine, baclofen and tocainide may be useful but all have unwanted effects that limit treatment. There is no specific treatment for the disease itself. Many patients with the disease show stubborn personality traits that make management difficult. The glucose intolerance is mild and unresponsive to insulin therapy. Cardiomyopathy may be severe, or even fatal. Cataracts may be severe enough to require surgical removal. In large families in which the disease occurs in three or more generations genetic counselling using chromosome markers associated with the locus on chromosome 19 is practicable.

Other myotonic syndromes

Myotonia congenita is a benign autosomal dominant trait in which myotonia and muscular stiffness, troublesome after rest and improved by exercise, are associated with pronounced muscular hypertrophy, and normal strength. A rare *recessive form* occurs in which mild myopathic weakness may be present. *Paramyotonia congenita* is an autosomal dominant form of myotonia in which exercise or cold may induce weakness and myotonia that may last several hours. These disorders are not associated with clinical features of myotonic dystrophy, and are genetically distinct from the latter disorder. The myotonia is more severe in these myotonic syndromes than in myotonic dystrophy.

Benign childhood myopathies

This term is used to describe a group of muscular disorders beginning in infancy and childhood, presenting with poor spontaneous movements or, in older children, with delayed motor development milestones. There is hypotonia (reduced resistance to passive movements) and an increased range of movement of joints. The child may be categorized by the paediatrician as suffering from 'floppy infant syndrome', a clinical syndrome of multiple causation (see Chapter 17).

Benign childhood myopathies (Table 14.2) are usually only slowly progressive, and most reach a stage of non-progression or may even improve during later childhood or adolescence. The palate is often highly-arched and there may be associated skeletal deformities, respiratory disturbances and impaired ocular movements in some cases. Most are inherited, but the pattern of inheritance is often uncertain. There is controversy as to the myopathic or neurogenic basis of some of these disorders. They are classified by their morphological features.

Table 14.2 *Benign childhood myopathies.*

Central core and multicore disease
Nemaline (rod body) myopathy
Myopathy with tubular aggregates
Congenital fibre type disproportion
Congenital muscular dystrophy

Metabolic myopathies

The clinical features of the metabolic myopathies, which are muscular diseases known to be due to specific metabolic disturbances, are variable, ranging from benign muscular cramps to a limb-girdle syndrome with marked muscular atrophy. Episodes of muscular weakness and muscle pain, or even myoglobinuria may occur e.g. in disorders of carnitine metabolism. In some there are characteristic structural changes in muscle, for example mitochondrial inclusions, and vacuoles of various types. They are classified by their underlying biochemical disturbance (Table 14.3).

Table 14.3 *Metabolic myopathies.*

Glycogenoses (glycogen storage myopathies)
   Type   II   acid maltase deficiency
   Type III debranching enzyme deficiency
   Type IV branching enzyme deficiency
   Type   V myophosphorylase deficiency (McArdle's disease)
   Type VII phosphofructokinase deficiency
Mitochondrial cytopathies
   disorders of electron transport
   lipid storage myopathies
Periodic paralysis
   hypokalaemic
   hyperkalaemic and normokalaemic
   thyrotoxic (hypokalaemic)
Malignant hyperpyrexia myopathy
Idiopathic rhabdomyolysis with myoglobinuria

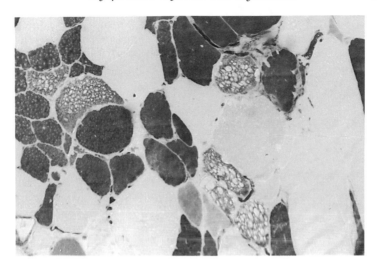

Fig. 14.6 Muscle biopsy in Type 2 glycogenosis (adult-onset type). There is a vacuolar myopathy. The vacuoles contain intra-lysosomal glycogen.

Glycogenoses

Late onset forms of glycogen storage often only affect muscle and are usually slowly progressive (Fig. 14.6). Infantile forms, on the other hand, e.g. *Pompe's disease* (Type II glycogenosis), are severe disorders of infancy or childhood with multisystem involvement, including brain, heart, liver and muscle. The muscular involvement in the adult-onset forms of these disorders is usually proximal but may be asymmetrical. Fatigue and exercise intolerance with cramp, and sometimes with severe involvement of respiratory muscles, are frequent problems. Patients with *adult-onset acid maltase deficiency* may develop diaphragmatic paralysis with fatal sleep apnoea. The muscle biopsy shows prominent lysosomal vacuoles with glycogen granules.

Myophosphorylase deficiency (McArdle's syndrome) presents with weakness, fatiguability and cramp after exercise. There is no weakness at rest, although in longstanding cases some muscular wasting may develop. The disease is diagnosed by the absence of a rise in venous blood lactate or pyruvate levels after exercise with the limb maintained ischaemic by means of a tourniquet. The muscle biopsy shows absence of myophosphorylase and accumulation of cytoplasmic glycogen.

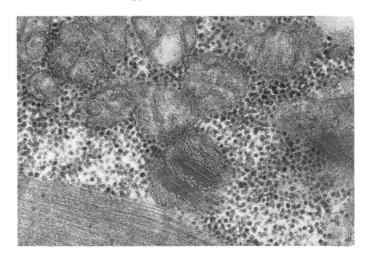

Fig. 14.7 Electron micrograph of muscle mitochondria in a metabolic myopathy, showing paracrystalline inclusions characteristic of a mitochondrial cytopathy.

Mitochondrial cytopathies

These myopathies were originally recognized by the presence of 'ragged-red fibres' in the muscle biopsy. These fibres consist of granular-appearing fibres containing a prominent red-staining rim consisting of accumulations of enlarged, complex mitochondria and glycogen granules. Electron microscopy reveals characteristic crystalline-like bodies between the two outer layers of the mitochondria (Fig. 14.7). This abnormality is associated with defects in electron transport in oxidative mitochondrial metabolism.

Clinically, there are several syndromes. Most patients have mild proximal weakness with fatiguability and abnormalities of ocular movement and retinitis pigmentosa, cerebellar ataxia, dementia, deafness and cardiomyopathy may occur. There is an increased venous blood lactate level after exercise and, rarely, at rest. The CSF protein is raised. The CT brain scan shows stippled calcification of the basal ganglia.

Carnitine deficiency is a related syndrome in which intermittent attacks of hypoglycaemia, vomiting and encephalopathy occur; this may sometimes be relieved by dietary supplements of L-carnitine. Both systemic and muscular forms occur.

Periodic paralyis

This is a rare autosomal recessive syndrome characterized by episodes of weakness of the limbs, usually occurring during a period of rest after exercise. The muscles of respiration and mastication are usually spared. The blood potassium level is either low or raised during attacks. In the hypokalaemic form attacks of muscle weakness can be provoked by insulin, or by fasting-induced hypoglycaemia, and the hyperkalaemic form may be induced by an oral glucose load. The latter syndrome is frequently accompanied by mild myotonia of peri-orbital muscles. The muscle biopsy shows characteristic vacuoles derived from the T tubular system. The heart is not affected. Treatment with acetazolamide reduces the frequency and severity of attacks.

In Oriental peoples hypokalaemic periodic paralysis may complicate thyrotoxicosis. Hypokalaemic muscle weakness also develops with diuretic-induced or liquorice-induced hypokalaemia, but only with potassium levels < 2.5 mmol/litre.

Malignant hyperpyrexia

This is a rare disorder in which sudden and sometimes fatal hyperpyrexia develops unexpectedly during anaesthesia. The skeletal muscles are rigidly and intensely contracted and there is hypertension, tachypnoea and a rapidly and uncontrollably increasing temperature, leading to death in a few hours. Hyperkalaemia and myoglobinuria may develop and the blood CK level is very high. Succinylcholine and halothane have been particularly associated with hyperpyrexia, but narcotics, barbiturates and pancuronium appear to be safe. The trait is often inherited as a dominant characteristic, but some cases are associated with myotonia congenita or with central core disease. It complicates 1 : 50 000 anaesthetics. An *in vitro* test is available on excised muscle samples to test for susceptibility.

Management consists of ventilation with 100% oxygen, cooling by sponging and with fans, reversal of metabolic acidosis with i.v. bicarbonate, and calcium gluconate infusion to reverse hypocalcaemia. Dantrolene is the treatment of choice; 2.5 mg/kg i.v. should be given with curare, to reverse the effect of succinylcholine. Renal failure may complicate the illness, secondary to myoglobinuria.

Alcohol and drug-induced myopathies

Alcoholic myopathy occurs as an *acute* painful form following a recent binge, as a *subacute* myopathy associated with alcoholic hypokalaemia, and as a *chronic* form in which proximal weakness and wasting develop during a period of several weeks or months.

The muscles are slightly painful. Recovery occurs gradually following alcohol withdrawal.

Drug-induced myopathies are relatively uncommon. Acute toxic myopathy, with extensive muscle necrosis, may follow treatment with emetine. Chronic painless muscular weakness is associated with treatment with diuretics, purgatives or steroids. Repeated muscular injections, mainly in drug addicts, may cause a focal myopathy. Perhexilene and chloroquine may cause a vacuolar myopathy.

Endocrine myopathies

Proximal muscle weakness is a common feature in endocrine disease (Table 14.4) and as a complication of treatment with certain hormones, especially steroid drugs. In most patients with endocrine disease myopathy is a minor part of the clinical syndrome but in thyroid disease myopathy may be a presenting feature. The endocrine myopathies are reversible with appropriate management of the endocrine disorder. These myopathies are not associated with structural changes in affected muscles.

Table 14.4   *Endocrine myopathies.*

Thyroid myopathies
hyperthyroidism
hypothyroidism
Osteomalacic myopathy
Adrenal disorders and steroid myopathy
Acromegalic myopathy

Thyroid myopathies

Most patients with thyroid disease have abnormalities in muscle, although these are often very mild.

Hyperthyroid myopathy

Proximal weakness, affecting upper and lower limb girdles, is the major muscular feature, but the typical features of hyper-thyroidism are always present. The weak muscles may be slightly atrophic. Fasciculations occur in a few patients and bulbar muscle weakness may be present. The tendon reflexes may be increased, so that the clinical features may erroneously lead to the suggestion of motor neuron disease as a diagnosis. Myasthenia gravis is rarely associated with hyperthyroidism. The blood CK level is

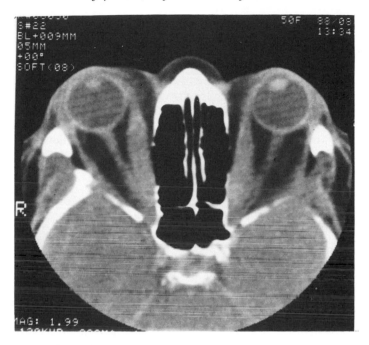

Fig. 14.8 CT scan of orbits in thyroid eye disease, showing exophthalmos and prominent thickening of the medial rectus muscles. The lateral rectus muscles are less markedly involved.

normal. The myopathy improves 1–3 months after commencing treatment of the thyrotoxicosis.

The presence of ocular signs of hyperthyroidism, or of thyroid eye disease (Fig. 14.8), i.e. exophthalmos, lid lag and external ophthalmoplegia, does not correlate with myopathic features in limb muscles. Indeed, severe thyroid eye disease may develop in the euthyroid state.

Hypothyroidism

Muscle pain occurs in up to half of patients with hypothyroidism, and proximal muscular weakness develops in about 25%. There may be atrophy or hypertrophy of muscles. The clinical features of hypothyroidism are present. *Myoedema*, consisting of a localized contraction of a muscle, persisting for up to a minute, induced by percussion, is often associated with myxoedema, but it may also occur in aged subjects and in cachexia. Two-thirds of patients with hypothyroidism show slowed relaxation of the Achilles reflex, due to changes in muscle metabolism of sufficient degree to be ascertainable clinically, but electrical timing of this phase of the reflex shows that it is always abnormal in this disorder. The blood CK level is usually modestly raised.

The diagnosis is confirmed by thyroid function tests and by blood TSH levels, showing low levels of thyroid hormone and raised TSH levels. There may be autoantibodies to thyroid tissue and a raised ESR in Hashimoto's thyroiditis. Treatment with l-thyroxine in gradually incrementing doses to provide replacement therapy (about 0.2–0.3 mg l-thyroxine daily maintenance therapy) results in improvement in muscular symptoms.

Osteomalacic myopathy

Proximal weakness occurs in 50% of patients with osteomalacia, but is relatively infrequent with hypercalcaemia due to hyperparathyroidism or malignant bone disease. Myopathy may be associated either with a low or a raised blood calcium level, and the muscular weakness probably results from disturbed vitamin D metabolism, as in steatorrhoea, renal failure or anticonvulsant drug toxicity. Calcium transport in the sarcoplasmic reticulum of muscle is dependent on the presence of active metabolites of vitamin D; thus abnormal vitamin D metabolism will lead to weakness. The blood CK level is normal. Improvement occurs with treatment of the underlying cause of the metabolic bone disease, and with vitamin D dietary supplements.

Adrenal disorders and steroid myopathy

Hyperadrenalism (Cushing's syndrome) and treatment with steroid drugs may be accompanied by painless progressive proximal weakness. Most cases are due to steroid therapy. When high doses of synthetic steroids are used, especially anti-inflammatory steroid drugs, myopathy may appear in 10 days. Fluorinated steroids are particularly likely to cause myopathy. Susceptibility to develop steroid myopathy is variable, but prednisone dosages in the range 15–100 mg daily for a month or more are commonly associated with myopathy. The CK level in steroid myopathy is normal, but there is evidence of increased protein breakdown and impaired synthesis of cell proteins by steroids thus accounting for the loss of contractile force. When steroid therapy is stopped there is gradual improvement in muscular strength. Steroid myopathy is sometimes a factor in muscle weakness in patients with polymyositis treated with moderately high-dose steroids.

Acromegalic myopathy

The muscles sometimes undergo mild hypertrophy in acromegaly, but despite this are weak. This feature is clinically evident only in relatively advanced cases and is a minor part of the syndrome of acromegaly. Recovery occurs with appropriate treatment.

Inflammatory myopathies

Inflammatory myopathy, due to idiopathic, autoimmune polymyositis, is the commonest form of muscle disease. The clinical features vary in relation to the extent of cutaneous involvement, as in *dermatomyositis*, involvement of other systems, e.g. *mixed connective tissue disease*, or other associated or causative factors (Table 14.5).

Table 14.5 *Inflammatory myopathies.*

Idiopathic polymyositis/dermatomyositis (adult-onset)
Childhood-type dermatomyositis
Dermatomyositis/polymyositis associated with autoimmune disorders
Dermatomyositis/polymyositis associated with malignancy
Sarcoid myopathy
Inclusion body myositis
Polymyositis due to infections and infestations

Idiopathic polymyositis and dermatomyositis

Polymyositis, with or without cutaneous involvement, is the commonest of the inflammatory myopathies. These disorders usually present with proximal weakness, more marked in upper limbs than in lower limbs. The patient complains of weakness, which particularly causes difficulty raising the arms, and getting up from low chairs. There is often difficulty supporting the neck because of weakness of neck extensors, and in getting up from, or turning over in bed. In addition, the muscles are usually painful, swollen and stiff, particularly after exercise. In some cases dysphagia is a feature, and these patients sometimes experience ventilatory difficulties.

Involvement of the skin causes a characteristic violaceous discoloration, particularly evident in regions exposed to light such as cheeks, nose, forehead, chin, knuckles and forearms. This rash may become scaly. Ulceration of the nailbeds, which appear shiny, reddened and oedematous, is sometimes present. Telangiectasia appear on the face and scleroderma-like inflexibility of facial and digital skin is seen. Some patients with dermatomyositis show predominant involvement of the skin, so marked that they present to the dermatologist.

Systemic features, including weight loss and fever, are common. More serious systemic complications, such as fibrosing alveolitis, myocardial involvement and oesophageal involvement may also occur. Other features of multi-system disorder are common, including arthralgias and Raynaud's phenomenon. These features merge into the syndrome of mixed connective tissue disease, in which polymyositis is a well-known component.

Childhood-type dermatomyositis

This serious disorder of childhood consists of a severe inflammatory myositis, almost invariably associated with a rash. The child presents with weakness, fever and lassitude, and proximal muscles are weak, swollen and tender. The cutaneous manifestations are not invariably present from the outset. Involvement of the gastro-intestinal tract with mucosal ulceration and perforation due to vasculitis is much more frequent in this childhood form than in adults. Subcutaneous calcinosis is characteristic, and without appropriate treatment joint contractures are almost invariable. The average age at presentation is 7 years, but some cases present up to 10 years later.

Polymyositis in other autoimmune diseases

Inflammatory myopathy is a component of many autoimmune diseases, e.g. polyarteritis nodosa, systemic lupus erythematosus, rheumatoid arthritis, scleroderma and Sjogren's syndrome, but it is rarely a major feature in these disorders. Primary involvement of muscle is uncommon in these diseases.

Polymyositis/dermatomyositis associated with malignancy

An association between malignant disease and inflammatory myopathy has been recognized for many years. This association is significant only for patients older than 50 years and it is generally not worthwhile to investigate patients with inflammatory myopathy younger than 40 years with this possibility in mind. The association is strongest for small cell carcinoma of the lung, and carcinoma of the gastro-intestinal tract in men, and for carcinoma of the breast or ovary in women, but lymphomas have also been recognized as associated with inflammatory myopathy.

Investigations. Almost all patients with inflammatory myopathies have increased blood CK levels, and this is a useful test in monitoring progress in the long-term management of the disease. The ESR is

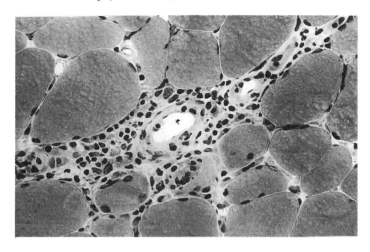

Fig. 14.9 Polymyositis, haematoxylin and eosin. There is infiltration with small lymphocytes, and scattered degenerating and regenerating muscle fibres are seen.

raised in more than half the cases. There may be abnormalities in blood IgG levels, especially in patients with associated autoimmune disease and other antibodies may be detected, e.g. anti Jo1 in patients with pulmonary involvement. The ECG may be abnormal in patients with cardiac involvement.

The diagnosis is usually evident clinically, but may be confirmed by EMG examination which reveals a characteristic combination of neurogenic and myopathic features. The muscle biopsy (Fig. 14.9) reveals muscle fibre necrosis and regeneration with a diffuse or multifocal inflammatory cell and macrophage infiltration. There may be evidence of vasculitis in the biopsy and, in chronic cases, fibrosis and fatty infiltration may be prominent. There are no specific features to the pathological changes in the different types of inflammatory myopathy, although in the *childhood type* vasculitis is prominent, and in *sarcoid myopathy* non-caseating granulomata may be found. Specific subgroups of *eosinophilic myositis*, and of *necrotizing myositis*, an acute severe and often fatal form, are recognized. Some patients show relatively little inflammatory reaction in the biopsy. There is controversy as to the relative contribution of humoral and cell-mediated immunological abnormalities in the aetiology of the disease.

Management. The objective of treatment is to suppress the autoimmune inflammatory process leading to muscle destruction. Initial treatment consists of high-dose steroid therapy, usually with prednisolone 60 mg daily as a single morning dose. Bed rest is necessary, but physiotherapy should be utilized from the earliest phase of treatment in order to prevent joint contractures. Analgesics and local heat are useful. The rare complications of ventilatory failure and cardiomyopathy should be borne in mind. If there is no response to 60 mg prednisolone daily after 4–6 weeks a maximal dose of 2 mg/kg should be tried. The dosage can be gradually reduced after 2–3 months, perhaps by changing to an alternate-day regime, but treatment will need to be continued for 1–2 years. In patients refractory to high-dose steroids azathioprine (50–150 mg daily) may be combined with steroids or a course of intravenous methotrexate may be used. The latter is effective but carries a risk of aplastic anaemia, and of non-bacterial cystitis. Similar treatment regimes are used in all forms of polymyositis, including the childhood-type, with appropriate adjustments of drug dosage. Despite treatment, there is a mortality of about 10%, and residual disability is a problem in about 20% of survivors.

Polymyalgia rheumatica and giant cell arteritis

Polymyalgia rheumatica forms part of the differential diagnosis of polymyositis. There is muscle pain and tenderness, fever and weight loss, but muscle strength is normal. Visual symptoms occur in about 10% of patients, consisting of transient blindness or even retinal infarction. This feature is associated with giant cell arteritis in temporal artery biopsies. Giant cell arteritis may also present with stroke, with claudication of the muscles of mastication, or with headache from ischaemia of the face and scalp.

The ESR is usually very high and there may be a polyclonal increase in IgG, with abnormalities in liver function. The blood CK is normal. In giant cell arteritis treatment with steroids, initially in high dose but later with a low maintenance dose (5–15 mg predisone daily) is effective. The disease is almost confined to people older than 55 years and most patients are women.

Myasthenia gravis

This uncommon disease has a prevalence of 1 in 25 000, and affects women more commonly than men. Myasthenia gravis is an autoimmune disease of the neuromuscular junction. The immunological target is the post-synaptic acetylcholine receptor protein at the motor end-plate. The axonal pre-synaptic component of the nerve terminal is not directly affected by this humorally-mediated, complement-dependent immune process, although it may undergo secondary proliferation in response to the destruction of the post-synaptic part of the end-plate as a compensatory response. The cause of the production of this acetylcholine receptor (AChR) antibody is unknown but presumably relates to abnormalities of the T-cell suppressor/helper system leading to dysregulation of the B cell lymphocyte system. The disease is therefore associated with production of a specific IgG antibody to the nicotinic AChR protein moiety. This antibody can cross the placental barrier leading to temporary myasthenia, of 1–3 weeks duration, in the children of myasthenic mothers.

Clinical features. The disease is characterized by fluctuating weakness and abnormal fatiguability during exercise, with improvement in strength after rest. The severity of these symptoms varies from week to week. The patient is stronger after waking from sleep and weaker at the end of the day. The severity of the symptoms is exacerbated by systemic illness, including common viral illnesses, and by heat so that weakness may be worsened by a hot bath, or by sunbathing.

The external ocular muscles are particularly susceptible; about 40% of cases present with ocular muscle involvement causing ptosis (Fig. 14.10) or diplopia. As the disorder progresses, as happens in most patients, involvement of limb muscles, especially hand and distal arm muscles, becomes prominent but in 16% of cases the disease remains restricted to the external ocular muscles. In 65% of cases symptoms reach their maximum intensity within a year of onset.

On examination there may be weakness of external ocular muscles, facial muscles and upper limb muscles, with ptosis. This weakness is usually asymmetrical. The most characteristic feature is fatiguability. This may be demonstrated by repetitive maximal contraction of an affected muscle group, e.g. by repeatedly clenching

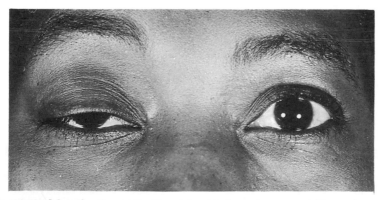

Fig. 14.10 Myasthenia gravis. The right-sided ptosis was variable, and more marked after prolonged upward gaze, illustrating the fatigability characteristic of the disease. Note the compensatory elevation of the right eyebrow denoting overaction of the right frontalis muscle.

the fist, abducting the outstretched arm against resistance, or maintaining full upward or lateral gaze. The observer can often readily detect increasing weakness in the tested muscles during only a minute or so of examination. The tendon reflexes are normal and there is no muscle wasting.

Diagnosis. The level of AChR IgG antibody in the blood is raised in more than 90% of patients with generalized myasthenia and in about 70% of patients with ocular myasthenia. The antibody level correlates only poorly with the severity of the disease.

Pharmacological investigation is useful in establishing the diagnosis and in demonstrating the possibility of treatment to the patient. This test depends on the inhibition of cholinesterase at the motor end-plate thus enhancing the effectiveness of neuromuscular transmission, a cholinergic process. A short-acting anticholinesterase

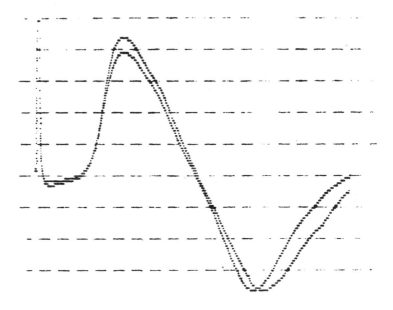

Fig. 14.11 Electromyogram (EMG) in myasthenia gravis. Stimulus artefact to left. After supra-maximal stimulation of the ulnar nerve at the wrist the evoked muscle action potential (MAP) is recorded from the abductor digiti mimin muscle. Stimuli are applied at 0.3 second intervals. The larger amplitude trace was the first MAP recorded, and the smaller was the fourth. The decrement in amplitude between the two traces in this case is 14%, a value consistent with a myasthenic transmission defect at the neuromuscular junctions in this muscle.

drug, edrophonium hydrochloride (Tensilon) is given by incremental intravenous dosage, using 2 mg initially. If no response develops in the muscle group chosen for assessment by another observer in 45 seconds another 2–8 mg is given slowly. If the response is uncertain the test should be repeated using a placebo saline injection so that the two responses can be compared directly.

Electrophysiological tests have high reliability in the diagnosis of myasthenia gravis. Repetitive nerve stimulation at 3 Hz is used to excite a supramaximal response in a muscle. Normally there is no reduction in the amplitude of the evoked muscle response, but in myasthenia gravis the fourth response is reduced in amplitude by 8% or more (Fig. 14.11), indicating progressive failure of successful neuromuscular transmission at diseased motor end-plates. The functional capacity of the neuromuscular junction can also be assessed more directly by measuring the variability in neuromuscular transmission in motor end plates belonging to individual motor units during voluntary contraction; the *neuromuscular jitter*. In addition, intermittent *failure* of neuromuscular transmission is shown by intermittent blocking of muscle action potentials. This test is sufficiently sensitive to reveal abnormalities in clinically normal limb muscles in most patients with ocular myasthenia.

Treatment. There are three components of treatment. Firstly, anticholinesterase drugs are used in order to increase the concentration of acetylcholine in the synaptic cleft, thus improving the effectiveness of neuromuscular transmission at diseased motor end plates. The two most commonly used drugs are neostigmine (15–30 mg), which has a short duration of action and is useful before meals, and pyridostigmine (Mestinon) 60–120 mg three to six times daily. Pyridostigmine has a longer duration of action (2–5 hours) and is therefore suited to regular use. These drugs cause cholinergic unwanted effects, including sweating, abdominal colic and cramps, bradycardia, salivation or urinary urgency, but these effects can be partially prevented with atropine and probanthine.

Secondly, the immunological abnormality can be suppressed with steroids or, on a more long-term basis, with immunosuppressant drugs. Azathioprine (100–150 mg daily) is the safest of the available immunosuppressant drugs. Its effect is delayed for some weeks or months but there is then gradual resolution of myasthenic symptoms. It is necessary to continue treatment indefinitely. Improvement can be followed using electrophysiological or IgG AChR antibody levels. Steroid therapy is useful in patients with severe weakness, particularly when there is respiratory embarrassment. The drug, usually prednisolone, is given in incrementing doses during a 7–14 day period to achieve a dose of 40–60 mg daily or on alternate days. It may be necessary to continue steroid therapy for several months while waiting for co-incident azathioprine therapy to take effect; long-term steroid therapy is rarely necessary except in the most severe cases.

Thirdly, plasma exchange is used to remove circulating anti-AChR antibodies. A course of 4–8 treatments is used and there is usually an improvement in strength within 7–10 days of commencing treatment. This is maintained for 4–8 weeks, providing a convenient window in which other treatments, for example immunosuppression with steroids and azathioprine, or thymectomy, may be undertaken. It is particularly useful in the pre-operative preparation of a patient for thymectomy.

Fourthly, thymectomy is effective in inducing remission, especially during the 2 years after onset of the disease in younger patients, and in improving the natural history of the disease. It is indicated in all patients at the time of diagnosis except, perhaps, those with only very mild ocular symptoms. It improves ocular myasthenia as well as generalized myasthenia. In 10% of patients overall, but in 60% of male patients, there is a thymoma. This is usually a benign tumour, but local spread in the mediastinum occurs occasionally. The prognosis for the myasthenia after excision of thymoma is less good than that of patients with the more common thymic hyperplasia but, clearly, the operation is indicated simply on the basis of the presence of the tumour. The mortality of thymectomy in established cardio-thoracic centres approaches zero.

Myasthenic crisis and cholinergic crisis

Exacerbations of myasthenic weakness (myasthenic crisis) require treatment with anticholinesterase drugs and with plasma exchange or steroids. They occur as a response to viral infection, pregnancy and emotional factors. *Cholinergic crisis* consists of blockade of the neuromuscular receptors by excessive dosage with cholinergic (anticholinesterase) drugs, or by interaction of these drugs with other drugs such as phenytoin and certain antibiotics. Treatment consists of withdrawing anticholinesterase drugs for a few days while recovery occurs. It is thus important to distinguish these two forms of crisis.

In cholinergic crisis fasciculation, sweating, pallor and diarrhoea may occur. The diagnosis, however, rests on the demonstration of a response to edrophonium, given intravenously by 2 mg incremental doses as described above, in patients with myasthenic crisis, and by the absence of response or even dramatic worsening including ventilatory failure, in patients with cholinergic crisis. This 'Tensilon test' should therefore always be carried out in the presence of an experienced assistant, with equipment for temporary, manual ventilation, including an airway, set out ready for use (not locked in a cupboard).

Lambert–Eaton myasthenic syndrome (LEMS)

This syndrome consists of weakness in proximal muscles, especially of the legs, improved initially by exercise, but accompanied by fatiguability during continued exercise. The reflexes are diminished at rest but become brisker after exercise or muscle contraction, and there is almost always a complaint of dry throat. Most cases are older than 40 years. Ocular muscles are invariably spared. The disease is particularly associated with small cell carcinoma of the bronchus. An association with cancer has been reported in 70% of men and 25% of women. Thus half the cases are not associated with malignant disease; there is evidence that these are due to an autoimmune disorder, with IgG antibody binding to an unspecified presynaptic ACh release receptor.

The diagnosis is established electrophysiologically. During repetitive nerve stimulation there may be a slight decrement in the evoked muscle action potential resembling that found in myasthenia gravis. However, at faster frequencies of stimulation, e.g. 20 Hz, there is a marked incrementing response, the amplitude of the evoked muscle action potential increasing severalfold. A similar effect is found after a short voluntary contraction. This response indicates fluctuating, stimulus-sensitive, release of ACh neurotransmitter from the preterminal axonal release sites in the motor end-plate.

Management. A search for underlying malignant disease, usually pulmonary neoplasm, is essential. Treatment of the neoplasm, however, has little or no effect on the LEMS, and anaesthetic management is difficult during surgery. Drug treatment of the end-plate disorder consists of guanidine or 3,4-diaminopyridine therapy, but both these drugs are potentially toxic, causing bone-marrow depression and epilepsy respectively. Plasma exchange and steroid therapy have shown encouraging results, especially in auto-immune cases, although the response is not as rapid as in myasthenia gravis. Azathioprine is also useful in the latter cases.

Congenital myasthenic syndromes

Several myasthenia-like syndromes have been described in which weakness and fatiguability, with prominent extraocular and facial weakness, with difficulty breathing, have been noted from birth. These disorders, associated with several different specific abnormalities in ACh receptor function, show varying responses to anticholinesterase drug treatment.

15

Spinal Cord and Nerve Root Disorders

The spinal cord extents from the foramen magnum to the second lumbar vertebra. Like the brain, it is surrounded by meninges. It retains its segmental anatomical organization, each segment having ventral motor and dorsal sensory roots. These segments are associated with vertebrae, as shown by the exit of the mixed sensorimotor nerve roots through the intervertebral foramina. The spinal cord receives a rich blood supply from aortic and vertebral artery feeder vessels, which anastomose along the spinal cord in the anterior and posterior spinal artery circulations.

The spinal cord is susceptible to diseases of the central nervous system, of which it is a part, and also to tumours arising in or metastatic to the vertebrae, or meninges. Disease of the vertebral column and intervertebral discs may cause disability from damage to the spinal cord, conus medullaris, cauda equina or nerve roots. This is the commonest cause of spinal or nerve root disorder. The disorders that affect the spinal cord and nerve roots are listed in Table 15.1. Many of these disorders affect both nerve roots and spinal cord and the localization of the nerve root lesion is thus particularly important in determining the level of the disease within the spinal column.

Root disease and vertebral pain syndromes

The clinical problem of root pain is inevitably related to that of low back pain, a disorder which accounts for 25% of consultations in general practice and which causes the loss of 30 million working days/year in the UK. More than half the adult population have experienced low back pain. Nerve pain is slightly less common, affecting 30% of the population. In management of painful root syndromes it is important to distinguish specific root disorders from non-specific pain in the spine or paravertebral regions. Pain syndromes from vertebral, intervertebral disc or root disease

Table 15.1 *Disorders of the nerve roots and spinal cord.*

Root disease
  spondylosis and disc prolapse syndromes
  tumours, e.g. neurofibroma, metastases
  trauma
  infection; H. zoster radiculopathy
         neuralgic amyotrophy (see Chapter 13)

Spinal compression syndromes
  cervical spondylosis
  canal stenosis
  intervertebral disc prolapse
  extra-medullary spinal tumours
    e.g. meningioma, neurofibroma, metastatic tumours
  infections, e.g. tuberculous extradural abscess
  spinal trauma
  congenital dysraphism
    e.g spina bifida, meningomyelocele

Intrinsic cord syndromes
  multiple sclerosis
  syringomyelia
  intrinsic spinal tumours,
    e.g. astrocytoma, ependymoma
  degenerative disorders,
    e.g. vitamin B_{12} deficiency, Friedreich's ataxia, motor neuron disease
  vascular lesions
    spinal infarction, spinal angioma
  infections
    e.g.post-viral myelopathy, syphilis, tropical paraplegia, AIDS
  radiation myelopathy
  decompression sickness

are most frequently cervical or lumbosacral; thoracic disc disease is relatively uncommon.

These syndromes result from spondylosis, osteophyte formation, degenerative joint disease and intervertebral disc degeneration and prolapse. In older people osteoporosis is also a contributory factor, and other acquired vertebral diseases, especially metastatic cancer or infection can produce similar symptoms. People with developmental stenosis of the vertebral canal (canal stenosis) are particularly susceptible to pain syndromes and cord compression as age-related degenerative changes further encroach on the spinal canal and intervertebral foramina. Canal stenosis is usually associated with short stature, short neck, shortness of the limbs and an unusually straight spine with loss of cervical and lumbar lordosis.

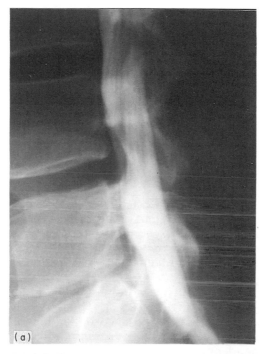

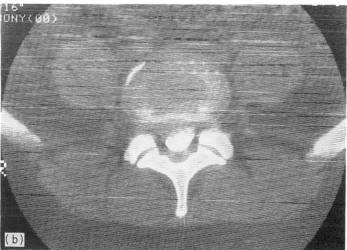

Fig. 15.1 Lumbar disc protrusion at L4/5. (a) Myelogram (radiculogram); there is indentation of the contrast column at the L4/5 disc interspace. (b) CT myelogram; the asymmetrical disc protrusion displaces the contrast posteriorly on the right, and is encroaching laterally on the nerve root as it exits the intervertebral foramen.

Achondroplasia, complete or partial, is frequently accompanied by canal stenosis, with neurological complications.

Spondylosis refers to degeneration of intervertebral discs, leading to narrowing of the intervertebral discs with osteoarthritis of the intervertebral and paravertebral joints. This radiological change is present in most people older than 50 years, especially at the C5/6, C6/7, L4/5 and L5/S1 disc interspaces. These interspaces are subject to particular mechanical stresses in relation to spinal movement and the upright posture, especially in manual labourers and nurses. The discs themselves carry most of the large forces acting through the spine during ordinary activities. This function depends on the water and proteoglycan content of the disc, which decreases with age, and on its ligamentous margins.

Low back pain results from osteoarthrosis of the spine, or from minor disc prolapse in which part of the nucleus pulposus herniates through the disc margin, projecting posteriorly into the spinal canal or posterolaterally toward the intervertebral foramen. This may produce local spinal pain and tenderness, with paravertebral muscle spasm. If the disc prolapse is more extensive, nerve root compression will result, causing radicular syndromes related to the distribution of the root compression (Fig. 15.1). Thus there will be pain, weakness, sensory loss and absence of tendon reflexes in the appropriate distribution. These features are often not all present together, dependent on the severity, suddenness and duration of the intervertebral disc prolapse, and also on the presence of other factors, especially severe pre-existing spondylosis and canal stenosis, both of which tend to cause more severe disability since there is less available space to accommodate the prolapsed disc material (Table 15.2).

Large or central disc protrusions in the cervical and thoracic spine may cause cord compression, with root syndromes at the level of the disc prolapse marking the clinical level. In the lumbosacral spinal canal central disc lesions may cause compression of the conus medullaris leading to numbness of the seat area with acute incontinence or retention of urine and faeces, and buttock pain, with extensor plantar responses; or to cauda equina compression causing acute sphincter disturbance with sensory loss in the perineum. These syndromes represent neurological emergencies since delay in treatment may often result in permanent, severe disability.

Sciatica and root pain

Sciatica is the commonest and best-known root pain. There is pain in the buttock and in the posterior aspect of the thigh, which may extend into the lower leg and lateral aspect of the foot. It is worsened by exercise and movement and, especially, by stretching the nerve,

Table 15.2 *Main features of root syndromes.*

	Pain	Sensory loss	Predominant weakness	Reflex loss
Cervical syndromes				
C5	Shoulder tip	Deltoid region	Deltoid	—
C6	Thumb and index	Lateral forearm and hand	Biceps Brachioradialis Wrist extension Abduction of wrist	Biceps
C7	Dorsal forearm	(Inconstant)	Triceps Metacarpo-phalangeal extension Flexion of wrist	Triceps
C8	Fourth and fifth fingers	Medial forearm and hand	Interphalangeal extension and flexion Adduction of wrist	Finger jerk
T1	Axilla	Medial upper arm	Intrinsic hand muscles	—
Thoracic syndromes				
	Radicular chest and back	Radicular	Often undetectable	—
Lumbo-sacral syndromes				
L4	Anterior thigh	Anteromedial thigh and knee	Quadriceps Dorsiflexion large toe	Knee jerk
L5	Lateral thigh and shin	Lateral shin and dorsal foot	Eversion of foot Foot drop and toe drop Inversion of foot	—
S1	Buttock, posterior thigh and leg	Lateral foot	Plantar flexion Eversion of foot	Ankle jerk
Lower sacral	Buttock and perineum	Perineal buttock and posterior thigh and calf	Pelvic floor and sphincter Intrinsic foot muscles	Anal reflex Cremasteric reflex

for example during active or passive hip flexion (Lasègue's sign). The pain consists of an aching discomfort together with a shooting, burning component that is exacerbated by movement. Sciatica is related to irritation of the L5 or S1 nerve roots. Similar pain arises in other roots, radiating in their distribution, and C5, C6 and C7 are particularly commonly affected because of the frequency of cervical spondylosis. Similar pains occur from root irritation due to diverse causes, e.g. disc prolapse, spondylosis, trauma, Herpes zoster infection, and metastatic neoplasm with nerve root encroachment. There is often sensory impairment, weakness and a reduced tendon reflex in the appropriate distribution (see Table 15.2).

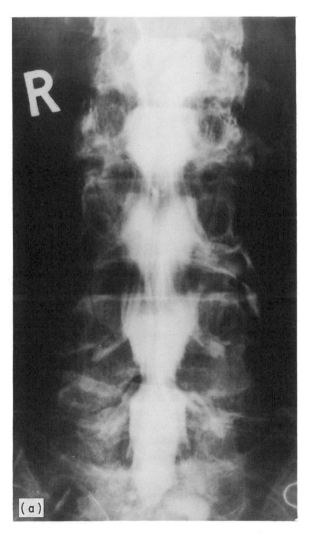

Fig. 15.2(a)

Canal stenosis and spondylosis

When the spinal canal is congenitally narrow, as occurs in achondroplasia, and in about 10% of normal subjects, the nerve roots and spinal cord are particularly vulnerable to compressive injury from additional narrowing of the canal and its lateral recesses near the intervertebral foramina (Fig. 15.2) due to spondylosis, trauma or other disease processes. Most affected people have a rather straight spine, and a strikingly short neck, and many are of short stature. There is often a history of heavy manual labour, or of cervical and lumbar disc or joint pain. In the lumbo-sacral region only nerve roots will be compressed but in the cervical canal both nerve roots and spinal cord may be affected, producing a combination of nerve root and cord symptoms (radiculomyelopathy).

In *lumbar canal stenosis* the commonest symptom is neurospinous claudication. This consists of cramp-like or aching pain induced by standing or walking, felt in the buttock, thigh or leg and relieved by rest. It is often bilateral. The pain may also be relieved by fully extending the spine. Investigation reveals radiological features of

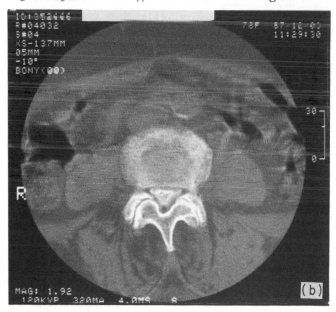

Fig. 15.2 Lumbar canal stenosis. (a) *(opposite)* Myelogram. There is segmental narrowing of the column of contrast adjacent to each intervertebral disc space, with general narrowing of the column more caudally. (b) *(above)* CT myelogram. The vertebral body appears normal, but the spinal canal is stenosed and triangular in cross-sectional area, with marked narrowing of the intervertebral foramina.

lumbo-sacral spondylosis, with a narrow canal in the sagittal plane, and often with lumbar disc prolapse. Clinically there may be features of radicular involvement, with reduced ankle or knee jerks.

In *cervical canal stenosis*, which is commonly associated with lumbo-sacral canal stenosis, there is a combination of root and cord features. Some patients, however, may have clinical problems restricted to radicular or cord involvement. The sagittal diameter of the cord is less than 15 mm at the C6 level, and there is often associated disc prolapse and narrowing. The radicular component usually involves C6, C7 and C8 nerve roots (see Table 15.3), but this is often minimal in relation to presentation with a slowly progressive paraplegia. The latter is often not associated with major sensory loss but, later, bladder involvement develops (see Table 15.2). Sometimes the cord syndrome may be greatly worsened or even initiated by trauma to the spine, as in a whiplash injury.

Cervical canal stenosis is also a feature of ankylosing spondylitis and rheumatoid arthritis, in which subluxation of the atlanto-occipital or atlanto-axial joints may encroach on the cord at the foramen magnum level. In many patients with cervical canal stenosis the whole cervical canal is narrowed, although the C5/6 and C6/7 levels are usually most severely affected.

The aetiology of cord involvement is controversial. Direct mechanical compression, repeated injury from compression in full flexion, impairment of arterial circulation and impairment of venous return from the cord have all been suggested as causative factors.

Investigation and management

The cause of root lesions is often evident from clinical examination, especially when trauma or H. zoster are implicated. Investigation requires plain X-rays of the spine, which may reveal narrowing of disc spaces, calcification of discs, and the features of osteoarthritis and canal stenosis. CT scanning has become increasingly used to demonstrate disc prolapse, both with and without CSF enhancement with intrathecal contrast agents (Fig. 15.1). Magnetic resonance imaging promises to supplant both these investigations and also to replace myelography since it demonstrates cord, roots and discs without invasive procedures or X-ray exposure. EMG evaluation can be useful in defining the extent of root involvement, both motor and sensory, by using needle EMG and sensory evoked potential techniques. X-ray evaluation remains important because it may reveal unexpected pathology such as tuberculosis or metastatic cancer.

Management of spondylotic or disc prolapse syndromes is usually conservative, consisting of rest, and immobilization of the neck by a collar and of the lumbar spine by bed rest on a firm mattress. This is followed, when there is resolution of pain, by progressive mobilization using passive range of motion exercises and active exercises to strengthen paraspinal muscles and encourage spinal mobility. This programme should be continued even when recovery has occurred. Exercises such as swimming may be particularly well tolerated. Analgesics are indicated during the early phase of treatment. Traction is used by some physiotherapists.

Surgical exploration is justified:
1. when medical treatment fails in the presence of motor and sensory signs of radicular involvement
2. when there is cauda equina compression
3. for neurospinous claudication
4. when there is progressive myelopathy associated with cervical canal stenosis
5. in some patients with instability of the spine, e.g. in C1/C2 rheumatoid arthritis or lumbo-sacral spondylolisthesis.
6. to explore suspected paravertebral abscess or cancer for diagnostic purposes.

Cord syndromes (myelopathies)

Intrinsic and extrinsic (compressive) cord syndromes may arise acutely or develop chronically. In assessing these myelopathies it is important to establish whether the disease process is intrinsic or extrinsic (see Table 15.3) and the upper level of the lesion. The latter is especially important since it enables investigation to be planned appropriately in terms of visualizing the likely cause by radiological means, and provides a baseline for assessing the progress of treatment. The upper level is determined clinically by sensory or motor examination. Less commonly, reflex changes may be useful. The sensory level itself may be misleading since the lamination of sensory fibres in the spinothalamic tracts and posterior columns is such that the level of sensory disturbance may be many segments caudal to the level of the lesion. Thus patients with a thoracic sensory

Table 15.3 *Clinical features of the development of intrinsic and extrinsic cord tumours.*

Intrinsic lesions	Extrinsic lesions
Incontinence/retention of urine	Root pain, worsened by movement
Dissociated sensory loss	Progressive asymmetrical paraparesis
Spinothalamic pain	Brown-Séquard syndrome
Bilateral pyramidal signs	Paraplegia with sensory level
Paraplegia and sensory level	Incontinence

level should be investigated by myelography extending to the cervical region.

Intrinsic and extrinsic spinal cord disease

The clinical features of intrinsic and extrinsic cord disease differ. Intrinsic disorders may be highly specific, affecting particular spinal pathways as in Friedreich's ataxia and subacute combined degeneration (vitamin B_{12} deficiency), in which the posterior columns and corticospinal tracts are selectively affected; or the corticospinal tracts and anterior horn cells, as in motor neuron disease.

When tumours arise intrinsically within the spinal cord, e.g. spinal cord astrocytoma, there is a typical sequence of symptoms and signs as the disease progresses that is, broadly, the converse of that found in patients with extrinsic compression syndromes. Both intrinsic and extrinsic spinal cord disorders may lead to spastic paraplegia but the mode of development of the clinical features is strikingly different in the two disorders (Table 15.3).

Intrinsic lesions tend to present with features of involvement of centrally-placed pathways, e.g. those subserving bladder function and the spinothalamic sensory system. Extrinsic lesions often involve nerve roots, causing root pain, a feature of localizing importance, together with asymmetrical paraparesis, or the syndrome of hemicompression of the cord described by Brown-Séquard. Paraplegia and incontinence develop in the last stages of compressive myelopathy (Table 15.2). The Brown-Séquard syndrome consists of contralateral impairment of pain and temperature sensation, (with an upper level marked by a zone of hyperpathia representing irritation of the compressed segment) and ipsilateral impairment of light touch and vibration sense (posterior column disturbance) and of corticospinal tract function below the level of the lesion.

Investigation of cord syndromes

Many of the disorders of the spinal cord listed in Table 15.1 can be recognized by their clinical features (see below). Investigation is needed to confirm this diagnosis, and to localize tumours or other surgically treatable conditions, e.g. prolapsed disc, extradural infection or rheumatoid spine with subluxation. Plain X-rays of the spine will often provide useful information, especially the presence of an extradural mass or bone destruction at the level of the lesion. Narrowing of the spinal canal in cervical myelopathy due to spondylosis with canal stenosis, and widening of the canal in syringomyelia can be recognized. In neurofibromatosis scalloping of the posterior margins of the vertebral bodies (Fig. 15.3), or

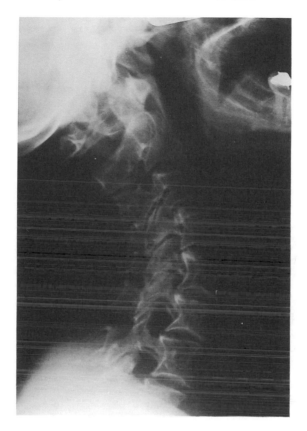

Fig. 15.3 Neurofibromatosis. Lateral X-ray of cervical spine. There is a scalloped outline to the anterior border of the vertebral bodies, with enlarged intervertebral foramina. The latter are indicative of the presence of neurofibromas arising from the posterior roots in these locations.

widening of intervertebral foramina associated with neurofibroma arising on a nerve root may be seen. Arteriovenous malformations of vertebrae, or Paget's disease may be evident and multiple metastases, e.g. from carcinoma of the prostate, may cause lytic or sclerotic lesions. Infections often involve intervertebral discs rather than the bodies of the vertebrae.

Exact localization of cord disorders can be achieved in the case of extrinsic, compressive lesions by myelography and CT scanning, before or after intrathecal contrast. MR imaging is useful in detecting extrinsic and intrinsic lesions (Fig. 15.4) especially syringomyelia and demyelination.

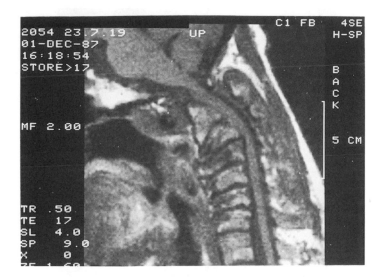

Fig. 15.4 MRI cervical spondylosis. The upper six cervical vertebrae are abnormal in shape, with loss of intervertebral disc space, and angulation in flexion at the C2/C3 and C4 levels. The cervical canal in this region is narrowed, causing deformity, angulation and focal thinning of the spinal cord. The patient had a paraplegia with features of a cervical lesion.

Spinal compression syndromes

Myelopathies due to spinal compression are relatively common (Table 15.1) and are important because surgical decompression by laminectomy, with removal of the cause of the compression, can be curative. The first successful such operation was carried out by Sir Victor Horsley in 1886 in a patient with spinal meningioma diagnosed by Sir William Gowers. In all cord compression syndromes early treatment is imperative. Cases with a slowly progressive onset generally recover more completely than those with a rapidly progressive course. Paraplegia accompanied by retention of urine with overflow is unlikely to recover completely. The progressive development of the typical syndrome (Table 15.3) is therefore particularly important in diagnosis.

Cervical myelopathy due to spondylosis

There are three common syndromes:
  1. Symmetrical quadriparesis with spasticity of the limbs, but with little weakness, and with intense paraesthesiae in the

hands. This syndrome is due to a high cervical lesion, often with multiple levels of cord compression about C5/6 level.

2. Brown-Séquard syndrome (see above).
3. Spastic paraparesis with wasting of muscles in the upper limbs, especially triceps and intrinsic hand muscles. These muscles are weak and the triceps tendon reflex is absent. Sensory loss in the upper limbs is inconstant but may be found in a root distribution, usually C6 or C8, or affecting both hands. The latter suggests compression of the posterior columns. In some patients wasting of the hands occurs with high cord compression as a result of interference with venous drainage from the lower cervical segments. Bladder symptoms are a late feature implying the need for immediate surgery.

These clinical syndromes develop insidiously and painlessly. In some patients there is a history of rapid deterioration following minor cervical trauma and in most patients there is marked reduction in the range of cervical movement to passive and active assessment. Cervical root pain is relatively infrequent unless the syndrome is due to cervical intervertebral disc protrusion rather than spondylosis and congenital spinal canal stenosis. Canal stenosis is present when the sagittal diameter is less than 15 mm at the C4–C7 level.

Management. In the early stages, or if the cord syndrome seems not to be progressive, conservative management by collar immobilization of the neck may be helpful. However, patients with significant disability, and especially those with a progressive course, should be treated by decompressive laminectomy at the appropriate level. Some patients, particularly those with localized disease, can be treated by an anterior surgical approach rather than by laminectomy. In this procedure (Cloward's operation) the disc material at the appropriate level is removed anteriorly via the neck, and the adjacent vertebral bodies are fused with a dowel of bone taken from the iliac crest.

Intervertebral disc prolapse

Central disc protrusions in the cervical or thoracic regions may lead to cord compression. Central lumbar disc lesions can cause conus compression. These lesions develop suddenly, in response to hyperextension or torsional trauma, but the causative trauma may be barely significant. In most patients the history of cord damage is shorter than 3 months. Sudden paraplegia associated with disc prolapse is usually painless and multiple sclerosis may be suggested as a more likely diagnosis, emphasising the importance of thorough investigation of patients presenting with paraplegia. Posterior column features may predominate over motor dysfunction.

Management. The diagnosis is established radiologically, by CT scanning and myelography, or by MR imaging (Fig. 15.4). Laminectomy, or anterior discectomy results in rapid improvement in most cases.

Extramedullary spinal tumours

Compression of the cord by tumour may occur with extradural or intradural tumours. Extradural tumours are usually metastatic, especially carcinoma, lymphoma or myeloma. Intradural tumours are more frequently benign, especially meningioma and neurofibroma, but metastases may also occur in the intradural space (Table 15.4).

Extradural compression by malignant tumour is often of rapid onset (Fig. 15.5), in a few days. There may be a prodromal period of a few weeks with localized spinal pain and root pain, but the sinister significance of these symptoms is often not appreciated until paraplegia develops. Surgical decompression of malignant metastatic cord compression often fails to relieve the paraplegia; the prognosis is largely determined by the distribution of metastases in other organs. Although biopsy may be required to establish the diagnosis, when the paraplegia is the presenting symptom treatment with steroids and high-dose, but short-course radiotherapy to relieve pain is more effective than surgery. Patients with paraplegia due to cord compression from lymphoma or myeloma, however, may improve rapidly with radiotherapy and this is the treatment of choice in these patients. Sometimes nerve roots may be infiltrated by metastatic tumour (Fig. 15.6).

Table 15.4   *Spinal tumours.*

Extramedullary tumours
  Extradural:
    metastases, especially lungs, breast,
      prostate, thyroid
    lymphoma and Hodgkin's disease
    plasmacytoma (myeloma)
  Intradural:
    neurofibroma
    meningioma
    sacral ependymoma and lipoma

Intramedullary tumours
  ependymoma
  astrocytoma
  oligodendroglioma
  teratoma
  metastases and lymphomas

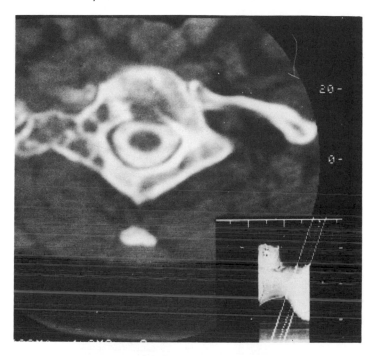

Fig. 15.5 CT myelogram of lower cervical spine in a woman with a painful right-sided brachial root syndrome. There is erosion of the lateral part of the vertebra by metastatic carcinoma. The primary tumour was in the breast.

Surgical removal of neurofibroma or meningioma is usually followed by virtually complete recovery, provided that the surgical treatment is carried out before the cord syndrome becomes complete, especially before bladder involvement develops. In patients with von Recklinghausen's syndrome there may be multiple spinal tumours, and further operations may be required. Meningiomas (Fig. 15.7) arise in the subarachnoid space from arachnoid cells and neurofibromas arise in the subdural space from the Schwann cells of the posterior nerve roots. The latter often present, therefore, with a long history of root pain before the tumour reaches a size sufficient to compress the spinal cord. Spinal meningiomas are mainly found in the thoracic spine of middle-aged women (Fig. 15.7), and neurofibromas in the cervical spine of patients with Type 1 neurofibromatosis.

Spinal compression due to infection

Tuberculosis of the spine (Fig. 6.4), arising in the intervertebral disc or vertebral plate, or in the extradural space, may cause spinal

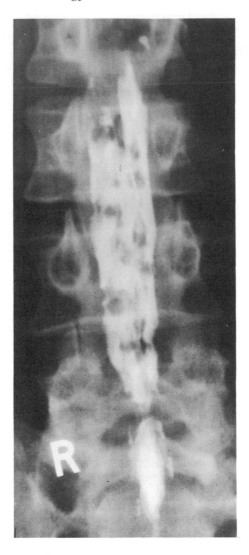

Fig. 15.6 Myelogram. Metastatic deposits on the cauda equina nerve roots.

cord compression. There is invariably an associated paraspinal mass, representing a tuberculous abscess. In the lumbar region this may track beneath the psoas muscle towards the inguinal ligament. In addition to cord involvement there is frequently subacute spinal tuberculous meningitis with tuberculous radiculopathy, producing a mixed neurological syndrome of spastic paraplegia with lumbosacral root involvement and local pain. Systemic features, with fever

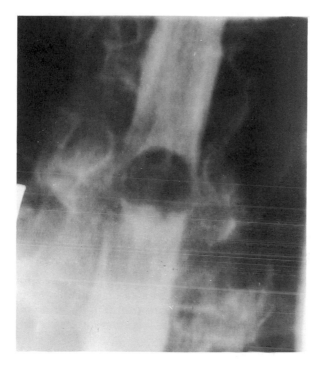

Fig. 15.7 Myelogram. Thoracic intraspinal meningioma in a middle-aged woman presenting with a slowly progressive paraparesis. The negative shadow of the meningioma is clearly seen, outlined against the column of contrast. Recovery followed surgical removal of the tumour.

and weight loss, develop. Tuberculous paraplegia (Pott's disease) is uncommon in Western countries but remains a serious problem in countries where tuberculosis is frequent.

Pyogenic spinal abscess and osteomyelitis is an acute disease. The abscess is usually metastatic from the lungs or from bacterial endocarditis. There is local pain and tenderness in the spine, with paraplegia when the cord becomes involved, together with features of a systemic infection.

Management. Early treatment of spinal tuberculosis with antituberculous chemotherapy or antibiotics as appropriate is indicated. Pyogenic spinal abscess is usually due to staphylococcal or streptococcal infection and responds to penicillin, chloramphenicol or cephalosporins. Surgical exploration and drainage is usually necessary and, if the spine is unstable, a fusion procedure is indicated during the healing phase, following a period of immobilization in a back support and bedrest. The prognosis for functional recovery is excellent.

Rheumatoid arthritis and ankylosing spondylitis

These two disorders cause marked spinal deformity. In *rheumatoid arthritis* the cervical spine becomes unstable from damage to intervertebral and paravertebral joints. This results in subluxation at multiple levels, including the atlanto-axial and atlanto-occipital joints, with cord compression that may lead to progressive quadriplegia or even to sudden irreversible quadriplegia. The latter may follow minor trauma. Surgical fixation of the unstable cervical spine requires complex orthopaedic and neurosurgical management and is often not followed by useful neurological improvement.

In *ankylosing spondylitis* the spine is rigid and vulnerable to trauma, leading to paraplegia or quadriplegia. A cauda equina syndrome may develop, probably due to arachnoiditis associated with the disease involving the lumbosacral nerve roots.

Achondroplasia and narrow canal syndrome

Patients with *achondroplasia* have congenitally narrow spinal canals and are likely to develop progressive paraplegia in adult life. Laminectomy, often very extensive, is useful in restoring movement, by relieving the cord compression. Trauma may precipitate sudden deterioration.

Spinal trauma

In the UK there are about 350 new cases of spinal cord injury causing paraplegia or quadriplegia every year; 80% of these are due to road traffic accidents or falls and 60% are younger than 30 years of age. Not all spinal cord injuries are associated with a spinal fracture, since the cord lesion can result from concussion or contusion of the cord, or from haemorrhage into the cord (haematomyelia). Concussive cord injuries are relatively common in contact sports, e.g. rugby, and are often associated with forced hyperextension (Fig. 15.8). Recovery, partial or complete, may occur in a few minutes or during several days.

Patients with unstable spinal fractures are vulnerable to cord injury *after* the initial injury if the neck or spine is moved, and care in lifting and moving such patients from the place of injury to hospital and during subsequent clinical and radiological investigation is essential. Patients with pre-existing spinal canal stenosis, spondylosis, rheumatoid disease or ankylosing spondylitis are especially at risk of cord injury.

Management. Little can be done to promote recovery. In some patients with unstable injuries surgical fixation may be important,

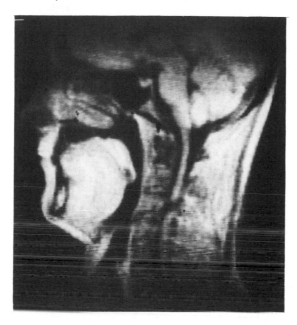

Fig. 15.8 MRI cervical spine in a traumatic cord injury. There is loss of continuity of the spinal cord at the C4 level. The patient sustained a quadriplegia in a rugby accident.

after initial evaluation, in preventing further spinal cord damage. Management consists of recognizing the inevitable paralysis and sensory loss and loss of bladder and bowel control, in preventing bedsores, and in promoting improved muscle strength in the upper limbs in patients with paraplegia in order to aid wheelchair mobility and self-caring. A long period of rehabilitation and re-education is necessary to achieve social independence and the capacity for earning.

Congenital dysraphism (see Chapter 18)

Intrinsic cord syndromes

Diseases of the spinal cord itself (Fig. 15.9) (Table 15.1) or of its blood supply causes a cord syndrome which develops in a different pattern from that typically occurring with extrinsic compressive cord syndromes (Table 15.3). When the intrinsic disease process is localized to a given segment the clinical features are referable to that level, but other conditions in which the disorder is more diffuse,

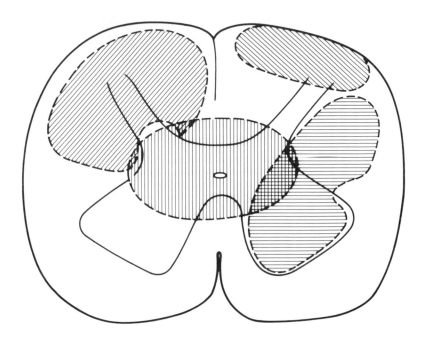

Friedreich's ataxia and subacute combined degeneration (B_{12} deficiency)

Syringomyelia

Tabes dorsalis

Amyotrophic lateral sclerosis (motor neuron disease)

Fig. 15.9 Cord syndromes. The diagram illustrates the sites of damage in five cord syndromes. These disorders are bilaterally symmetrical.

e.g. subacute combined degeneration of the cord, or post-viral myelopathy, cause clinical features without clearly defined motor or sensory upper level and consistent with extensive rather than localized disease.

Myelopathy in multiple sclerosis (Chapter 9)

The cord is frequently involved in multiple sclerosis. The demyelinating lesion is most commonly located in the cervical cord. Lesions in the conus medullaris and sacral cord are probably more frequent than has so far been recognized, presenting with retention or incontinence of urine or faeces. The most frequent syndrome is chronic progressive myelopathy with paraparesis, bladder disturbance and variable involvement of the upper limbs. An acute transverse myelitis, in which demyelination develops rapidly in one or two contiguous segments of the cord, is also a feature of the disease, although it may also occur as an isolated syndrome without clinical features of multiple lesions, or in association with optic neuritis (Devic's syndrome). These syndromes are discussed in Chapter 9.

Syringomyelia

In this condition a cyst-like cavity forms in the spinal cord, lined by glia and often extending rostrally into the medulla (syringobulbia). The cavity lies close to the central canal and is usually situated in the cervical cord, extending into the upper thoracic cord in many cases (Figs 15.9 and 15.10). This cavity is often associated with malformations in the brain at the foramen magnum and in the posterior fossa, especially with congenital extension of the cerebellar tonsils into the foramen magnum (Chiari type 1 malformation), cerebellar ectopia and communicating hydrocephalus (Arnold–Chiari malformation), occult hydrocephalus with or without aqueductal

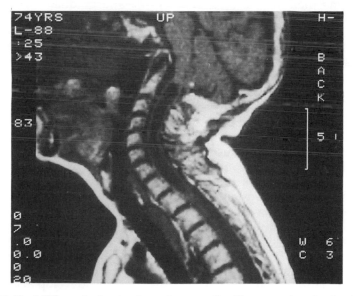

Fig. 15.10 MRI cervical spine in syringomyelia. The central cavity (syrinx) extends from the cervico-medullary junction to the C8/T1 level. The cerebellum is of an abnormal configuration, with herniation of the abnormal tonsils into the foramen magnum.

stenosis, and acquired hydrocephalus due to basal arachnoidal adhesions. The cavity in the cord communicates with the CSF pathway in the fourth ventricle and it is believed that the cyst develops as a consequence of transmitted vascular pressure waves in the CSF acting upon the spinal cord substance, which has low resistance to such forces. In another form of the condition a similar cystic cavity develops in association with cord trauma, intrinsic cord tumours and spinal arachnoiditis. A 'non-communicating' syrinx can also be due to a local ischaemic, exudative or degenerative process.

Clinical features. The clinical features can be related to the site of the cord cavity. Since this lesion is located paracentrally in the cord, the patient often notices wasting of one hand from loss of anterior horn cells in the ventral horn. There is impaired sensation to pinprick and temperature in the opposite limb, but normal touch, vibration and position sense. This 'dissociated sensory loss' is due to interruption of the decussating spinothalamic fibres at the level of the cavity. As the lesion extends in the transverse plane of the cord the area of dissociated sensory loss affects approximately homologous zones of skin on the two sides of the body and begins to affect the lower limbs by involvement of the spinothalamic tracts, affecting the lumbosacral segments first and gradually ascending toward the upper zone of radicular dissociated sensory loss. The sacral segments are represented mesially in the spinothalamic tracts. As the cavity becomes bigger, involvement of posterior columns and corticospinal tracts occurs, causing spastic paraplegia and impaired position and vibration sense in the legs and, to a lesser extent, in the hands. Involvement of the descending fibres in the spinal tract of the trigeminal pathway leads to dissociated sensory loss on the face beginning around the nose. Horner's syndrome, and wasting of the tongue are features of syringobulbia. This may also involve cerebellar pathways, causing nystagmus and limb ataxia.

In the classical syndrome examination will thus disclose a patient with nystagmus, wasting of the tongue, Horner's syndrome, dissociated facial sensory loss, wasting of the hands with absence of upper limb reflexes, a 'cape-like' zone of dissociated sensory loss involving at least the C4–6 segments, and spastic paraplegia. The disorder is usually asymmetrical and most cases do not show this fully developed syndrome. Pain is common in the early stages from irritation of the spinothalamic pathways, and this may be very severe. Trophic joint and cutaneous lesions may develop in affected regions.

Management. The diagnosis can most easily be confirmed by MR imaging of the cord in the sagittal plane (Fig. 15.10). Surgical treatment, by shunting CSF into the peritoneum, helps some patients by controlling pain and preventing progression of the disorder. When there is hydrocephalus this should be treated by ventriculo-atrial or ventriculo-peritoneal CSF shunting with a Pudenz or Holter valve. Posterior fossa decompression has also been advocated. These procedures may halt progression and result in some improvement, especially in pain. Other features are rarely relieved.

Intrinsic cord tumours

Intrinsic tumours of the cord are uncommon but there are many different types. Primary tumours, e.g. ependymoma, astrocytoma and epidermoid tumours, are usually located in the sacral cord, perhaps representing the result of defective neural crest migration. They are slowly progressive lesions during several years, causing lumbosacral weakness and sensory loss with prominent bladder, anorectal and sexual problems. Treatment by surgical excision and radiotherapy can arrest progression of symptoms and result in improvement. These tumours are histologically benign but tend to recur. Intrinsic tumours also occur more rostrally and metastases, e.g. from carcinoma of the breast or lymphomas, may also present with progressive cord syndromes.

Arteriovenous malformations

Spinal angiomas are uncommon. They are usually situated in the dura overlying the cord, but may extend into the cord circulation itself, or involve the cord by compression from large, tortuous, arterialized veins, or by shunting blood away from the cord, thus causing patchy infarction of segments of the cord. The thoracic cord is the commonest region to be affected. There is a slowly progressive paraplegia punctuated by episodes of deterioration usually associated with pain and incontinence. This syndrome is often attributed to demyelination but the recurrent symptoms *at the same spinal level* should suggest angioma as the likely diagnosis. In a few patients spinal subarachnoid haemorrhage with sudden, severe, persistent spinal pain and paraspinal muscle spasm occurs. The diagnosis is made by recognition of the malformation during myelography and CT scanning, by the presence of xanthochromic CSF with a raised CSF protein level, and by selective spinal angiography. Many such lesions can be satisfactorily removed surgically since the arteriovenous connection is dural, rather than intramedullary, in location. Considerable clinical recovery from neurological deficit may follow surgical excision of the lesion.

Spinal infarction

The spinal circulation is derived from anastomotic circumferential vessels, consisting of branches from the anterior and posterior spinal arteries. The anterior circulation is larger than the posterior, supplying all the spinal cord apart from the posterior columns and posterior horns. The anterior spinal artery circulation in the cervical and upper thoracic region is derived from the vertebral arteries and from small branches arising from inferior thyroid and costocervical arteries. The lower thoracic and lumbar cord is perfused by intercostal and lumbar branches of the aorta. This circulation is dependent on a major tributary in the lower thoracic region, the artery of Adamkiewicz. The lowest part of the spinal circulation is derived from internal iliac branches.

This complex, segmental arrangement of cord circulation implies susceptibility to perfusion failure in its various parts. Thus, vertebral occlusion can cause an anterior spinal artery sydrome in the cervico-thoracic region; aortic dissection may infarct the thoracic cord; iliac occlusion may damage the sacral cord; and perfusion of the Adamkiewicz vessel is crucial to the thoraco-lumbar spinal circulation, e.g. during aortic surgery or during balloon assist pump treatment for circulatory failure after myocardial infarction. The prognosis of cord infarction is poor.

Infarction in the anterior cord circulation causes spastic or flaccid paraplegia; the latter develops if the cord is infarcted in length so that no voluntary or reflex function is possible. There is loss of spino-thalamic sensation and of bladder and of anorectal sphincter control, but posterior column sensation, including touch, position and vibration sense, is preserved. There is usually a clearly demarcated sensory level to pinprick in the lower thoracic or cervico-thoracic region, depending on the level of the circulatory impairment. The outcome is dependent on systemic factors, for example if there is visceral infarction due to mesenteric occlusion death is virtually inevitable.

Major contributory factors include anaemia, hyperviscosity states, sustained hypotensive shock, embolism, diabetes and hypertension. Sickle cell disease can also cause spinal infarction.

Degenerative myelopathies (see Chapter 12)

Degenerative disorders of the spinal cord are a component of the system degenerations, which may be hereditary or acquired. The best known acquired system degeneration of the cord is subacute combined degeneration, in which degeneration of the posterior columns and corticospinal tracts occurs (see Chapter 13).

Radiation myelopathy

Radiotherapy is directed toward eradicating cancer cells. The spinal cord, in common with other tissues, is susceptible to damage from this form of energy, and care is necessary to avoid exposing the cord to more than about 4000 Rads during treatment of neoplasms in the chest, neck, breast or abdomen. An *acute syndrome*, consisting of a transient myelopathy characterized by tingling in affected dermatomes, especially in the hands after radiation therapy to the neck, develops a few weeks after treatment and resolves in 6–8 weeks. A *progressive myelopathy* with paraparesis, spinothalamic and posterior column sensory loss and sphincter dysfunction may develop 9–15 months after exposure to radiation in a dose of more than about 6000 Rads. The syndrome slowly progresses during several weeks or months and then remains unchanged. It is associated with degeneration of neurons and fibre tracts, with pronounced thickening of blood vessels. The latter is perhaps the major causative mechanism. There is no effective treatment. Diagnosis depends on exclusion of neoplastic compression or invasion of the cord.

Decompression sickness (Caisson disease)

Myelopathy was recognized in early times in pearl divers in the South Seas, causing paraplegia and, especially, urinary retention. Haldane recognized that this, and a similar syndrome occurring in men involved in tunnel construction under conditions of increased atmospheric pressure, was due to nitrogen bubble formation in the arterial circulation during decompression following several hours' work under pressure. This condition has become of considerable importance with the contemporary emphasis on deep-sea diving in oil exploration, in military and scientific application, in the construction industry and in spaceflight technology. It can be prevented by careful, slow decompression according to established tables of time to be spent at gradually ascending levels, either underwater or in a pressure chamber. The occurrence of bubbles is determined by physical principles in relation to compressed air, oxygen and 'heliox', a mixture of helium and oxygen suitable for sustained, very deep dives (200–1000 metres).

Brain involvement may occur, as well as myelopathy, causing dysarthria, dysphasia, hemiparesis, sensory loss and visual impairment or even decerebrate coma. There is often associated barometric damage to the vestibular system and eardrums, and bubble formation in the skin. Pulmonary damage from gas efflorescence, and bone and joint involvement, with pain and haemorrhage, may occur. Severe syndromes such as these may be fatal.

Treatment consists of immediate recompression, usually in an oxygen enriched atmosphere, and dexamethasone, intravenous fluid and circulatory support. Anticonvulsant drugs are indicated. If the neurological deficit rapidly reverses, decompression is gradually accomplished using one of the modified Haldane tables. Additional oxygen recompression treatments may be helpful if there is residual neurological deficit.

Divers, whether amateur or professional, who have suffered a 'neurological bend' (Type 2 decompression sickness) should be advised not to dive again since there is electrophysiological and neuropathological evidence of residual cord damage even when clinical recovery is complete, and the functional capacity to withstand any future event is thus reduced.

Myelopathies associated with infection

Most of these disorders are uncommon (Table 15.5). AIDS myelopathy occurs in 30% of patients with AIDS; it is usually of insidious onset, unlike the other opportunistic pulmonary, gastro-intestinal and CNS infections that characterize this syndrome.

Table 15.5 *Myelopathies associated with infection.*

AIDS vacuolar myelopathy
Poliomyelitis
H. zoster myelopathy
Lyme disease myelopathy
Syphilitic myelopathy
Tropical spastic paraplegia (HTLV-I infection)

In *poliomyelitis* there is viral invasion of anterior horn cells leading to cell death and rapid paralysis and neurogenic atrophy. This condition is now virtually unknown in developed countries, since widespread immunization was introduced in the 1950s. Myelopathy with spastic paraparesis and sensory loss is an uncommon complication of *H. zoster*, associated with persistent pain, and only slow and partial recovery from the myelopathy. Myelopathy may also complicate *Lyme disease*, a spirochaetal infection (*Borrelia burgdorfi*) spread by a tic in temperate climes. *Syphilitic myelopathy* is now an uncommon complication of the disease (see Chapter 6); the commonest form is tabes dorsalis, but a spastic paraplegia may also develop (Erb's paraplegia). *Tropical spastic paraplegia* is a progressive condition that has been associated with infection with a retrovirus HTLV-I.

Post-viral myelopathy is a rapid-onset, ascending paralysis with bladder and anorectal sphincter involvement, which follows a viral infection, usually an exanthem, about 2–3 weeks later. The paralysis develops in a period of a few hours and progresses during 12–48 hours. It may ascend to involve brain stem and more rostral parts of the CNS, leading to respiratory failure and death, but in other cases the disorder arrests and recovery occurs during several weeks or months. This condition is associated with swelling of the cord, seen on myelography and CT scanning, and with a raised CSF protein, and a lymphocytosis or pleocytosis, but with a normal CSF sugar level. Treatment with steroids, 60–150 mg prednisolone daily, or methylprednisolone 1 g i.v. ×5 days, may produce rapid improvement, or arrest the progressive phase of the disorder. This syndrome thus resembles post-viral encephalitis in representing an allergic reaction to previous viral infection. It is not recurrent and, although often termed 'transverse myelitis', is not a form of multiple sclerosis.

Brain Tumours and Raised Intracranial Pressure

Brain tumours are common. About 50% of all brain tumours are primary tumours of the brain, its coverings, the cranial nerves, or of the pituitary gland; the other 50% are metastases. In neurological and neurosurgical practice there is selection, due to referral patterns, so that the proportion of metastases is relatively low, consisting of patients in whom the metastatic disease is the presenting or overwhelmingly important feature. About 2% of all necropsies reveal a brain tumour, but many brain metastases are not clinically important in relation to the extent of involvement of other organs such as the liver or lungs.

Primary brain tumours represent 2% of all malignancies, but in children 25% of all neoplasms arise in the brain, only leukaemias being commoner. In adults 75% of tumours are supratentorial; in children 60% are infratentorial. Brain tumours are commonest in the first decade, and in the fifth and sixth decades. Of patients presenting with brain tumours, about 40% are gliomas, 25% are metastases, 15% meningiomas and pituitary and acoustic neurilemmomas represent about 5% each. Other tumours (Table 16.1) are relatively uncommon.

Pathogenesis of brain tumours

Little is known about the causation of primary brain and other intracranial tumours. Meningiomas are slightly more common in women, and these tumours, neurofibromas, neurilemmomas and gliomas are particularly associated with neurofibromatosis. The latter is one of a group of developmental disorders of neuroectoderm and mesoderm that are also called phakomatoses, a term referring to other 'mother lesions' seen in the retina (see below). Other phakomatoses, e.g. tuberose sclerosis, are also associated with an increased incidence of brain tumours. Radiation exposure has been shown to be a factor initiating the growth of brain tumours but trauma,

Table 16.1 *Classification of brain tumours (modified from WHO classification 1979).*

Neuroepithelial tumours
  astrocytomas
  oligodendroglioma
  ependymal and choroid plexus tumours
    ependymoma
    choroid plexus papilloma
  pineal tumours
  neuronal tumours
    e.g. neuroblastoma
  poorly differentiated and embryonal tumours
    glioblastoma
    medulloblastoma
Nerve sheath tumours
  neurilemmoma (Schwannoma)
  neurofibroma and sarcoma
Meningeal tumours
  meningioma and meningosarcoma
Primary malignant lymphoma of brain
Blood vessel tumours and vascular malformations
  haemangioblastoma
  arteriovenous malformations
Malformative tumours and tumour-like lesions
  e.g. craniopharyngioma
    colloid cyst
    dermoid and epidermoid cysts
    lipoma
Pituitary tumours
  pituitary adenomas and microadenomas
Local invasion from neighbouring tumours
  chondrosarcoma
  chordoma
  glomus jugulare tumour
  salivary and nasal sinus tumours
Metastases from other organs
  e.g. breast, lung, thyroid, kidney cancers
    lymphoma
    melanoma

infection and exposure to industrial and environmental toxins has not been shown to be relevant. Nonetheless certain industrial substances, such as the nitrosourea compounds are potent carcinogens, particularly leading to brain tumours in animal experiments. In addition primary brain tumours, particularly primary cerebral lymphomas, develop more frequently in immuno-compromised patients, such as patients immunosuppressed for renal or bone marrow transplantation, and in AIDS. There is a slightly increased risk of meningioma and glioma associated with breast cancer.

Clinical presentation

There is a combination of features of general brain dysfunction, focal disturbances and raised intracranial pressure. The clinical syndrome depends on the location of the tumour, whether it is intrinsic, e.g. glioma, or extrinsic, e.g. meningioma, its relation to the ventricular system, and its rate of growth. Thus tumours in the non-dominant frontal lobe may attain considerable size before causing sufficient disability to cause presentation, whereas a small tumour in the motor cortex, or in the fourth ventricle may cause severe disability. Rapidly growing, malignant, primary or secondary tumours may present with a relatively abrupt course that sometimes mimics stroke, presumably because of secondary changes in perfusion of neighbouring brain, or from the effects of haemorrhage or necrosis of the tumour causing a sudden increase in size of the mass lesion.

General features. These consist of mental deterioration and changes in personality, with irritability, fatigue and impairment of memory. These features may occur with tumours in any location in the brain, but are only found in the presence of large tumours that cause displacement of the brain from side to side or into the tentorial notch. Generalized convulsions also occur with supratentorial tumours as a presenting, non-focal feature. Suspicion of a cerebral tumour is particularly important in patients with epilepsy of late onset. About 10% of patients with generalized epilepsy beginning after the age of 20 years are eventually found to have a cerebral tumour, especially meningioma, astrocytoma or metastases. Focal seizures in adults are particularly commonly associated with cerebral tumours.

Focal features. These are common features of brain tumour. They consist of progressive hemiparesis, visual disturbance, cranial nerve palsies or ataxia, depending on the location of the lesion. A stuttering course is not uncommon. Higher-level deficits, such as aphasia, parietal sensory and orientation disorders, and frontal lobe features also occur with tumours intrinsic or extrinsic to the relevant portions of the brain. Progressive deafness with vertigo is a feature of acoustic Schwannoma. Focal seizures are often associated with these progressive focal cortical deficits and may commonly precede them.

Raised intracranial pressure. Headache, vomiting and papilloedema are the classical features of raised intracranial pressure. However, brain tumours are diagnosed at an earlier stage than formerly and the fully-developed features of raised intracranial pressure are a relatively uncommon presentation of brain tumours in adults. In children, posterior fossa tumours are common and these often present with raised intracranial pressure. Raised intracranial pressure occurs also in patients with the syndrome of *benign intracranial hypertension* (see below), and in other space-occupying disorders, e.g. cerebral abscess, intracranial and intracerebral haemorrhage, and intracranial thrombophlebitis.

The *headache* of raised intracranial pressure (Chapter 5) is of variable severity, usually throbbing in character, but is diffuse and inconstant, although characteristically worse on waking in the morning. It is sometimes associated with pain in the root of the neck and may be aggravated by coughing, sneezing or bending down and by other manoeuvres that increase intracranial venous pressure. It may rarely be accompanied by transient loss of vision from retinal ischaemia. *Vomiting* is usually associated with changes in head posture, and is particularly likely to occur when intracranial pressure is at its highest, i.e. in the morning. The term projectile vomiting is used to describe the sudden occurrence of vomiting due to raised intracranial pressure, often without a warning period of nausea. Vomiting is particularly common with posterior fossa tumours.

Papilloedema is not always found in patients with raised intracranial pressure associated with brain tumours since it develops only when the intracranial pressure has been raised for some time. It may be bilateral or asymmetrical.

Raised intracranial pressure is associated with cerebral oedema. Oedema associated with cerebral tumours is typically white matter in location, a point of difference from cerebral oedema associated with stroke, in which the oedema involves both white and grey matter. The oedema extends widely in the white matter around the tumour causing extensive brain swelling and herniation.

Special features of common brain tumours

Certain clinical features are characteristic of individual types (Table 16.1) of brain tumours. These are useful in clinical diagnosis and in planning investigation and management. For example, medulloblastomas are common in children and are almost always cerebellar in location. Gliomas occur mainly in adults, and meningiomas almost entirely in older people. Pituitary and other localized tumours produce clinical features that are characteristic in relation to their endocrine effects, and to involvement of neighbouring structures, e.g. the optic chiasm.

Gliomas

In adults gliomas arise mainly in the cerebral hemispheres (Fig. 16.1) but in children they are commoner in the cerebellum and brain stem. The peak incidence is at about the age of 50 years. Gliomas are

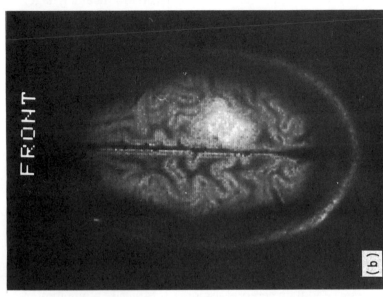

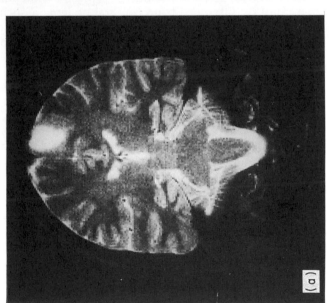

Fig. 16.1 (a and b) MRI scan, showing a low-grade tumour, an astrocytoma, in the left parasagittal region. The patient, a young man, presented with focal seizures, without other neurological findings.

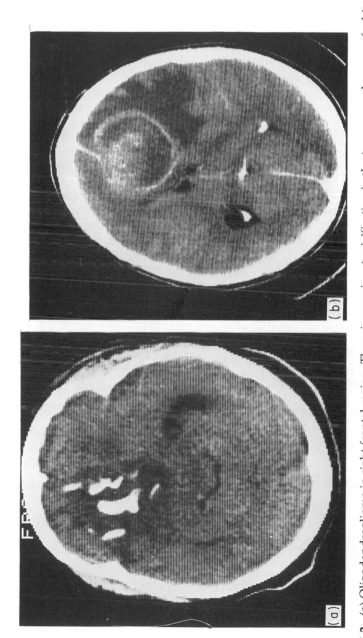

Fig. 16.2 (a) Oligodendroglioma in right frontal region. There is prominent calcification in the tumour, and a zone of white matter oedema is visible. (b) Malignant glioma left frontal region. This enhanced CT scan shows a tumour mass in a zone of oedema and swelling, with a prominent, capsule-like edge, indicating impairment of the blood–brain barrier. There is marked mass effect.

always locally invasive, representing a variable degree of malignancy. Younger patients tend to have less malignant tumours and thus a longer history before presentation. Symptoms have often been present for up to 2 years before the diagnosis is established. The more benign gliomas often present with focal symptoms, without raised intracranial pressure. Cyst formation is not infrequent. Calcification is particularly a feature of oligodendrogliomas (Fig. 16.2a). In some tumours anaplastic change develops and the mass lesion begins to expand relatively rapidly (Fig. 16.2b). Malignant gliomas (glioblastoma multiforme) may run a rapid course leading to death in a few weeks or months (Fig. 16.2b). The first symptom may be a focal or generalized seizure, or a stroke-like syndrome with hemiparesis and recovery. Investigation shortly after the initial episode may be normal and the recurrence of symptoms in a patient suspected to be suffering from glioma should prompt reinvestigation. Progressive neurological deficit, e.g. hemiparesis, with focal seizures and features of raised intracranial pressure is particularly characteristic. When the tumour is frontal, personality changes predominate.

Meningiomas

These slow-growing, extra-axial neoplasms arise from arachnoidal cells and compress and distort the brain without directly invading

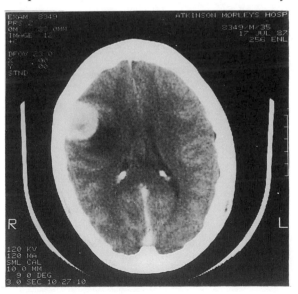

Fig. 16.3 CT scan. Right frontal meningioma. There is a spherical, enhancing mass applied to the meninges of the calvarium, with some local white matter oedema.

it (Fig. 16.3). They arise frequently from the sphenoid wing, tuberculum sellae, olfactory groove and falx cerebri, but may occur in any location. Thus, oculomotor palsies may be a feature of sphenoid wing tumours, visual defects of tuberculum sellae lesions, anosmia and frontal lobe syndromes of subfrontal meningiomas and motor syndromes from falx tumours. Posterior fossa meningiomas also occur. Generalized seizures are a relatively frequent presentation, often with a focal, Jacksonian onset. Surgical treatment is sometimes difficult because of the location of the tumour, with local invasion of dura and bone around the margins of the tumour so that complete excision may not be possible. Sarcomatous change, with local invasion, may develop.

Acoustic Schwannomas

These neurilemmomas arise from the vestibular part of the eighth nerve in the internal auditory meatus (Fig. 16.4). In patients with Type 2 neurofibromatosis bilateral acoustic neuromas are a characteristic feature. The tumour presents with progressive sensorineural deafness, and with tinnitus and episodic vertigo. As the tumour enlarges it may produce ipsilateral cerebellar ataxia and nystagmus, ipsilateral facial numbness from trigeminal involvement, and symptoms of brain stem compression, with hydrocephalus. Rarely, Schwannomas may arise on the sensory roots of the trigeminal or facial nerves. Early diagnosis is important for effective surgical removal, without residual neurological deficit, especially facial palsy, and this is achieved by electrophysiological assessment of cochlear, vestibular and eighth nerve function and, especially, by nuclear magnetic resonance imaging (MRI) which delineates the tumour without interference from neighbouring petrous temporal bone. X-ray CT scanning is less discriminating. Meningiomas may also develop in the cerebello-pontine angle, mimicking the features of acoustic Schwannoma.

Pituitary tumours

Pituitary adenomas (Fig. 16.5) may be functioning, secreting hormone inappropriately, or non-functioning. Non-functioning tumours present with features of compression of neighbouring structures, especially of the optic chiasm. This causes bitemporal paracentral scotomas, progressing to bitemporal hemianopia (often asymmetrical), or blindness, with primary optic atrophy. There may be panhypopituitarism. Occasionally, large pituitary tumours extend beyond the confines of the suprasellar region causing temporal lobe seizures and hemiparesis, and such tumours may undergo infarction

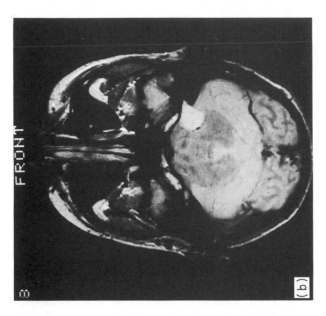

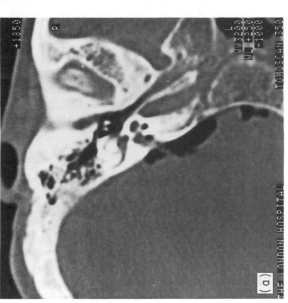

Fig. 16.4 (a) CT scan of right internal and middle ear, taken with air in the sub-arachnoid space. The normal eighth nerve is clearly seen as it leaves the internal auditory meatus; a semicircular canal can be seen in the inner ear. (b) MRI scan showing an acoustic neuroma on the left, arising within the internal auditory meatus, and impressing into the cerebellum in the cerebello-pontine angle.

(*pituitary apoplexy*), resulting in coma with bilateral ophthalmoplegia. The prognosis in this syndrome is poor.

Functioning tumours are small, or even microscopic in most cases, especially in the case of prolactin-secreting adenomas (*prolactinomas*) that cause galactorrhoea with amenorrhoea. Prolactinomas account for about 25% of cases of infertility, and cause reduced libido in men. Adenomas that secrete ACTH or growth hormone are more frequently larger. Thyrotoxicosis may also result from pituitary adenomas. Prolactinomas and growth-hormone secreting tumours, causing *acromegaly*, respond both endocrinologically, and in terms of reduction in tumour size and recovery of visual fields, to treatment with bromocryptine (20–60 mg daily) or other dopaminergic agonists such as pergolide and lisuride that, like bromocryptine, are ergot derivatives. Surgical removal by the transnasal route is also safe and effective, and is preferred for smaller tumours. Pituitary tumours may increase rapidly in size during pregnancy, even leading to marked impairment of vision, and thus these adenomas may present acutely in pregnancy.

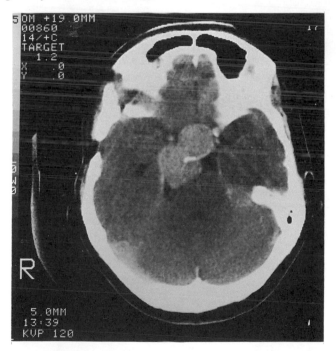

Fig. 16.5 Pituitary tumour. There is an enhancing mass arising from the sella turcica, extending posteriorly to displace the brain stem and right temporal lobe. The tumour was a chromophobe adenoma.

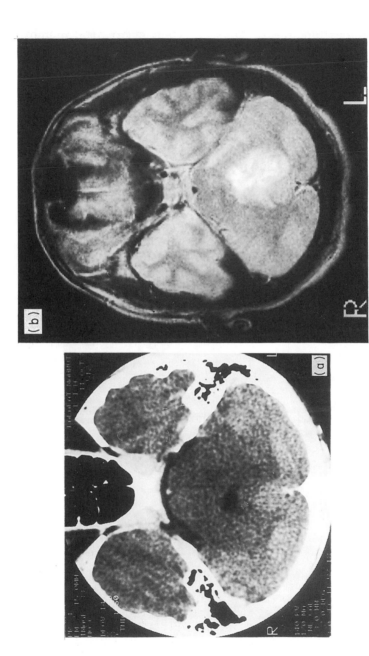

Fig. 16.6 Malignant glioma of cerebellum invading the brain stem. (a) CT scan. There is low attenuation in the brain stem and cerebellar peduncle, with displacement of the fourth ventricle to the right. (b) MRI scan. The tumour is shown as a white mass consisting of the tumour and its associated oedema.

Craniopharyngioma

This tumour arises from remnants of Rathke's pouch in the suprasellar region, i.e. in the floor of the third ventricle. It presents with panhypopituitarism, including diabetes insipidus, chiasmal compression and hydrocephalus. It is the most common supratentorial tumour in children, and is recognized by its clinical features, its location and the radiological appearances, including cyst formation and calcification. Complete surgical removal is feasible if the tumour is relatively small.

Posterior fossa tumours of childhood

These tumours include medulloblastoma, ependymoma, cerebellar astrocytoma and brain stem glioma. *Medulloblastoma* presents with truncal ataxia and features of raised intracranial pressure. The tumour is highly malignant and frequently metastasizes to other parts of the CNS and treatment requires local excision and radiation therapy to the whole neuraxis, including spinal cord and cauda equina. *Ependymoma* usually arises in the fourth ventricle; the tumour presents with hydrocephalus and with nausea, vomiting and nystagmus. The tumour is relatively benign. *Astrocytomas of the cerebellum* involve the cerebellar hemisphere (Fig. 16.6) and present with limb ataxia rather than truncal ataxia before the development of hydrocephalus and raised intracranial pressure. These tumours are cystic and histologically benign. *Brain stem glioma* is a tumour of young people that is often pontine in location, leading to cranial nerve palsies, long tract signs and dysarthria. Hydrocephalus is a late feature. Surgical treatment is impossible but radiotherapy may prolong survival in some cases. *Optic nerve gliomas* also have a predilection for children, presenting with unilateral or bilateral impairment of vision.

Other brain tumours

Pinealomas are rare. They cause complex endocrine disorders, including precocious puberty, hydrocephalus and disturbances of sleep, with cutaneous pigmentation from secretion of melanocyte-stimulating hormone (MSH). Boys predominate 20 : 1. *Colloid cysts* occur particularly in the third ventricle and may cause hydrocephalus with attacks of akinetic coma due to ventricular obstruction. The diagnosis is readily made by CT scanning. *Haemangioblastomas* are benign cystic tumours derived from blood vessels, particularly found in the cerebellum, that cause ataxia and hydrocephalus. They may be associated with *von Hippel–Lindau syndrome*, including retinal angiomatosis and renal carcinoma, and often secrete erythropoietin,

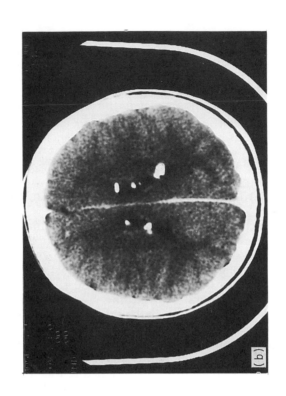

Fig. 16.7 Tuberous sclerosis. (a) Typical facies, with paranasal lesions resembling acne. (b) CT brain scan showing paraventricular calcified masses (tubers).

causing increased red cell mass and a raised haemoglobin level. *Chordomas* are malignant tumours of the clivus or sacrum derived from notochordal remnants. Cerebral astrocytomas or glial nodules, with epilepsy, mental deficiency and adenoma sebaceum, an acne-like nodular facial rash, are features of *tuberose sclerosis* (Bourneville's disease) (Fig. 16.7), a dominantly-inherited phakoma of variable penetrance. *Glioblastoma multiforme* is a common, highly malignant tumour, almost always supratentorial in location, usually associated with marked cerebral oedema, and with a rapidly progressive course. *Primary lymphomas* of the brain are relatively uncommon. They may be multifocal and are associated with immunosuppression, presenting with seizures, raised intracranial pressure, mental changes and focal neurological signs.

Metastases

Secondary cancer of the brain is usually multiple (Fig. 16.8), but may be solitary. In the latter instance the tumour presents like a malignant astrocytoma, or may resemble cerebral abscess. Clinical diagnosis

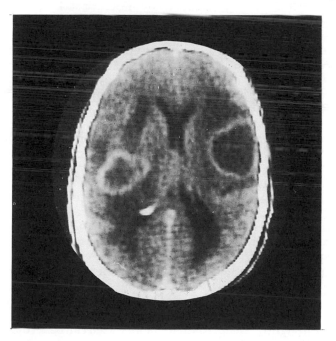

Fig. 16.8 Cerebral metastases. This enhanced CT scan shows two large masses, with several smaller lesions, each delineated by a capsule-like margin. These lesions may be difficult to distinguish from abscesses on radiological criteria.

is unreliable without clear evidence of a primary tumour, and the CT appearances are so variable as also to be unreliable for diagnosis without histological verification by biopsy.

Carcinoma or lymphoma may extend widely through the meninges, causing a clinical syndrome resembling meningitis (Chapter 6) but associated with multiple cranial nerve palsies and radicular lesions, especially involving the cauda equina. Neoplastic cells can usually be identified in the centrifuged CSF sediment, and the CSF glucose level is low, and the protein level raised.

Investigation of suspected brain tumour

The suspicion of brain tumour is almost always first raised by the clinical features, particularly by focal symptoms or signs with a progressive course, often including seizures, and by features of raised intracranial pressure. A history of previous or present malignant tumour in a patient with cerebral problems clearly also suggests that intracranial tumour is a likely diagnosis. In some patients, however, investigation by EEG or CT scanning for suspected epilepsy or stroke reveals an unexpected tumour. Rarely, skull X-rays carried out after a minor head injury may reveal features consistent with longstanding increased intracranial pressure, or focal calcifications in the brain suggestive of occult glioma, craniopharyngioma, meningioma or arteriovenous malformation.

CT scanning and MR imaging are the initial investigations of choice in evaluating a tumour suspect. These investigations reveal the tumour, its surrounding oedema and any resultant cerebral herniation or hydrocephalus. MR imaging is particularly helpful in posterior fossa lesions, including both intrinsic and extrinsic tumours, and in perichiasmatic tumours. In many instances the nature of the tumour can be surmised from these appearances. CT brain scans provide a 90% predictive value for gliomas and meningiomas but are less reliable in characterizing solitary metastases. These figures indicate the necessity for tissue diagnosis in virtually all patients with CT appearances consistent with tumour; a few such patients will be found to have other, readily treatable, lesions such as brain abscess, Herpes simplex encephalitis or cerebral infarction. Brain biopsy is often carried out after CT scanning alone, but if a vascular tumour is suspected, or if meningioma or benign tumour is likely, angiography is helpful in planning possible total excision through a cranioplastic flap. Biopsy itself can be accomplished through a burr hole with a biopsy needle, or by a stereotactic method which allows precise control of the area to be biopsied.

Other investigations are indicated in particular problems. In pituitary and suprasellar tumours endocrinological evaluation is essential in documenting the tumour type and in arranging hormone replacement therapy and appropriate medical techniques for suppressing inappropriate hormone production, e.g. growth hormone, ACTH and prolactin. Blood electrolyte and urea levels should be checked. The ESR, Hb and WBC count are all important, e.g. in excluding infection, and in recognizing polycythaemia in patients with haemangioblastoma. When metastatic disease is suspected, e.g. in patients with multiple tumours at the grey/white matter junction, extensive investigation may be justified in order to achieve tissue diagnosis without craniotomy. Chest X-ray and cytological examination of the sputum, examination of the breasts, and ultrasound or CT examination of abdominal organs are often useful. Lumbar puncture is not indicated in the investigation of intracranial neoplasms unless meningeal carcinomatosis is suspected, when malignant cells may be found in the CSF (see Chapter 8).

During management serial CT scanning is often used to assess the outcome and effectiveness of treatment.

Treatment of brain tumours

The results of treatment of malignant brain tumours are unsatisfactory, and benign tumours may also prove refractory to treatment if total primary excision proves impossible for technical reasons, e.g. proximity to vital structures such as the carotid arteries. In all patients with brain tumours the essential aspect of treatment is to establish the tissue diagnosis by biopsy of the tumour, and to attempt as complete removal of the tumour as possible without increasing the patient's disability.

At the very least, raised intracranial pressure requires effective management. The latter can be accomplished by steroid therapy and this is usually given for several days prior to operation, as well as during the phase of post-operative recovery. Dexamethasone is usually used (2–4 mg qds) in gradually decreasing dosage. This drug may cause serious complications if used in large doses for more than a few weeks, including avascular necrosis of bone, diabetes mellitus, psychosis, vertebral collapse, weight gain and myopathy; not all these complications are reversible. Most patients require prophylactic anticonvulsant drug therapy during surgery and for at least several months afterwards.

In patients with hydrocephalus, due to posterior fossa and intraventricular tumours it may be best to relieve the hydrocephalus by CSF shunting (ventriculo-atrial or ventriculo-peritoneal CSF shunt operations) rather than to attempt surgical excision of the tumour.

Radiotherapy is indicated post-operatively for most malignant brain tumours, including gliomas, and for some benign tumours, e.g. some meningiomas, incompletely removed. This is given in 10–25 fractionated doses in a period of 2–6 weeks. Medulloblastomas, pineal germinomas and lymphomas are highly sensitive, and cure may be achieved provided whole-neuraxis treatment schedules are used. Radiotherapy for gliomas is helpful in the less malignant tumours but has little or no useful effect in more malignant forms. Glioblastomas respond poorly, and the 1 year survival, even with aggressive treatment, is only about 5%. Cytotoxic chemotherapy has so far not been shown to have practical value in the treatment of primary brain tumours. Malignant infiltration of the meninges and metastatic tumours such as melanoma may respond to this treatment. Prolactin-secreting and growth hormone-secreting pituitary tumours usually decrease in size and endocrinological activity with bromocryptine therapy (see above).

Prognosis and outcome

Most benign tumours can be cured by total excision but will inevitably recur if any tumour is left at the original operation. Meningiomas recur in about 10% of cases during 10 year follow-up, and pituitary tumours in about 40% of cases. Radiotherapy improves these figures and is thus usually recommended. Prolactinomas can be successfully treated with a combination of bromocryptine and radiotherapy; fertility is restored in as many as 90% of women with this tumour. If prolactin levels return to normal for some years, treatment with bromocryptine may be stopped without recurrence of the tumour. Medulloblastoma responds in many patients to radiotherapy, sometimes supplemented by cytotoxic chemotherapy given intravenously and intrathecally, and survival figures of 50% at 10 years are attainable, although at the cost of some impairment of cerebral function and of growth impairment. Glioblastoma has a poor prognosis, with death in 3–6 months untreated, and perhaps 6–10 months treated. Cerebral gliomas in adults vary in outcome dependent on histological type, and degree of malignancy; some patients survive as long as 20 years, particularly in the case of oligodendrogliomas. Cerebellar astrocytomas of childhood have an excellent outcome provided total excision is followed by radiotherapy. Metastatic carcinoma, if multiple, usually leads to death in less than 3 months, but some patients with solitary metastases survive for many years after excision and radiotherapy. Intracranial lymphomas can be satisfactorily managed by radiotherapy and systemically administered cytotoxic chemotherapy with haematological and steroid support.

Benign intracranial hypertension
(pseudotumour cerebri)

This condition consists of a syndrome of raised intracranial pressure causing morning headache with papilloedema, but without cerebral tumour or other demonstrable focal cause after full investigation. The CSF pressure is raised (200–300 cm water) but is otherwise normal. The CT scan shows small or normal-sized lateral ventricles. Sometimes the CT scan reveals an unexpected cause for the clinical syndrome, for example a clinically unsuspected frontal or posterior fossa tumour, or angiographic features suggestive of lateral sinus thrombosis. Focal neurological symptoms or signs exclude the diagnosis but sixth nerve palsies and visual disturbances may occur as non-specific consequences of the raised CSF pressure. Indeed, transient or even permanent blindness from retinal infarction due to compression of the optic nerves by CSF under increased pressure, or due to the effects of papilloedema itself, may occur. These secondary effects are the main reason for treatment.

There are many causes of this syndrome but, in some patients, no cause is evident despite extensive investigation (Table 16.2). Most cases occur in young women at menarche; there are also associations with obesity, menstrual dysfunction and pregnancy.

Management. Weight reduction, salt restriction and diuretic treatment are all useful. Acetazolamide is often used because of its direct effect in reducing intracranial pressure. Repeated lumbar puncture, at first at daily and then weekly intervals, is also effective treatment but not easily tolerated. Steroid therapy, initially with full doses of dexamethasone and then with the smallest effective maintenance dose of prednisolone, is effective but may need to be continued for many months before the condition spontaneously resolves. During follow up, assessment of visual fields and visual acuity, and

Table 16.2 *Causes of benign intracranial hypertension.*

Young obese women
Menstrual irregularity, and Stein–Leventhal syndrome
Pregnancy
Steroid withdrawal
Systemic lupus erythematosus
Oral contraceptive therapy
Other medications:
   tetracycline
   nalidixic acid
   vitamin A excess
Behçet's disease
Lateral sinus thrombosis ('otitic hydrocephalus')

measurement of intracranial pressure by lumbar puncture, are essential to ensure effectiveness of treatment. Very rarely, subtemporal decompression may be needed to control raised intracranial pressure but before this is contemplated reinvestigation by CT scanning, CSF examination and cerebral angiography should be carried out to exclude a focal cause missed during initial evaluation. About a third of cases recur when steroid therapy is stopped, and treatment should then be recommenced.

17

Pain Syndromes

Pain is the commonest symptom encountered in clinical practice. In most patients this is due to local disease, with destruction of tissue but, in others, pain is caused by disease in the sensory pathways in the nervous system itself, either in the peripheral or central nervous system, and occasionally pain seems to be a feature of depression.

Physiology of pain

Pain is a subjective sensation, consisting of an unpleasant sensory and motor experience, associated with actual, potential or imagined tissue damage. The emotional component is associated with anxiety, depression and aggression and these factors are important in determining the patient's description of and reaction to pain. The neuronal circuitry of pain is still incompletely understood.

Nociceptive stimuli, for example, needle pricks, burning, intense cold and chemical or electrical injury, cause pain by exciting terminal, unmyelinated nerve endings, mainly C fibres, and small A-delta thinly myelinated afferent fibres. These stimuli also excite other specialized endings but these probably do not subserve the sensory input responsible for the perception of a stimulus as painful. The role of locally produced substances such as histamine, bradykinin and prostaglandins in firing C fibre and A-delta fibre input is imprecisely defined. These inputs synapse in the dorsal horn in the outer and middle layers respectively, including the substantia gelatinosa. Sensory terminals in these layers consist of small neurons; deeper, larger neurons are activated by mechanical, thermal and other cutaneous stimuli such as light pressure and touch. The small nociceptive neurons in the substantia gelatinosa contain neurotransmitter peptides, including substance P, cholecystokinin, somatostatin and vasoactive intestinal peptide (VIP), which are important in the relay of nociceptive input into the contralateral anterolateral quadrant (spinothalamic tracts) of the spinal cord that project to the ventral, postero-lateral, posterior and intralaminar thalamic nuclei, and thence to the post-central gyrus of the cerebral cortex. Opioid peptides of several classes in the dorsal horn of the spinal cord, e.g. enkephalins, appear to regulate nociceptive information by modulating activity in the nociceptive neurons in the superficial layers of the dorsal horn. Similar enkephalin-containing neurons and terminals are found in the periaqueductal grey matter, amygdala, hypothalamus and ventro-medial medulla (raphé nuclei). These opioid peptides resemble morphine in their analgesic properties, and are probably responsible for CNS control of pain and for the beneficial effects of CNS stimulation in the management of intractable pain.

The gate control theory of Melzack and Wall predicted that stimulation of large, rapidly-conducting afferents of low threshold would inhibit pain induced by bombardment of the dorsal horn by the activity of small, slowly-conducting, nociceptive afferents. This theory was confined to an interpretation of the function of dorsal horn neuronal circuits. More recent ideas involve control mechanisms, both synaptic and humoral, functioning at multiple levels in the CNS. These ideas imply therapeutic approaches at several levels other than spinal cord. They are also consistent with the development of pain in zones of skin partially deafferented by disease of the peripheral or central nervous system.

Clinical types of pain syndrome

Persistent, remittent or intractable pain may arise from disease of the pain pathways in the nervous system, or from destruction of tissues of the body. There are many different types of pain, ranging from low-grade, dull, continuous pain to lancinating paroxysms of brief, severe, sharp, shooting pain. The clinical description of pain is important in diagnosis, particularly in suggesting a neurological or non-neurological cause (Table 17.1). Shooting, burning, sharp pain is often neurological in origin. Dull aching pain is associated with chronic arthropathies, or with local disease in a tissue; colicky pain is usually visceral in origin, throbbing pain is vascular or inflammatory. Pain may be referred from a local source to the dermatome of the nerve innervating the diseased area, or from a visceral location into a related cutaneous zone (via spinal cord connections). In chronic pain syndromes, whether of neurological or non-neurological origin, pain may extend locally or diffusely from the original site. Such extended pain distributions imply increasing excitability in pain pathways in the CNS, and are often associated with the development of intractable, remorseless, severe pain that is difficult to manage effectively.

Table 17.1 *Pain syndromes.*

Neurological causes
  Peripheral nervous system disorders
    Neuralgias
      trigeminal neuralgia
      other focal neuralgias, e.g. glossopharyngeal, occipital
      post-herpetic neuralgia
      focal neuropathies, e.g. entrapment syndromes
      generalized neuropathies, e.g. alcoholic neuropathy
      root lesions, e.g. sciatica
      plexus lesions, e.g. causalgia
      phantom limb pain
    Central nervous system disorders
      thalamic pain
      spinothalamic pain
      tabes dorsalis
  Pain of psychological origin
  Depression
  Muscle spasm, e.g. flexor spasms, overuse syndromes, cramp

Non-neurological causes
  cancer
  ischaemia
  referred pain
  joint disease, etc.

Neuralgia

Neuralgia means pain referred along a nerve distribution, usually originating in a focal zone of damage in the nerve. Thus neuralgia may be a symptom of damage to any sensory nerve (Table 17.2). However, the term is particularly associated with a characteristic painful syndrome of the fifth cranial nerve; trigeminal neuralgia.

Table 17.2 *Common neuralgias.*

Trigeminal neuralgia
Occipital neuralgia
Post-herpetic neuralgia
Glosso-pharyngeal neuralgia
Meralgia paresthetica
Sciatica
Entrapment neuropathies
Root and plexus lesions
Painful peripheral neuropathies
Migrainous neuralgia
Neuralgic amyotrophy
Causalgias and painful neuromas

Sciatica, pain referred into the distribution of the sciatic nerve, is also a form of neuralgia. Thus, there are many possible causative disease processes.

Trigeminal neuralgia. This syndrome, often excrutiatingly painful, consists of frequent paroxysms of severe shooting pain in the face, lasting only a few seconds at a time. It may recur every few minutes or only a few times a day and tends to wax and wane so that exacerbations and remissions occur during several weeks or months. The pain is nearly always unilateral and involves the second or third division of the nerve, but not the first division. Examination is difficult since even light contact or movement, as in talking, eating or sitting in a light draught, may be sufficient to trigger the paroxysm of pain. There is often a dull, intense discomfort in the lower face between the paroxysmal attacks of pain. No sensory or motor abnormality can be detected in the trigeminal distribution to conventional testing, but there are usually one or more trigger points on the face, lips, gums or tongue from which painful paroxysms can be initiated. The pain is so severe that the patient will suddenly stop moving, with a quick inward breath, while waiting for it to subside.

Idiopathic trigeminal neuralgia, the common form of the syndrome, is uncommon under the age of 60 years. In young people trigeminal neuralgia is usually due to a focal lesion in or adjacent to the sensory root of the trigeminal nerve. Multiple sclerosis is the commonest cause in young people and this may be bilateral. Acoustic or trigeminal tumours, and other neoplasms in this region may also cause trigeminal neuralgia. The cause of idiopathic, late-onset trigeminal neuralgia is controversial; recent evidence supports the concept put forward by Dandy in 1934 that it results from irritation of the sensory root due to compression in the cerebello-pontine angle by a loop of the superior cerebellar artery.

Treatment: Carbamazepine is effective in two-thirds of cases. It should be begun in a small dose (100 mg bd) and slowly increased until a response is achieved or toxic effects preclude further increases in dosage. Some patients respond to small doses but others require much larger doses. When a remission has been achieved the drug can be gradually withdrawn, but it may need to be reinstituted when the pain recurs. Other drugs, for example phenytoin, are much less effective. If medical treatment fails, alcohol or phenol injection of the nerve root at the foramen rotundum is often tried. This can be achieved through the cheek under X-ray control. Injections sufficient to relieve pain also produce variable sensory loss in the second and third divisions, and this may also affect the first division, producing a hypoaesthetic cornea and thus leading to corneal abrasion. Lateral tarsorrhaphy may be necessary to protect the cornea in such patients.

Radiofrequency thermocoagulation of the Gasserian ganglion is more easily controlled, and can be delivered by a stereotactically directed probe, reducing the risk of extensive facial anaesthesia.

Trigeminal neuralgia can also be treated by exploration and mobilization of the nerve, freeing it from entrapment in vascular loops; this is often effective and permanent. Craniotomy is indicated if a focal cause can be demonstrated radiologically. Trigeminal neuralgia associated with multiple sclerosis usually responds to carbamapezine, and resolves spontaneously after several weeks.

Other neuralgias. Neuralgia may present in the distribution of other nerves, especially in the head and face. Thus pain may be restricted to the distribution of a *dental nerve*, usually in relation to dental abscess, cyst, root disease or neoplasm, or in a *supra-orbital nerve*, due to local injury. *Occipital neuralgia* is probably due to local injury to an occipital nerve from pressure, trauma or spondylosis. *Glosso pharyngeal neuralgia*, a very rare syndrome, resembles trigeminal neuralgia in its idiopathic origin. It is felt in the back of the throat radiating down the side of the neck, in front of the ear and into the lateral jaw. Other neuralgic syndromes in the face are probably related to migrainous neuralgia, and are vascular in causation.

Nerve entrapments in the limbs also cause neuralgia. Thus *sciatica* is due to entrapment of lumbo-sacral nerve roots by a prolapsed intervertebral disc and similar pain occurs in the arms or thorax from cervical or thoracic root lesions. Ulnar nerve entrapment at the elbow can cause ulnar neuralgia (tennis elbow). *Meralgia paresthetica* is due to entrapment of the lateral femoral cutaneous nerve of the thigh under the inguinal ligament or by fat at this region, usually in obese women. There is pain in the lateral thigh with disturbed sensation in this region. The pain resolves with weight reduction but occasionally a local steroid injection or nerve section may be necessary.

Post-herpetic neuralgia consists of pain resembling that of other neuralgias, with a continuous deep component and a lancinating, stimulus-sensitive component that develops after the acute phase of H. zoster radiculitis. The pain may persist for months or even indefinitely. Post-herpetic neuralgia is more likely to develop in old people than in the young, and can be limited by early anti-viral treatment of the infection at the onset of the eruption. About 10% of patients with H. zoster develop this syndrome. Most patients are reluctant to allow any skin contact in the affected area, but examination usually reveals some impairment of sensation in the zone marked by the vesicular scars and there may also be some motor involvement in the same root distribution (see Chapter 6). Treatment is difficult, requiring antidepressant drugs, nerve blocks and transcutaneous nerve stimulation. Analgesics are ineffective, but carbamazepine may be helpful.

Causalgia. Trauma to a nerve, nerve plexus or nerve root may be followed by the development of constant, spontaneous burning pain of variable sensitivity. At its most severe it may be extreme and associated with numbness, tingling and coldness in the affected skin. There is marked hyperpathia so that all contact is avoided. The pain is intensified by all forms of stimulation, including movement and emotion. The pain is initially limited to the distribution of the affected nerve developing days or weeks after the injury, but it may spread to involve the distal parts of the limb, or even the whole limb and other proximal parts. In most cases causalgia improves within a year of the onset. Causalgia is particularly common after lesions of the brachial plexus, or brachial roots, cauda equina or peripheral nerves such as the median or sciatic nerves.

Examination is difficult because the patient will not allow contact with the affected skin. The limb appears pink and vasodilated, and oedema, perhaps associated with disuse, may be present. Trophic changes in the limb, including atrophy of the subcutaneous tissue with decalcification of bones, may develop (Sudeck's atrophy).

Treatment: Analgesics are ineffective. Carbamazepine is rarely useful. Antidepressants may be indicated and chlorpromazine is helpful. Nerve exploration or proximal nerve section is also ineffective, but sympathetic nerve block by alcohol injection or by surgical sympathectomy may relieve the pain. Transcutaneous nerve stimulation is effective in about 40% of cases and this should be used in the first instance since the causalgia will resolve in many patients in about a year. Intrathecal opiates cause short-lived relief and radiofrequency lesions in the CNS (in thalamus or periaqueductal grey matter) are rarely indicated.

Sympathectomy is probably effective because it decreases *efferent* nervous traffic in the peripheral nerve; this efferent activity is transferred ephaptically to afferent fibres at the site of nerve damage leading to chaotic afferent activity transmitted to the dorsal horn. Causalgia thus arises from abnormal pain discharges in afferent pathways, associated with central oversensitivity to the de-afferented state caused by the nerve lesion.

Phantom limb pain. Pain resembling causalgia may develop in a phantom limb after amputation. This probably arises from disordered afferent activity initiated in the nerve stump or neurons at the site of the amputation. It occurs in about 30% of patients, but is unremitting in only about 5%. Sympathectomy may be helpful in some cases, but transcutaneous electrical stimulation is the treatment of choice. In addition, treatment with chlorpromazine and simple analgesics such as paracetamol is often useful.

Painful polyneuropathies. In alcoholic neuropathy and diabetic neuropathy burning, dysaesthetic pain in the distal parts of the limbs can be severe and unremitting. It is often associated with features of autonomic involvement and has been associated with damage to small myelinated fibres and unmyelinated fibres. It seems particularly likely to develop when the neuropathy is progressive and improves when the neuropathy is treated adequately, e.g. by withdrawal from alcohol or by control of diabetes mellitus. Painful neuropathy may also be a feature of para-neoplastic sensory neuropathy and of Guillain–Barré syndrome.

Central pain syndromes

Pain may arise from disordered function in the CNS, especially with lesions near the thalamus, in the spinothalamic tract or in the dorsal horn of the spinal cord, as in tabes dorsalis, i.e. at any site in the afferent pathways in the CNS.

Thalamic pain. After infarction in the posterior cerebral artery territory severe, persistent pain may develop in the hemiparetic and hemi-anaesthetic limbs. This syndrome of spontaneous pain is accompanied by over-reaction to ordinary superficial and noxious stimuli with poor localization of the stimulus and a tendency for the evoked painful response to be perceived as a spreading unpleasant sensation, often mislocalized and proximally located. There is often a delay before the stimulus is perceived and repeated stimuli cause both spatial and temporal perseveration so that the stimulus seems to be present for some seconds after it has ceased. In most cases this sensory disturbance is temporary but in other patients it remains as a permanent and unpleasant disability. Partial forms, consisting of dysaesthesiae in response to cutaneous stimuli, are more common. The infarct is located in the ventral part of the thalamus or in the subparietal white matter overlying the thalamic nuclei. Similar symptoms may arise with tumours in this location.

Treatment: Drug therapy, including analgesics, carbamazepine and major tranquillizers such as chlorpromazine, is only partially effective. Transcutaneous and CNS electrical stimulation are also often ineffective.

Spinothalamic pain. Burning dysaesthesiae, exacerbated by cutaneous stimuli, but without the characteristic spatial mislocalization found in thalamo-parietal lesions, may occur in patients with lesions, usually due to infarction, in the spinothalamic, small-fibre, afferent pathways through the spinal cord, brain stem and diencephalon. Infarction, trauma, syringomyelia, encephalitis and neoplasms may all cause this symptom. Carbamazepine and chlorpromazine are often helpful.

Tabes dorsalis. In tabes dorsalis there is degeneration and gliosis in the dorsal horn, involving the substantia gelatinosa and associated white matter in the spinal cord. Lancinating pains, paraesthesiae and aching pain become persistent and continuous in the limbs, epigastrium and pelvis in association with loss of position and vibration sense, ataxia, sphincter disturbance and, in some cases, spastic paraparesis. This is a late manifestation of tertiary syphilis. The ankle jerks and knee jerks are absent and other features of neurosyphilis, especially Argyll Robertson pupils, may be present.

The underlying syphilitic infection should be treated with penicillin and steroids (Chapter 6). The pain may respond to carbamazepine or phenytoin, and chlorpromazine and antidepressants may also be useful.

Pain of psychological origin

Pain may be a feature of major depressive illness, or the presenting feature of patients with depression in whom pain appears to be the major symptom. In the latter there is often a migrainous background and the patient presents with migrainous neuralgia, atypical facial pain or with disseminated aches and pains, especially involving the neck, low back or limbs. Pain in the perineum and genitalia is also often associated with overt depressive symptoms, for example feelings of inadequacy, misery, sleeplessness, tearfulness, social isolation and suicidal ideation. Interpretation of these syndromes is complicated by the common occurrence of depressive symptoms as a reaction to unrelieved organic pain. It is therefore appropriate to treat patients with intractable pain and depressive symptoms with tricyclic antidepressant drugs while assessing underlying causes. Other poorly-defined syndromes such as temporo-mandibular joint pain (Costen's syndrome) are additional examples of this clinical conundrum and empirical treatment with antidepressant drugs is often effective.

Complementary medicine in pain syndromes

Many patients derive comfort and support from acupuncture, manipulation, vibration, physiotherapy, spa treatment, psychotherapy, hypnotherapy, special exercise and postural regimes and quasi-religious techniques such as meditation. All pain is subjective and the influence of mental set and attitude on the interpretation is profound, and culturally and educationally determined. These alternative treatment methods are, therefore, likely to benefit certain patients and are to be encouraged provided that proper diagnosis of any underlying cause has been achieved.

Non-neurological pain

Intractable pain is a major feature of cancer, severe trauma, arthropathy, inflammatory disease and ischaemic disease. Direct treatment of these disorders may be ineffective and palliative treatment, e.g. radiotherapy to metastases, or opiate analgesia, should be offered as needed. Localized pain can be relieved by nerve block, regional opiate infusion, intrathecal opiates, transcutaneous electrical stimulation, CNS electrical stimulation at thalamic, periaqueductal or posterior column locations or, in regional cancer, especially of the lower limbs and pelvis, by spinothalamic tractotomy. These neurosurgical techniques are nowadays carried out by stereo-tactic methods without the need for major surgery and can be remarkably effective, without risk of serious complications.

Spinothalamic tractotomy is carried out in the thoracic or cervical cord as a unilateral or bilateral procedure. It results in contralateral loss of pain and temperature sensation, but spares posterior column sensation and strength, so that motor control and sphincter function are unaffected. Small fibre input to the thalamus is interrupted but large fibre input is not involved; the phylogenetically older, nociceptive input that enters the brain through the spinothalamic system is especially important in generating the psychological state we call pain.

Muscle spasm pain and frozen shoulder. In patients with neurological dis-ability, e.g. hemiparesis, pain may arise from muscle spasms, e.g. in flexor spasms, spasticity and dystonia, or from fibrosis or joint contrac-tures associated with abnormal postures or reduced mobility. *Frozen shoulder* is a common example of the latter problem. It consists of spontaneous onset of shoulder pain accompanied by increasingly severe limitation of shoulder movement without locally identifiable abnormality in the joint. It is associated with severe local pain on active or passive movement, particularly in external rotation, and in a painful arc of movement during the early phase of shoulder abduction. It is attributed to stiffness and thickening of the shoulder joint capsule ('capsulitis') and responds to a programme of mobilization by physio-therapy or by recovery of the underlying weakness. An injection of steroid into the joint is often helpful in initiating improvement. It is a common and rather neglected complication of hemiparesis due to stroke and is important since it may retard rehabilitation.

Paediatric Neurological Problems

Neurological disorders in children pose special problems. Many of the neurological diseases that affect infants and children also affect adults, e.g. infections, peripheral neuropathies, inflammatory muscle disease and epilepsy, but in children malformations and genetically-determined disorders are especially important since most of these disorders present during the period of development. Further, the process of maturation, especially during the first few years of life, modifies assessment of the neurological status and introduces culturally and socially-determined variables into the neurological examination. Childhood consists of four periods of development: *neonatal*, consisting of the first 4 weeks of life, *infantile*, consisting of the first year, *juvenile* and *adolescent*. Prematurity implies that gestational and chronological age do not necessarily coincide, an important factor in assessing neurological status in newborn infants. For descriptive purposes it is helpful to combine neonatal and infantile periods, and juvenile and adolescent periods.

Maturation

Following birth the child undergoes development and maturation so that functional milestones of motor and mental ability can be recognized and used to assess development in relation to expected levels of achievement. The neurological status in the newborn child has implications for future development and can be used to assess the likelihood of brain injury possibly sustained during or shortly after birth. The Apgar score (Table 18.1) is in general use in this assessment. An Apgar score of 6 or less at 5 minutes after birth is associated with neurological deficit in about 10% of cases, but a low score 1 minute after birth is much less predictive of brain damage. A high Apgar score, on the other hand, is not necessarily associated with a good outcome since it is not accurately predictive of cerebral palsy due to focal brain infarction or haemorrhage. Premature infants of less than 32 weeks gestation have a 30% chance of severe neurological handicap, but this risk is probably lessening with better

Table 18.1 *The Apgar score.*

In each of the five categories a score of 0, 1, or 2 is awarded giving a maximum score of 10. A score of 7–10 is good, 3–6 moderate CNS depression and 0–2 severe CNS depression.

Heart rate
Respiratory effort
Muscle tone
Reflex irritability
Colour

care of premature neonates. Neonates showing jitteriness, disturbances in arousal, an incomplete Moro startle response and the persistence of tonic neck reflexes have a relatively high probability of mental or physical handicap.

In assessing the neurological status of neonates three categories must be considered. These consist of *tonus*, a term used to describe active and passive muscular reactions to stretch of the limbs and trunk, *automatic reactions* and the *conventional neurological examination*, especially assessment of strength, tone, reflexes, reaction to sensory testing and plantar responses. The *automatic reactions* consist of walking and stepping, foot placement, crossed extensor, and traction and grasp responses. These are normal features of newborn infants. The *Moro reflex* consists of a flexion response to a sudden startle provoked by noise or movement; the thighs flex and the arms extend transiently. Asymmetrical Moro responses occur with unilateral weakness, e.g. brachial plexus or hemisphere lesions. The *tonic neck reflexes* consist of extension of an arm and flexion of the other in response to rotation of the neck; the arm to which the face looks extends. These reflexes are easily elicitable from 2 to 4 months of age, but usually disappear at about 7 months. Persistence or dominance of these responses implies cerebral palsy or developmental retardation.

The normal milestones of social and motor behaviour are important aspects of developmental assessment (Table 18.2). Delay in achieving these milestones must be interpreted with caution since there is wide variability between individuals, and much depends on the social environment. For example, some children walk after a long period of sitting and shuffling whereas others crawl on all fours before starting to walk. Language acquisition is particularly dependent on experience of language in the home.

Disorders of the first year of life

The major neurological problems of the first year of life are shown in Table 18.3.

Table 18.2 *Developmental milestones.*

Weeks	Social	Motor
4	Watches mother	Hands mainly closed
6	Social smiling	Sits with help; holds head up in ventral suspension
12	Responsive smiles Looks at objects	Easily holds head and trunk in ventral suspension Grasp reflex disappears Holds toes Vocalizes freely in consonants
16	Responsive with toys Listens	Sits with some help
26	Socializes readily Learns to play	Can roll prone to supine Sits alone Bears weight if stood passively
52	Can make tower with 2 or 3 cubes Holds cup	Stands and takes a step with support Jargon speech; a few real words Obeys some commands
2 years	Bladder control in 50% of children	Phrases spoken Clear comprehension Toddling, or even running Can climb stairs

Table 18.3 *Neurological disorders of the first year of life.*

Neonatal seizures
Cerebral infarction and haemorrhage
Infections of the brain
Trauma
Malformations
Metabolic disorders

Neonatal seizures

The incidence of seizures in neonates is related to prematurity as shown by birth weight. About 5% of newborns weighing less than 1500 g have fits, mostly in the first 48 hours of life. In these children there is a mortality of 30%, 30% of survivors have mental handicap and 20% develop epilepsy later. The seizures may be focal, multifocal, clonic, tonic, myoclonic or apnoeic in type, but only rarely resemble the typical tonic/clonic seizures of adults or older children. Neonatal seizures have many different causes; seizures occurring in the first 3 days are usually due to cerebral ischaemia, cerebral hypoxia, intraventricular or subarachnoid haemorrhage or to infection, especially bacterial meningitis. Seizures occurring after the first week are more likely to be due to metabolic disorders whether inherited or acquired, including hypocalcaemia and hypoglycaemia. Management consists of recognition and correction of the underlying cause; the seizures should be managed with phenobarbitone given as a loading dose (15–20 mg/kg) followed by maintenance therapy with 3–3.8 mg/kg/day. Phenytoin should be avoided because there is a risk of cerebellar damage and diazepam is usually reserved for older infants. In most neonates seizures cease in 3–10 days. Pyridoxine is often given (100 mg i.v.) in order to exclude the rare syndrome of pyridoxine-dependent seizures. Infantile spasms usually begin in the first year of life (see Chapter 2).

Infarction and haemorrhage

Both periventricular haemorrhage and cerebral infarction are relatively common problems in newborn premature infants. Periventricular haemorrhage is due to arterial bleeding into the subependymal plate (germinal matrix) cells, associated in premature babies with respiratory distress syndrome and arterial hypertension. Haemorrhage also occurs into the brain itself. Hydrocephalus may complicate this brain lesion, necessitating ventricular drainage; this presents with increasing head size, loss of tone and reflexes and pupillary abnormalities. Seizures may complicate the illness. The prognosis is dependent on the extent of the haemorrhage; 75% of infants develop normally after slight haemorrhage but more severe haemorrhages may cause death or severe subsequent neurological disability (cerebral palsy syndrome).

Neonatal infections

Cerebral infection may be due to a number of different organisms (Table 18.4). Meningitis in the first week of life is most commonly due to *E. coli* or Type B. streptococcal infection. Later in infancy, *N. meningitidis*, *H. influenzae* and *S. pneumoniae* are the common causes. Meningitis is commoner in the first week of life than at any subsequent time throughout life. The disease presents as irritability, nausea, and fever, but seizures and coma may supervene in a few

Table 18.4 *Neonatal cerebral infections.*

Meningitis: *E. coli*, streptococcus
Rubella
Toxoplasmosis
Cytomegalovirus
H. simplex (types 1 and 2)
HIV infection

hours or days. Diagnosis is made by lumbar puncture and by blood culture. Treatment with intravenous ampicillin 75–150 mg/kg daily, and intravenous gentamicin 4–8 mg/kg/day with intrathecal gentamycin 1 mg/day for 10–14 days is effective. Cefotaxime may also be used.

Rubella is acquired *in utero* and causes growth retardation, cataract, sensorineural deafness, acute and chronic meningoencephalitis, mental retardation and epilepsy. This disorder is preventable by immunization of women before conception. Toxoplasmosis may be acquired *in utero* by trans-placental infection from the mother. The infection causes chorioretinitis, ependymitis with intracranial calcification and hydrocephalus. There is drowsiness, raised intracranial pressure and seizures, and the prognosis for normal development is very poor. *Cytomegalovirus* infection is a congenital infection that can be detected in urine. The clinical features include skin rash, hepatosplenomegaly with jaundice, chorioretinitis, microcephaly and cerebral calcification, and there is frequently severe retardation. Milder infections are more common, with less marked consequences. *HIV infection* may also be acquired *in utero*. The outcome is uncertain but a major proportion of affected children develop AIDS and succumb to infective and neoplastic complications during the first decade of life.

Toxoplasmosis responds poorly to treatment with pyrimethamine and sulphadiazine. H. simplex infections respond to acyclovir.

Trauma

Physical injury to the peripheral or central nervous system may occur in the perinatal period, in infancy (Table 18.5) or later in life. Injury *in utero* is uncommon. Injuries in childhood are similar to those of adult life.

Table 18.5   *Trauma during the perinatal period, and the first year.*

Perinatal (birth) injuries:
  trauma to skull and scalp
  intracranial haemorrhage
    subdural and intracerebral haemorrhage
  spinal cord injury
  brachial plexus injuries
  peripheral and cranial nerve injuries
Injuries in the first year of life:
  accidental
  non-accidental (battered baby syndrome)

Perinatal injuries

Trauma to the scalp during delivery may be caused by forceps or vacuum extractor manipulations, consisting of scalp haematoma, scalp oedema (caput succedaneum), or sub-periosteal haemorrhage. These are minor problems not requiring treatment. *Linear skull fractures*, sometimes with a depressed component to the fracture, may be caused by the force of uterine contraction pushing the head against the pelvic brim, or by forceps delivery. These heal within 3 months, and are only rarely associated with subdural haematoma of fluid collections. Fractures depressed more than 0.5 cm should be surgically elevated to avoid injury to the underlying brain.

The trauma of childbirth may lead to *extradural haemorrhage*, due as in adults to rupture of the middle meningeal artery, *subdural haemorrhage* or *intracerebral haemorrhage*. Extradural haemorrhage is rare in infancy and subdural haemorrhage appears less common than formerly, perhaps because it is particularly associated with breech and forceps deliveries which are themselves less frequent now than in the past. Intracerebral haemorrhage is associated with forceps delivery in 50% of cases. The newborn child is hemiplegic, focal seizures occur and the CSF is blood-stained; the CT scan is diagnostic. The prognosis for functional recovery is poor.

Trauma to the *brain stem* or *spinal cord* is a serious event that is frequently associated with a fatal outcome. It is due to traction injuries associated with forceps or breech deliveries. Spinal cord injuries are usually cervical or thoracic. The diagnosis of cord injury is suggested by flaccid, motionless legs, or flaccid quadriplegia with diaphragmatic breathing. The bladder is distended. The prognosis for recovery is virtually hopeless.

Facial palsy is found in 6% of all cephalic presentations; it is usually unilateral. Most recover within a month of birth. Bilateral facial palsy is usually due to congenital facial muscle aplasia, perhaps due to nuclear dysgenesis in the brain stem (Möbius syndrome).

Brachial plexus palsies are due to traction during birth, occurring in 0.7/1000 live births. They occur when the head and shoulder are forcibly separated or rotated away from each other. The upper plexus (C5 and C6 roots) are most commonly involved (Erb–Duchenne palsy), resulting in weakness in shoulder and biceps muscles. Lower plexus (C8 and T1 roots) lesions (Klumpke palsy) cause weakness of forearm and intrinsic hand muscles with ipsilateral Horner's syndrome. Complete plexus palsy also occurs. Complete recovery occurs in 80% of cases in 4 months, and in 95% after 4 years, leaving a minority of cases with permanent deficit. Palsies of individual peripheral nerves are rare in the perinatal period.

Accidental trauma

Injuries of this type can result in syndromes resembling those of perinatal trauma.

Non-accidental injury

Physical assault in infancy (*battered baby syndrome*) occurs in a setting of social deprivation, parental behavioural disorder or mental illness, or rejection of the baby. It is sometimes associated with other features of inadequate care, e.g. lack of hygiene, malnutrition and concern on the part of other family members, friends or social agencies, but may consist in the presentation of the child with the consequences of trauma, allegedly due to a fall. Examination discloses evidence of recent and previous trauma, with superficial bruising, limb or rib fractures, and frequently signs of cerebral and cranial trauma. These features are indications for hospitalization for appropriate treatment of the child and for arrangements for future care. The latter necessitates an order for care, so that the child can be removed to a place of safety and out of the parental situation that led to the trauma. Such arrangements may sometimes need to be permanent.

Malformations

There are many varieties of nervous system malformation, of minor and major degree, consisting of disorders of development and migration of neural tissue during ontogeny. These are classified in Table 18.6.

Table 18.6 *Malformations of the CNS.*

Anencephaly and microcephaly
Hydrocephalus
Dysraphic states (neural tube disorders)
spina bifida
meningomyelocele
encephalocele
Cranio-facial malformations
Hydranencephaly
Porencephaly
Craniosynostosis

Anencephaly occurs in 1/1000 births. Death nearly always occurs before the first month. The disorder is due to failure of closure of the anterior neuropore early in development resulting in a major failure of development of the brain and cranial vault. Levels of α fetoprotein, a protein specific to the CSF of the developing child that leaks into the amniotic fluid when the neuraxis has not fused, may be raised in maternal venous blood when the fetus is anencephalic or has a dysraphic malformation. This test, if positive, should be followed by amniocentesis since amniotic fluid α feto-protein levels are raised in 95% of cases of anencephaly. The test should be carried out between the 14th and 16th week in mothers with a family or past history of neural tube disorders. Ultrasound examination of the foetus *in utero* is also a useful screening test. *Microcephaly*, consisting of a head circumference more than two standard deviations smaller than normal, is usually due to brain disease acquired *in utero* or perinatally rather than to congenital factors. This may consist of viral or other infections, such as congenital rubella, or toxoplasmosis, or to metabolic disorders such as fetal alcohol syndrome.

Dysraphism means failure of fusion of the neural tube. Anencephaly is one such disorder but spinal dysraphism and encephaloceles are about twice as common as anencephaly. The developmental error in these neural tube disorders often occurs at more than one level of the neuraxis as, for example, children with sacral meningomyelocele in whom an associated Arnold–Chiari malformation leads to hydrocephalus. In *meningomyelocele* there is a defect in the spinal cord and in its mesodermal covering. This may result in a complex malformation with a cystic mass of meninges, spinal cord and CSF. In the most severe cases the malformation is not covered by muscle or skin, leading to infection and death. In other cases the lesion consists of a subcutaneous swelling, the vertebral arches and muscles being defective at the level of the lesion. In *spina bifida occulta* the abnormality is occult, being discovered radiologically by failure of fusion of the neural arches. Most of these lesions occur in the lumbosacral region and many are associated with some degree of Arnold–Chiari malformation (see below). *Encephalocele* is a protrusion of brain and meninges through an anterior or posterior defect, most commonly in the midline in the occipital region. Meningoceles consists of a CSF-filled sac protruding through a skull or spinal defect, without involvement of neural tissue.

Arnold–Chiari malformation consists of elongation of the cerebellar vermis, and herniation of this tissue and of the cerebellar tonsils and medulla, downward into the foramen magnum. The fourth ventricle is displaced downwards and hydrocephalus results from obstruction of the outlets of the fourth ventricle, or from associated atresia and functional obstruction of the Sylvian aqueduct. In *Dandy–Walker malformation* the cerebellum is hypoplastic and the fourth ventricle is occluded and distended causing enlargement of the posterior fossa, and hydrocephalus.

Hydrocephalus in infancy, or at birth, is usually non-communicating in type, due to obstruction to the flow of CSF. It is most commonly due to obstruction of the aqueduct or fourth ventricle, due to congenital malformations, especially Arnold–Chiari malformation and aqueductal stenosis. Hydrocephalus presents with progressive enlargement of the head, widening of the cranial sutures, irritability and drowsiness. The head bulges frontally and temporally. In severe, untreated hydrocephalus tonic downward deviation of the eyes may occur (setting-sun sign) and delayed developmental milestones or seizures may be features. *Aqueductal stenosis* may occur without other abnormalities, perhaps associated with viral infection, and with toxoplasmosis. The diagnosis of hydrocephalus is readily made by CT brain scanning, which demonstrates the ventricular enlargement.

Hydranencephaly consists of virtual absence of the cerebral hemispheres in a cranium of normal size. The skull readily transilluminates. The disorder is thought to be due to obstruction of flow in the carotid circulation in fetal life leading to carotid territory infarction; the child has a normal brain stem and appears developmentally normal at first, but fails to make progress in the first weeks of life. *Porencephaly* consists of multiple or single cyst-like spaces in the brain, sometimes continuous with a lateral ventricle, due to traumatic, infective or vascular destructive lesions. It may be associated with signs of focal brain disease, with mental retardation or with epilepsy.

Chromosomal disorders

Developmental retardation associated with chromosomal abnormality is a relatively frequent cause of mental retardation. These disorders often present in the first year of life since the clinical features are characteristic. The commonest is Down's syndrome.

Down's syndrome occurs with abnormalities of chromosome 21, consisting of trisomy or translocation. Trisomy 21 occurs in 1 : 600 live births. Two-thirds survive to school age, and Down's syndrome accounts for 60% of all mentally subnormal children. There is developmental delay, hypotonia, shortness of stature, short square hands and stubby fingers, brachycephaly, prominent epicanthic folds, close-set eyes, smallness of the nose, thick fissured lips, and a tongue too large for the rather small mouth. Ear development is simplified. The degree of mental retardation varies from severe to moderately subnormal. Cardiac abnormalities are frequent and a transverse 'simian' palmar crease is characteristic. In adult life atlanto-axial dislocation with paraplegia may develop due to congenital anomalies at the C1 level. Dementia, resembling Alzheimer's disease both clinically and pathologically, may become a problem even as early as the 4th decade. Seizures are common.

The occurrence of an Alzheimer-like-dementia in Down's syndrome has led to the speculation that Alzheimer's disease itself may be due to an abnormality of the genome in relation to chromosome 21. Other chromosomal disorders involving autosomal translocations are uncommon. Certain X chromosome disorders, eg fragile X syndrome may also be associated with mental retardation.

Management of spinal dysraphism and hydrocephalus

Fully epithelialized meningomyeloceles do not require treatment. However, in some such cases progressive neurological deficits, particularly bladder disturbance, lumbosacral radiculopathy, spinal cord syndrome or hydrocephalus may develop. Lumbosacral syndromes may be due to associated intraspinal lipoma, dermoid tumour or ependymoma Cord syndromes rarely develop in association with tethering of the cord to the sacral malformation, with a higher malformation such as Arnold–Chiari malformation, or due to a cord malformation itself, e.g. diastematomyelia (division of the cord into two separate components around a congenital intraspinal bony spur). These complications necessitate investigation by myelography and CT scanning, and exploration by laminectomy; however, all such cases should have a CT brain scan before other investigations in order to exclude the commonly associated problem of hydrocephalus. Open, or ulcerated meningomyeloceles pose difficult practical and ethical dilemmas in management. A conservative approach is usually followed although, in some cases, primary closure of a lesion may be followed by a reasonable functional result. The mortality in patients managed without surgical closure of open lesions is about 90%.

Hydrocephalus is managed by CSF shunting. The principal objective of surgery is to drain CSF from the dilated ventricular system into the peritoneum or into the right atrium using a system of silastic tubing with a subcutaneous cranial reservoir and a valve opening at approximately 60–100 mm CSF. The major complication is bacterial colonization of the shunt tubing leading to chronic ventriculitis or septicaemia; subdural haematoma may also develop from sudden changes in brain volume associated with ventricular drainage. The ventriculo-atrial or ventriculo-peritoneal shunt requires revision during growth, and many treated children become 'shunt-dependent', so that it is not possible at a later stage to remove the shunt.

Metabolic disorders

Inborn disorders of metabolism are always present at birth, although many do not present clinically until later in life. Of those causing problems in neonates, thyroid disorders, and disturbances of carbohydrate and amino acid metabolism are the most frequent.

Hypothyroidism is a feature of 1 in 4000 live births. Early features are jaundice, poor temperature control, slow feeding, lethargy and a hoarse cry. Coarse features and mental retardation, with enlargement of the tongue, develop later. There is a low blood T_4 level, with high TSH levels. Treatment is indicated as early in life as possible in order to prevent retardation of growth, and of mental development; it consists of 25–50 μg thyroxine daily. The cause is unknown, but some cases are familial. *Hyperthyroidism* occurs in 1% of children of mothers with Graves' disease. There is goitre, hyperactivity, exophthalmos and tachycardia. There is a substantial risk of craniosynostosis, and of intellectual impairment, despite early treatment.

Disorders of carbohydrate metabolism are relatively uncommon but are important since some, e.g. galactosaemia and phenylketonuria, are reversible if treated adequately, and early enough. Many cause hypoglycaemic convulsions, e.g. hereditary fructose intolerance, galactosaemia and glucose-6-phosphatase deficiency (von Gierke's glycogenosis), and others present with lactic or metabolic acidosis causing lethargy, vomiting, irritability, seizures and coma. These disorders are characterized by hepatomegaly and sometimes splenomegaly and cardiomegaly, and by hypoglycaemia, hyperammonaemia or acidosis. The latter should lead to specific enzyme assay in carbohydrate pathways in white blood cells or other suitable tissue. In some of these disorders clinical presentation may be delayed into infancy or childhood, e.g. acid maltase deficiency (Pompe's disease), and presentation may be precipitated by extraneous events; thus, viral infection often induces symptoms in galactosaemia. Non-specific 'failure to thrive' is an important indicator of the possibility of an inborn error of metabolism.

Disorders of amino acid metabolism usually present in the newborn after the first protein feeding, characteristically with acidosis, hypoglycaemia, vomiting and convulsions. *Phenylketonuria*, a preventable cause of mental retardation and developmental delay, is now recognized shortly after birth by a screening test. The clinical manifestations are prevented by excluding phenylalanine from the diet during infancy, childhood and adolescence. The amino acid disorders are almost all associated with hyperammonaemia and with aminoaciduria, and the latter is useful in recognition of the precise metabolic disorder. Most can be treated by appropriate dietary management.

Disorders of ganglioside metabolism are rare, especially in newborns, but G_{M1} *gangliosidosis*, due to β galactosidase deficiency, and *Gaucher's disease* (sphingolipidosis) may present at birth. The former presents with facial anomalies, oedema, hepatosplenomegaly and failure to thrive, and the latter with the triad of hepatosplenomegaly, progressive neurological deterioration and hyperextension of the neck. These disorders are inexorably fatal. *Tay–Sach's disease* (G_{M2} gangliosidosis) begins in the first year of life, with slowed development, deterioration of behaviour after the age of 6 months, blindness, spasticity and seizures. Death usually occurs before the third birthday. *Batten's disease* (ceroid lipofuscinosis) like other lipid storage disorders, presents with infantile, late infantile and juvenile forms. There are seizures, myoclonic jerks, and progressive dementia with optic atrophy, but the cherry-red spots and visceromegaly found in G_{M1} and G_{M2} gangliosidosis are absent. *Niemann–Pick disease*, associated with sphingomyelin storage, is also heterogenous, with neurovisceral and visceral forms. Hepatosplenomegaly may be prominent, and intellectual deterioration develops, leading to death in early childhood. All these disorders are autosomal recessive traits, and the carrier state can be recognized in many susceptible individuals by leucocyte enzyme assay. Genetic counselling is thus relatively reliable.

In the *leucodystrophies* there is a hereditary disorder of myelin metabolism, leading to spasticity, ataxia and retardation, but without the seizures and progressive dementia characteristic of the lipid storage disorders. *Metachromatic leucodystrophy*, like many other inborn metabolic errors, may present in infantile, childhood or adult onset forms. There is a combination of upper and lower motor neuron disturbance with a prominent sensorimotor neuropathy, associated with enlargement of peripheral nerves in some cases. Diagnosis is suggested by finding sulphatides, consisting of metachromatic granules, in the urine, and confirmed by finding arylsulphatase A deficiency in cultured leucocytes. *Krabbe's disease* (galactocerebrosidosis) presents in infancy with vomiting, apathy, retardation and peripheral neuropathy. *Adrenoleucodystrophy* is an X-linked disorder, presents between the ages of 5 and 10 years with the clinical picture of Addison's disease, learning difficulties, corticospinal and extrapyramidal features and optic atrophy. It is associated with accumulation of long-chain fatty acids in the tissues and in the plasma.

The *mucopolysaccharidoses* are a group of diseases characterized by storage of acid mucopolysaccharides in various organs, due to lysosomal enzyme deficiencies. These disorders are characterized by mental retardation, hepatosplenomegaly, dysmorphic facial features, deafness, corneal clouding, enlargement of the tongue, bony deformities, dry skin and carpal tunnel syndromes. Spinal compression may develop, and hydrocephalus also occurs. There is a prospect of treatment by bone marrow transplantation.

Disorders of childhood

The neurological disorders of childhood in many respects resemble those of adults. For example infections, neoplasms and Guillain–Barré syndrome all occur in childhood. It is a period of development, however, in which seizures develop in patients with idiopathic epilepsy, and in which certain tumours may develop, e.g. cerebellar astrocytoma and haemangioblastoma. Certain metabolic disorders, for example late-onset glycogenoses or lipid storage disorders, also present at this time. Developmental disorders presenting in childhood may be due to brain lesions sustained in the perinatal or infantile periods, recognition being delayed until it is evident that attainment of intellectual or physical development is abnormal. Thus, problems in acquisition of motor or intellectual skills, such as reading and writing, may be the presenting feature of such a disorder. Some metabolic disorders, e.g. Wilson's disease and Lesch–Nyhan syndrome, present in childhood. In *Lesch–Nyhan syndrome* there is mental retardation, choreo-athetosis and self-mutilation, associated with hyperuricaemia due to a deficiency of hypoxanthine-guanine phosphoribosyl transferase (HG-PRT). Treatment with allopurinol may be helpful.

Development disorders not known to be associated with structural or metabolic disease also present in childhood; the developmental dyslexia syndrome, autism (Kanner's syndrome) and childhood psychoses are examples. The terms 'clumsy child syndrome' and 'hyperkinetic syndrome' describe children with poor motor skills and learning disabilities, and excessive distractibility respectively. These are thought to be due to subclinical brain damage, perhaps associated with hypoxic or other birth injuries. Drugs such as phenobarbitone may cause a similar syndrome in infancy and childhood.

Cerebral palsy

Cerebral palsy is a syndrome of movement and posture due to a non-progressive disorder of the immature brain. It occurs in about 3/1000 births, and is usually due to perinatal or neonatal injury, although a similar clinical syndrome may result from brain damage sustained in infancy. The underlying cause ranges from cerebral haemorrhage or infarction, to developmental defects of cerebral maturation. The cerebral palsy syndrome is particularly associated with prematurity, postmaturity, prolonged labour, forceps delivery, fetal distress and fetal apnoea.

The clinical syndrome is relatively uniform at birth, but shows marked differences during the first year, as increasing brain maturity allows expression of the disorders associated with the lesions in the brain. Thus, in the first few weeks of life, there may be flaccid weakness or asymmetrical movement of the limbs. The infant may suffer seizures or show lethargy and failure to feed adequately, leading to poor weight gain. Head control is poor and primitive reflexes, especially tonic reflexes, may be unusually persistent. Reflex stepping and standing responses are poorly or asymmetrically developed. Grasp reflexes are persistent and one or both plantar responses remain extensor.

Table 18.7 *Clinical types of cerebral palsy.*

Spastic cerebral palsy	65%
hemiplegia	
diplegia	
quadriplegia	
Dyskinetic (athetoid) cerebral palsy	20%
Mixed forms	15%

In older children the clinical manifestations can be classified into different forms (Table 18.7). Athetoid cerebral palsy, now uncommon, was particularly associated with kernicterus due to Rhesus incompatibility, and with perinatal anoxic encephalopathy. The involuntary movements and postures are not fully evident until the age of 2 or 3 years. In spastic diplegia the disorder affects both legs, relatively sparing the arms. In spastic quadriplegia, the most severe form, all four limbs are involved. In the latter type of cerebral palsy there is often severe mental retardation, and epilepsy, but in spastic hemiplegia and spastic diplegia intellectual functions are frequently normal. The spasticity and dystonia found in the limbs in these children develops during the first 2 years of life, evolving from the initial flaccidity as myelination and maturity of the nervous system develops. Speech is often abnormal, with poor co-ordination of speech and respiration leading to an explosive quality to spoken speech. This is not necessarily accompanied by a disorder of underlying language capacities, so that the dysarthric, disabled patient with cerebral palsy may be able to comprehend spoken and written language normally, and to communicate by using computer-aided techniques.

Management. Treatment of associated disorders such as strabismus is important in order to prevent disturbed vision. Education, with attention to methods of communication, is vital. Treatment of spasticity itself is disappointing, and requires physiotherapy and drug treatment. Orthopaedic procedures to maintain or restore joint mobility may be necessary if peri-articular fibrosis develops; the latter can be prevented by appropriate daily range-of-motion exercises.

Attempts at intensive physiotherapy or re-educative programmes, although attractive, are generally difficult to follow since they are so time-consuming, and there is no evidence that the ultimate outcome of such programmes justifies the time and effort they require. Nonetheless, careful attention to mental and physical well-being is very rewarding for patient and family. Epilepsy should be managed with anticonvulsant drug therapy, if indicated.

Further Reading

Chapter 1

Bannister, R. (1988) *Autonomic Failure: a Textbook of Clinical Disorders of the Autonomic Nervous System*, 2nd ed. Oxford: Oxford University Press.

Breuer, J. & Freud, S. (1956) *Studies on Hysteria*. London: Hogarth Press. (German Edition first published 1895.)

Brodal, A. (1981) *Neurological Anatomy in Relation to Clinical Medicine*, 3rd ed. Oxford: Oxford University Press.

Kandel, E. R. & Schwartz, J. H. (1986) *Principles of Neural Science*, 2nd ed. Amsterdam: Elsevier-North Holland.

Kinnier Wilson, S. A. (1940) *Neurology* 2 vols. London: Edward Arnold.

Nathan, P. (1982) *The Nervous System*. Oxford: Oxford University Press.

Patten, J. (1977) *Neurological Differential Diagnosis*. London: Springer-Verlag.

Rottenberg, D. A. & Hochberg, F. G. (1977) *Neurological Classics in Modern Translation*. London: Hafner Press.

Slater, E. (1965) Diagnosis of hysteria. *Brit. Med. J. 1*: 1395–1399.

Swash, M. (1989) Examination of the nervous system. In: *Hutchison's Clinical Methods* 19th ed. London: Baillière-Tindall.

Swash, M. & Kennard, C. ed. (1985) *Scientific Basis of Clinical Neurology*. Edinburgh: Churchill-Livingstone.

Walton, J. (1985) *Brain's Diseases of the Nervous System*, 9th ed. Oxford: Oxford University Press.

Chapter 2

Commission on classification and terminology; International League Against Epilepsy: Proposal for classification of epilepsies and epileptic syndromes (1985). *Epilepsia 26*: 268–278.

Currie, S., Heathfield, K. W. G. & Henson, R. A. *et al.* (1971) Clinical course and prognosis of temporal lobe epilepsy—a survey of 666 patients. *Brain 94*: 173–190.

Delgado-Escueta, A. V., Westerlain, C., Freiman, D. M., *et al.* (1982) The management of status epilepticus. *New Engl. J. Med. 306*: 1337–1340.

Eadie, M. J. (1976) Plasma level monitoring of anticonvulsants. *Clin. Pharmacokinetics 1*: 52–66.

Elwes, R. D. C., Johnson, A. L., Sharon, S. D. *et al.* (1984) The prognosis for seizure control in newly diagnosed epilepsy. *New Engl. J. Med. 311*: 944–947.

Hopkins, A. H. ed. (1987) *Epilepsy*. London: Chapman and Hall Medical.

Jackson, H. J. (1931) On epilepsy and epileptiform convulsions. In: *Selected Writings of Hughlings Jackson*, Vol 1, (ed. J. Taylor). London: Hodder and Stoughton.

Jennett, B. (1975) *Epilepsy after Non-missile Head Injuries*. Chicago: Year Book.

Neidermeyer, E. & Lopez da Silva, G. (1987) *Electroencephalography*. Baltimore: Urban and Schwarzenberg.

Nelson, K. B. & Ellenberg, J. H. (1978) Prognosis in children with febrile seizures. *Pediatrics 61*: 720–727.

Parkes, J. D. (1985) *Sleep and its Disorders*. Philadelphia: W. B. Saunders.

Parkes, J. D. & Marsden, C. D. (1974) Narcolepsy. *Brit. J. Hosp. Med. 22*: 325–334.

Reynolds, E. H. (1975) Chronic antiepileptic drug toxicity—a review. *Epilepsia 16*: 315–352.

Scambler, G. & Hopkins, A. (1986) Being epileptic: coming to terms with stigma. *Soc. Health Illness 8*: 26–43.

Theodore, W. H., Porter, R. J. & Penry, J. K. (1983) Complex partial seizures: clinical characteristics and differential diagnosis. *Neurology 33*: 1115–1121.

Chapter 3

Antiplatelet Trialists Collaborative Study: Secondary prevention of vascular disease by prolonged antiplatelet therapy (1988). *Brit. Med. J. 296*: 320–331.

Autret, A., Pourcelot, L. & Sandeau, D. *et al.* (1987) Stroke risk in patients with carotid stenosis. *Lancet 1*: 888–890.

Beal, M. F., Williams, R. S. & Richardson, E. P. *et al.* (1981) Cerebral embolism as a cause of transient ischaemic attacks and cerebral infarction. *Neurology 31*: 860–865.

Easton, J. D. & Sherman, D. G. (1980) Management of cerebral embolism of cardiac origin. *Stroke 2*: 433–441.

Fisher, C. M. (1982) Lacunar strokes and infarcts: a review. *Neurology 32*: 871–876.

Fisherr, C. M., Picard, E. & Polak, A. (1965) Acute hypertensive cerebellar haemorrhage: diagnosis and surgical treatment. *J. Nerv. Ment. Dis. 140*: 38–57.

Foltz, E. L. & Ward, A. A. (1956) Communicating hydrocephalus from subarachnoid bleeding. *J. Neurosurg. 13*: 546–566.

Furlan, A. J., ed. (1987) *The Heart and Stroke*. London: Springer-Verlag.

Graham, E., Holland, A. & Avery, A. *et al.* (1981) Prognosis in giant cell arteritis. *Brit. Med. J. 282*: 269–271.

Little, J. R., Tubman, D. E. & Ethier, R. (1978) Cerebellar haemorrhage in infarcts: diagnosis by computerised tomography. *J. Neurosurg. 48*: 595–599.

Marshall, J. (1982) The cause and prognosis of strokes in people under 50 years. *J. Neurol. Sci. 53*: 473–488.

McKissock, W., Richardson, A. & Taylor, J. (1961) Primary intracerebral haemorrhage; a controlled trial of surgical and conservative treatment in 180 unselected cases. *Lancet 2*: 221–226.

Ojemann, R. G. & Heros, R. C. (1983) Spontaneous brain haemorrhage. *Stroke 14*: 468–475.

Ross Russell, R. W., ed. (1983) *Vascular Disease of the Central Nervous System*, 2nd ed. Edinburgh: Churchill-Livingstone.

Sacco, R. L., Wolff, P. A. & Kannel, W. B. *et al.* (1982) Survival and recurrence following stroke; the Framingham study. *Stroke 13*: 290–295.

Spetzler, R. F. & Zabramski, J. M. (1986) Surgery of intracranial aneurysms. In: *Stroke*, ed. H. J. M. Barnett, J. P. Mohr, B. M. Stein & F. M. Yatsu, vol 2. New York: Churchill-Livingstone.

Stein, B. M. & Wolpert, S. M. (1980) Arteriovenous malformations of the brain: current concepts and treatment. *Arch. Neurol. 37*: 1–5, 69–75.

Uttley, D. (1978) Subarachnoid haemorrhage. *Brit. J. Hosp. Med. 19*: 138–154.

Wiechers, D. O., Whisnant, J. P. & Sundt, T. M. *et al.* (1987) The significance of unruptured intracranial saccular aneurysms. *J. Neurosurg. 66*: 23–29.

Winn, H. R., Richardson, A. E. & Jane, J. A. (1977) The long term prognosis in untreated cerebral aneurysms. I. The incidence of late haemorrhage in cerebral aneurysm: a 10 year evolution of 364 patients. *Ann. Neurol. 1*: p. 358.

Wolf, P. A., Dawber, T. R. & Thomas, H. E. *et al.* (1978) Epidemiologic assessment of chronic atrial fibrillation and risk of stroke: the Framingham study. *Neurology 28*: 973–977.

Chapter 4

Cawthorne, T. E. & Hinchcliffe, R. (1961) Positional nystagmus of the central type as evidence of subtentorial metastases. *Brain 84*: 415–426.

Dix, M. R. & Hood, J. D. (1984) *Vertigo*. Chichester: John Wiley.

Drachman, D. A. & Hart, C. W. (1972) An approach to the dizzy patient. *Neurology 22*: 323–337.

Hallpike, C. S. (1950) Ménières disease. *Proc. Roy. Soc. Med. 43*: 288.

Harrison, M. S. (1962) Vestibular neuronitis. *Brain 85*: 613–620.

Harrison, M. S. & Ozahinoglu, C. (1972) Positional vertigo: aetiology and clinical significance. *Brain 95*: 369–372.

Rudge, P. (1982) *Clinical Neuro-otology*. Edinburgh: Churchill-Livingstone.

Chapter 5

Blau, J. N. (1988) *Headache*. London: Chapman and Hall.

Drummond, P. D. & Lance, J. W. (1984) Clinical diagnosis and computer analysis of headache symptoms. *J. Neurol. Neurosurg. Psychiatry 47*: 128–133.

Ekbom, K. (1970) A clinical comparison of cluster headache and migraine. *Acta Neurol. Scand. 46*: Suppl 41, 1–48.

Feinmann, C., Harris, M. & Cawley, R. (1984) Psychogenic facial pain: presentation and treatment. *Brit. Med. J. 288*: 436–438.

Graham, E., Holland, A. & Avery, A. *et al.* (1981) Prognosis in giant cell arteritis. *Br. Med. J. 282*: 269–271.

Hockaday, J. M. (1982) Headache in children. *Brit. J. Hosp. Med. 27*: 383–341.

Johnston, I. & Paterson, A. (1974) Benign intracranial hypertension. *Brain 97*: 289–300 and 301–312.

Kelly, R. (1981) The post-traumatic syndrome. *J. Roy. Soc. Med. 74*: 242–245.

Merskey, H. & Woodforde, J. M. (1972) Psychiatric sequelae of minor head injury. *Brain 95*: 521–528.

Pearce, J. M. S. (1980) Chronic migrainous neuralgia—a variant of cluster headache. *Brain 103*: 149–159.

Peatfield, R. (1986) *Headache*. Springer-Verlag, London.

Whitty, C. W. M. (1953) Familial hemiplegic migraine. *J. Neurol. Neurosurg. Psychiatry 16*: 172–177.

Chapter 6
Booss, J. & Esiri, M. M. (1986) *Viral Encephalitis.* Oxford: Blackwell Scientific.
Brown, P., Cathala, F. & Castaigne, P. *et al* (1986) Creutzfeldt–Jakob disease: clinical analysis of a consecutive series of 230 neuropathologically-verified cases. *Ann. Neurol. 20*: 597–602.
Carne, C. A. (1987) ABC of AIDS: neurological manifestations. *Br. Med. J. 294:* 525–526.
Chun, C. H., Johnson, J. D., Hofstetter, M. & Raff, M. J. (1986) Brain abscess: a study of 45 consecutive cases. *Medicine 65*: 415–431.
Kennard, C. & Swash, M. (1981) Acute viral encephalitis: its diagnosis and outcome. *Brain 104*: 129–148.
Kennedy, P. G. E. & Johnson, R. T. (1987) *Infections of the Nervous System.* London: Butterworths.
Kocen, R. S. & Parsons, M. (1970) Neurological complications of tuberculosis; some unusual manifestations. *Quart. J. Med. 39*: 17–30.
Retroviruses in the nervous system (1988) *Ann. Neurol. (Suppl.) 23*: 1–217.
Parke, A. (1987) From New to Old England: the progress of Lyme disease. *Br. Med. J. 294*: 525–526.
Salaki, J. S., Louria, D. B. & Chinel, H. (1984) Fungal and yeast infections of the central nervous system. *Medicine 63*: 103–132.
Sande, M. A., Smith, A. L. & Root, R. K., ed. (1985) *Bacterial Meningitis.* New York: Churchill-Livingstone.
Storm-Mathiesen, A. (1978) Neurosyphilis. In: *Handbook of Clinical Neurology,* ed. P. J. Vinken & G. W. Bruyn, vol 33. New York: Elsevier.
Stutman, H. R. & Marks, M. I. (1987) Therapy for bacterial meningitis: which drugs and for how long? *J. Pediat. 110*: 812–814.
Swartz, M. N. & Dodge, P. R. (1965) Bacterial meningitis: a review of selected aspects. *New Engl. J. Med. 272*: 725–779, 842–898.
Traub, M., Colchester, A. C. F. & Kingsley, D. P. C. *et al.* (1984) Tuberculosis of the central nervous system. *Quart. J. Med. 209*: 81–100.
What Science Knows About AIDS. *Scientific American* (1988) pp. 24–112.
Whitley, R. J., Alvord, C. A. & Hirsch, M. S. *et al.* (1986) Vidarabine versus acyclovir therapy in Herpes simplex encephalitis. *New Engl. J. Med. 314*: 144–149.

Chapter 7
Bates, D. (1985) Predicting recovery from medical coma. *Br. J. Hosp. Med. 33*: 276–280.
Cairns, H. (1956) Disturbances of consciousness with lesions of the brain stem and diencephalon. *Brain 75*: 109.
Jennett, B. & Bond, M. (1975) Assessment of outcome after severe brain damage: a practical scale. *Lancet 1*: 480–484.
Jennett, B., Teasdale, G. & Braakman, R. *et al.* (1979) Prognosis in a series of patients with severe head injury. *Neurosurgery 4*: 283–300.
Karp, J. S. & Hurtig, H. I. (1974) 'Locked-in' state with bilateral mid-brain infarcts. *Arch. Neurol. 30*: 176–178.

Plum, F. & Posner, J. B. (1980) *The Diagnosis of Stupor and Coma*, 3rd ed. Philadelphia: F. A. Davis.

Royal Colleges and Faculties (1976) Diagnosis of brain death. *Lancet 2*: 1069–1070.

Teasdale, G. M. & Jennett, W. B. (1974) Assessment of coma and impaired consciousness. *Lancet 2*: 81–84.

Chapter 8

Cameron, M. M. (1978) Chronic subdural haematoma: a review of 114 cases. *J. Neurol. Neurosurg. Psychiatry 41*: 834–839.

Cartlidge, N. E. F. & Shaw, D. A. (1981) *Head Injury*. London: W. B. Saunders.

Corsellis, J. A. N., Bruton, C. J. & Freeman-Browne, D. (1973) The aftermath of boxing. *Psychol. Med. 3*: 270–303.

Dikmen, S., McLean, A. & Tempkin, N. (1986) Neuropsychological and psychosocial consequences of minor head injury. *J. Neurol. Neurosurg. Psychiatry 49*: 1227–1232.

Field, J. H. (1976) *Epidemiology of Head Injuries in England and Wales*. London: HMSO.

Graham, D. I. & Adams, J. H. (1971) Ischaemic brain damage in fatal head injuries. *Lancet 1*: 265–266

Jamieson, K. G., Yelland, J. D. N. (1968) Extradural haematomas; report of 167 cases. *J. Neurosurg. 29*: 13–23.

Jennett, B. (1975) *Epilepsy after Non-missile Head Injury*, 2nd ed. London: W. Heinemann.

Jennett, B. & McMillen, R. (1981) Epidemiology of head injury. *Br. Med. J. 282*: 101–104.

Jennett, B. & Teasdale, G. (1977) Aspects of coma after severe head injury. *Lancet 1*: 878–887.

Miller, J. D., ed. (1987) *Northfield's Surgery of the Central Nervous System* Oxford: Blackwell Scientific.

Roberts, A. H. (1969) *Brain Damage in Boxers*. London: Pitman Medical.

Rose, J., Valtonen, S. & Jennett, B. (1977) Avoidable factors contributing to death after head injury. *Br. Med. J. 2*: 615–618.

Russell, W. R. & Smith, A. (1961) Post-traumatic amnesia in closed head injury. *Arch. Neurol. 5*: 4–17.

Strich, S. J. (1956) Diffuse degeneration of the cerebral white matter in severe dementia following head injury. *J. Neurol. Neurosurg. Psychiatry 19*: 163–185.

Teasdale, G., Galbraith, S. & Murray, L. *et al.* (1982) Management of traumatic haematoma. *Br. Med. J. 205*: 1695–1697.

Chapter 9

Kurtzke, J. F. (1965) Further notes on disability evaluation in multiple sclerosis with scale modifications. *Neurology 15*: 654–661.

Laureno, R. (1983) Central pontine myelinolysis following rapid correction of hyponatraemia. *Ann. Neurol. 13*: 232–242.

McDonald, W. I. (1974) Pathophysiology in multiple sclerosis. *Brain 97*: 179–196.

McDonald, W. I. & Silberberg, D. H. (1986) *Multiple Sclerosis*. London: Butterworths.

Matthews, W. B., Acheson, E. D. & Batchelor, J. R. *et al.*, ed. (1985) *McAlpine's Multiple Sclerosis.* Edinburgh: Churchill-Livingstone.

Mehta, P. D., Miller, J. A. & Tourtelotte, W. W. (1982) Oligoclonal IgG bands in plaques from multiple sclerosis brains. *Neurology* 32: 372–376.

Miller, D. H., Rudge, P., Johnson, G. *et al.* (1988) Serial gadolinium-enhanced magnetic resonance imaging in multiple sclerosis. *Brain* 111: 927–940.

Milligan, N. M., Newcombe, R. & Compston, D. A. S. (1987) A double-blind controlled trial of high-dose methylprednisolone in patients with multiple sclerosis. I. Clinical effects. *J. Neurol. Neurosurg. Psychiatry* 50: 511–516.

Moser, H. W., Naidu, S. J., Kumar, A. J. *et al.* (1987) The adrenoleuco-dystrophies. *CRC Crit. Rev. Clin. Neurobiol.* 3: 29–88.

Parkin, P. J., Hierons, R. & McDonald, W. I. (1984) Bilateral optic neuritis: a long-term follow up. *Brain* 107: 951–964.

Paty, D. W., Oger, J. J. & Kastrukoff, C. F. *et al.* (1988) MRI in the diagnosis of MS. *Neurology* 38: 180–184.

Poser, S., Raun, N. E. & Poser, W. (1982) Age of onset, initial symptomatology and course of multiple sclerosis. *Acta Neurol. Scand.* 66: 355–362.

Swingler, R. J. & Compston, D. (1986) The distribution of multiple sclerosis in the United Kingdom. *J. Neurol. Neurosurg. Psychiatry* 49: 1115–1124.

Chapter 10

Folstein, S. E., Leigh, R. J. & Parhad, I. M. *et al.* (1986) The diagnosis of Huntington's disease. *Neurology* 36: 1279–1283.

Hachinski, V. C., Lassen, C. A. & Marshall, J. (1984) Multi-infarct dementia: a cause of mental deterioration in the elderly. *Lancet* 2: 207–209.

Hakim, S. & Adams, R. D. (1965) The special clinical problem of symptomatic hydrocephalus with normal cerebrospinal fluid pressure. *J. Neurol. Sci.* 2: 307.

Hayden, M. R. (1981) *Huntington's Chorea.* Berlin: Springer-Verlag.

Katzman, R., Terry, R. D. & Bick, K. L. (1978) *Alzheimer's Disease, Senile Dementia and Related Disorders.* New York: Raven Press.

Kowall, N. W., Ferranti, R. J. & Martin, J. B. (1987) Patterns of cell loss in Huntington's disease. *Trends Neurosci.* 10: 24–29.

Lees, A. J. & Smith, E. (1983) Cognitive deficits in the early stages of Parkinson's disease. *Brain* 106: 257–270.

Lishman, W. A., Jacobson, R. R. & Acker, C. C. (1987) Brain damage in alcoholism; current concepts. *Acta. Med. Scand.* (Suppl 717) 5–17.

Marsden, C. D. & Harrison, M. J. G. (1972) Outcome of investigation of patients with presenile dementia. *Br. J. Med. J.* 1: 249–252.

Mayeux, R., Stern, Y. & Spanton, S. (1985) Heterogeneity in dementia of the Alzheimer type: evidence of subgroups. *Neurology* 35: 453–461.

Pitt, B., ed. (1987) *Dementia.* Edinburgh: Churchill-Livingstone.

Rinne, J. O., Poljarvi, L. & Rinne, U. K. (1987) Neuronal size and density in the nucleus basalis of Meynert in Alzheimer's disease. *J. Neurol. Sci.* 79: 67–76.

Selzer, B. & Sherwin, I. (1983) A comparison of clinical features in early and late onset primary degenerative dementia: one entity or two? *Arch. Neurol.* 40: 143–146.

Tomlinson, B. E., Blessed, G. & Roth, M. (1970) Observations on the brains of demented old people. *J. Neurol. Sci.* 11: 205–242.

Victor, M., Adams, R. D. & Collins, G. H. (1971) *The Wernicke–Korsakoff Syndrome.* Philadelphia: F. A. Davis.
Wade, J. P. H., Mirsen, T. R. & Hachinski, V. C. *et al.* (1987) The clinical diagnosis of Alzheimer's disease. *Arch Neurol* 44: 24–29.
Williams, F. J. B. & Walshe, J. M. (1981) Wilson's disease: an analysis of the CT appearances in 60 patients, and the changes in response to treatment with chelating agents. *Brain* 104: 735–752.

Chapter 11
Bannister, R. (1979) Chronic autonomic failure with postural hypotension. *Lancet* 2: 405–406.
Bannister, R. (1988) *Autonomic Failure.* Oxford: Oxford University Press.
Burke, R. E., Fahn, S., Jankovic, J. *et al.* (1982) Tardive dystonia: late onset and persistent dystonia caused by antipsychotic drugs. *Neurology* 32: 1335–1341.
Cooper, I. S. (1976) Twenty year follow-up study of the neurosurgical treatment of dystonia muscularum deformans. *Advances in Neurology,* vol. 14, New York: Raven Press. pp. 423–452.
Diamond, S. G., Markham, C. H. & Hoehn, M. M. *et al.* (1987) Multi-center study of Parkinson mortality with early vs late dopa treatment. *Ann. Neurol.* 22: 8–12.
Findley, L. & Koller, W. C. (1987) Essential tremor: a review. *Neurology* 37: 1194–1197.
Hakim, A. M. & Mathieson, G. (1979) Dementia in Parkinson's disease: a neuropathologic study. *Neurology* 29: 1209–1214.
Hallett, M. (1987) The pathophysiology of myoclonus. *Trends Neurosci.* 10: 69–73.
Halliday, A. M. (1967) The electrophysiological study of myoclonus in man. *Brain* 90: 241–284.
Langston, J. W., Irwin, I. & Ricaurte, G. A. (1987) Neurotoxins, parkinsonism and Parkinson's disease. *Pharmacol. Ther.* 32: 19–50.
Lees, A. J. (1985) *Tics and Related Disorders.* Edinburgh: Churchill-Livingstone.
Marsden, C. D. & Fahn, S. (1986) *Movement Disorders 2.* London: Butterworths.
Marsden, C. D. & Parkes, J. D. (1976) On-off effects in patients with Parkinson's disease on chronic levodopa therapy. *Lancet* 1: 292–295.
Parkinson, J. (1817) *An Essay on the Shaking Palsy.* London.
Sacks, O. (1973) *Awakenings.* London: Duckworth.
Sheehy, M. P. & Marsden, C. D. (1982) Writer's cramp: a focal dystonia. *Brain* 105: 461–480.
Wilkins, R. B., Byrd, W. A. & Hofmann, J. (1987) Effectiveness of botulinum toxin therapy for essential blepharospasm. *Ophthalmology* 94: 971–975.

Chapter 12
Appenzeller, O. (1982) *The Autonomic Nervous System,* 3rd ed. Amsterdam: Elsevier.
Harding, A. E. (1981) Friedreich's ataxia: a clinical and genetic study of 90 families with an analysis of early diagnostic criteria and intra-familial clustering of clinical features. *Brain* 104: 589–620.

Harding, A. E. (1983) Classification of the hereditary ataxias and paraplegias. *Lancet 1*: 1151–1155.

Harding, A. E. (1984) *The Hereditary Ataxias and Related Disorders.* Edinburgh: Churchill-Livingstone.

Johnson, R. H., Lee, C. J. & Oppenheimer, D. R. *et al.* (1966) Autonomic failure due to intermediolateral column degeneration. *Quart. J. Med. 35*: 276–292.

Ludolph, A. C., Hugon, J. & Dwivedi, M. P. *et al.* (1987) Studies on the aetiology and pathogenesis of motor neuron disease. 1. Lathyrism: clinical findings in established cases. *Brain 110*: 149–166.

Mulder, D. W. (1982) Clinical limits of amyotrophic lateral sclerosis. In: *Human Motor Neuron Diseases*, ed. L. P. Rowland. New York: Raven Press.

Pearn, J. (1980) Classification of spinal muscular atrophies. *Lancet 1*: 919–921.

Spokes, E. G., Bannister, R. & Oppenheimer, D. R. (1979) Multiple system atrophy with autonomic failure. *J. Neurol. Sci. 43*: 59–82.

Swash, M. & Ingram, D. A. (1988) Preclinical and subclinical events in motor neuron disease. *J. Neurol. Neurosurg. Psychiatry 51*: 165–168.

Swash, M. & Schwartz, M. S. (1988) *Neuromuscular Diseases—a Practical Approach to Diagnosis and Management*, 2nd ed. London: Springer-Verlag.

Chapter 13

Asbury, A. K. & Gilliatt, R. W., ed. (1984) *Peripheral Nerve Disorders.* London: Butterworths.

Dyck, P. J., Thomas, P. K. & Lambert, E. H. *et al.*, ed. (1984) *Peripheral Neuropathy*, 2nd ed. Philadelphia: W. B. Saunders.

Fisher, C. M. (1956) An unusual variant of acute idiopathic polyneuritis (syndrome of ophthalmoplegia, ataxia and areflexia). *New Engl. J. Med. 233*: 57–65.

Greene, D. A. & Browne, M. J. (1987) Diabetic polyneuropathy. *Semin Neurol 7*: 18–19.

Guillain–Barré Syndrome Study Group (1985) Plasmapheresis and acute Guillain–Barré syndrome. *Neurology 35*: 1096–1104.

Hughes, R. A. C. & Winer, J. B. (1984) Guillain–Barré syndrome. In: *Recent Advances in Clinical Neurology*, vol 4, ed. W. B. Matthews & G. H. Glaser. Edinburgh: Churchill-Livingstone.

Kori, S. H., Foley, K. M. & Posner, J. B. (1981) Brachial plexus lesions in patients with cancer. *Neurology 31*: 45–50.

Layzer, R. B. (1985) *Neuromuscular manifestations of systemic disease.* Philadelphia: F. A. Davis.

Low, P. A. (1987) Recent advances in the pathogenesis of diabetic neuropathy. *Muscle Nerve 10*: 121–128.

Nakano, K. K. (1978) The entrapment neuropathies. *Muscle Nerve 1*: 264–279.

Parry, G. J. G. (1985) Mononeuropathy multiplex. *Muscle Nerve 8*: 493–498.

Schaumberg, H. H. & Spencer, P. S. (1987) Recognising neurotoxic disease. *Neurology 37*: 276–278.

Swash, M. & Schwartz, M. S. (1988) *Neuromuscular Diseases: a Practical Approach to Diagnosis and Management*, 2nd ed. London: Springer-Verlag.

Chapter 14

Dalakas, M. C., ed. (1988) *Polymyositis and Dermatomyositis.* Boston: Butterworths.

Dubowitz, V. (1980) *The Floppy Infant*. London: W. Heinemann.

Harper, P. S. (1979) *Myotonic Dystrophy*. Philadelphia: W. B. Saunders.

Hoffman, E. P., Brown, R. H. & Kunkel, L. M. (1987) Dystrophin: the protein product of the Duchenne muscular dystrophy locus. *Cell 51*: 919–928.

Morgan-Hughes, J. A. (1986) Mitochondrial diseases. *Trends Neurosci 9*: 15–19.

Newsom-Davis, J. (1987) Myasthenia. In: *Recent Advances in Clinical Neurology* vol 4, ed. W. B. Matthews & G. H. Glaser. Edinburgh: Churchill-Livingstone.

O'Neill, J. H., Murray, N. M. F. & Newsom-Davis, J. (1988) The Lambert–Eaton myasthenic syndrome: a review of 50 cases. *Brain 111*: 577–596.

Rowland, L. P. (1988) Clinical concepts of Duchenne muscular dystrophy: the impact of molecular genetics. *Brain 111*: 479–496.

Swash, M. & Schwartz, M. S. (1984) *Muscle Biopsy Pathology* London: Chapman and Hall.

Swash, M. & Schwartz, M. S. (1988) *Neuromuscular Diseases: a Practical Approach to Diagnosis and Management*, 2nd ed. London: Springer-Verlag.

Walton, J. N. (1988) *Disorders of Voluntary Muscle*, 5th ed. Edinburgh: Churchill-Livingstone.

Chapter 15

Alter, M. (1975) Statistical aspects of spinal cord tumours. In: *Handbook of Clinical Neurology*, vol 19, ed. P. J. Vinken & G. Bruyn. Amsterdam: Elsevier N. Holland.

Barnett, H. J. M., Foster, J. B. & Hudgson, P. (1973) *Syringomyelia*. London: W. B. Saunders.

Bedbrook, G. M. (1987) The development and care of spinal cord paralysis (1918–1986) *Paraplegia 25*: 172–198.

Blau, J. N. & Logue, V. (1961) Intermittent claudication of the cauda equina. *Lancet 1*: 1081–1086.

Hall, S., Bartleson, J. D., Onofrio, B. M. et al. (1985) Lumbar spinal stenosis: clinical features, diagnostic procedures and results of surgical treatment in 68 patients. *Ann Intern Med 103*: 271–275.

Henson, R. A. & Parsons, M. (1967) Ischaemic lesions of the spinal cord: an illustrated review. *Quart. J. Med. 36*: 205–222.

Logue, V. & Edwards, M. R. (1981) Syringomyelia and its surgical treatment: an analysis of 75 patients. *J Neurol Neurosurg Psychiatry 44*: 273–284.

Munro, P. (1984) What has surgery to offer in cervical spondylosis? In: *Dilemmas in the Management of the Neurological Patient*, ed. C. Warlow & J. Garfield. Edinburgh: Churchill-Livingstone.

Nurick, S. (1972) The pathogenesis of the cervical cord disorder associated with cervical spondylosis. *Brain 95*: 87–100.

Palmer, J. J. (1972) Radiation myelopathy. *Brain 95*: 109–122.

Shutz, H. & Watson, C. P. N. (1987) Microsurgical discectomy: a prospective study of 200 patients. *Can. J. Neurol. Sci. 14*: 81–83.

Stark, R. J., Henson, R. A. & Evans, S. J. W. (1982) Spinal metastases: a retrospective study from a general hospital. *Brain 105*: 189–213.

Williams, B. (1969) Hypothesis: the distending force in the production of 'communicating syringomyelia'. *Lancet 2*: 189–193.

Chapter 16

Barber, S. G. & Garvan, N. (1980) Is benign intracranial hypertension really benign? *J. Neurol. Neurosurg. Psychiatry* 43: 136–138.

Cushing, H. & Eisenhardt, L. (1938) *Meningiomas, their classification, regional behaviour, life history and surgical end results.* Springfield: C. C. Thomas.

Fryer, A. E., Chalmers, A. & Connor, J. M. *et al.* (1987) Evidence that the gene for tuberous sclerosis is on chromosome 9. *Lancet* 1: 659–661.

Henson, R. A. & Urich, H. (1982) *Cancer and the Nervous System.* Oxford: Blackwell Scientific.

House, W. F. & Hitselberger, W. E. (1974) Acoustic tumours. In: *Handbook of Clinical Neurology,* vol 17, ed. P. J. Vinken & G. W. Bruyn. Amsterdam: Elsevier N. Holland.

Kostereljanetz, M. (1987) Intracranial pressure: CSF dynamics and pressure–volume relations. *Acta Neurol. Scand.* 75, Suppl 111: 1–23.

Leibel, S. A. & Sheline, G. E. (1987) Radiation therapy for neoplasms of the brain. *J. Neurosurg.* 66: 1–22.

Martuza, R. L. & Eldridge, R. (1988) Neurofibromatosis 2 (bilateral acoustic neurofibromatosis). *New Engl. J. Med.* 318: 684–688.

Post, K. D. & Muraszko, K. (1986) Management of pituitary tumours. *Neurol. Clin. N. Amer.* 4: 801–832.

Russell, D. S. & Rubinstein, L. (1977) *Pathology of Tumours of the Nervous System,* 4th ed. London: Edward Arnold.

Salcman, M. (1980) Survival in glioblastoma: historical perspective. *Neurosurgery* 7: 435–439.

Todd, N. V., McDonagh, T. & Miller, J. D. (1987) What follows diagnosis by computed tomography of solitary brain tumour? Audit of one year's experience. *Lancet* 1: 611–612.

Wilkinson, I. M. S., Anderson, J. R. & Holmes, A. E. (1987) Oligodendroglioma: an analysis of 42 cases. *J. Neurol. Neurosurg. Psychiatry* 50: 304–312.

Chapter 17

Carlen, P. L., Wall, P. D. & Nadvorna, M. D. *et al.* (1987) Phantom limbs and related phenomena in recent traumatic amputations. *Neurology* 28: 211–217.

Culp, W. J. & Ochoa, J., ed. (1982) *Abnormal Nerves and Muscles as Impulse Generators.* Oxford: Oxford University Press.

Jannetta, P. J. (1967) Structural mechanisms of trigeminal neuralgia: arterial compression of the trigeminal nerve at the pons in patients with trigeminal neuralgia. *J. Neurosurg.* 26: 159–162.

Lehmann, T. R., Russell, D. W. & Spratt, K. F. *et al.* (1986) Efficacy of electro-acupuncture and TENS in the rehabilitation of chronic low back pain patients. *Pain* 26: 277–290.

Melzack, R. & Wall, P. D. (1965) Pain mechanisms: a new theory. *Science* 150: 971–979.

Portenoy, R. K., Duma, C. & Foley, K. M. (1986) Acute herpetic and post-herpetic neuralgia: clinical review and current management. *Ann. Neurol.* 20: 651–664.

Schott, B., Laurent, B. & Mauguire, F. (1986) Thalamic pain: a critical review of 43 cases. *Rev. Neurol. 142*: 308–315.

Wall, P. D. (1978) The gate control theory of pain mechanisms: a re-examination and re-statement. *Brain 101*: 1–18.

Wall, P. D. & Melzack, R. (1984) *Textbook of Pain*. Edinburgh: Churchill-Livingstone.

Wester, K. (1987) Dorsal column stimulation in pain treatment. *Acta Neurol Scand 75*: 151–155.

Chapter 18

Bell, W. O., Charney, E. B. & Bruce, D. A. *et al.* (1987) Symptomatic Arnold–Chiari malformation: review of experience of 22 cases. *J. Neurosurg. 66*: 812–816.

Brett, E. M., ed. (1983) *Paediatric Neurology*. Edinburgh: Churchill-Livingstone.

Brocklehurst, G. (1976) Spina bifida for the clinician. *Clinics in Developmental Medicine, No. 57*. Spastics International Med. Pub. London: W. Heinemann.

Chudley, A. E. & Haggerman, R. J. (1987) Fragile X syndrome. *J. Pediat. 110*: 821–831.

Fenichel, G. M. (1985) *Neonatal Neurology*. Edinburgh: Churchill-Livingstone.

Menkes, J. H. (1974) *Textbook of Child Neurology*. Philadelphia: Lea and Febiger.

Patterson, D. (1987) The causes of Down's syndrome. *Sci. Amer. 257*: 52–61.

Stone, D. H. (1987) The declining prevalence of anencephaly and spina bifida; its nature, causes and implications. *Dev. Med. Child Neurol. 29*: 541–555.

Warkany, J. (1975) *Congenital Malformations*. Chicago: Year Book.

Some addresses for patients, to obtain information and advice

Alzheimer's Disease
Alzheimer's Disease Society,
3rd Floor, Bank Buildings,
Fulham Broadway, London SW6 1EP
Tel: (01) 381 3177

Dystonia
The Dystonia Society,
Unit 32,
Omnibus Workspace,
29–41 North Road,
London N7 9DP
Tel: (01) 700 4594

Epilepsy
British Epilepsy Association,
Crowthorne House, New Wokingham Road,
Wokingham, Berks RG11 3AY
Tel: (0344) 773122

Friedreich's Ataxia
Friedreich's Ataxia Group,
Burleigh Lodge, Knowle Lane,
Cranleigh, Surrey GU6 8RD
Tel: (0483) 272741

Huntington's Chorea
Association to Combat Huntington's Chorea,
34a Station Road, Hinckley, Leics LE10 1AP
Tel: (0455) 615558

Migraine
British Migraine Association,
178a High Road, Byfleet, Weybridge,
Surrey KT14 7ED
Tel: (09323) 52468

Motor Neurone Disease
Motor Neurone Disease Association,
38 Hazelwood Road, Northampton NN1 1LN
Tel: Hazelwood (0604) 22269/22339

Multiple Sclerosis
The Multiple Sclerosis Society,
25 Effie Road, London SW6 1EE
Tel: (01) 736 6267/6278

Muscular Dystrophy
Muscular Dystrophy Group,
Nattrass House, 35 Macaulay Road, London SW4 0QP
Tel: (01) 720 8055

Myasthenia Gravis
The British Association of Myasthenics,
BAM Central Office,
Keynes House, 77 Nottingham Old Road,
Derby DE1 3QS
Tel: (0332) 290 219

Myalgic Encephalomyelitis
Myalgic Encephalomyelitis Association (post-viral syndrome)
PO Box 8,
Stanford-le-Hope,
Essex SS17 8EX

Neurofibromatosis
The Neurofibromatosis Association,
LINK, 1 The Alders, Hanworth, Middlesex TW13 6NU

Parkinson's Disease
Parkinson's Disease Society,
36 Portland Place, London W1N 3DG
Tel: (01) 323 1174

Spasticity (Cerebral Palsy)
The Spastics Society,
12 Park Crescent, London W1N 4EQ
Tel: (01) 636 5020

Spina Bifida and Hydrocephalus
Association for Spina Bifida and Hydrocephalus,
22 Upper Woburn Place, London WC1H 0EP
Tel: (01) 388 1382

Spinal Injuries
Spinal Injuries Association,
Yeoman House, 76 St James's Lane,
London N10 3DF
Tel: (01) 444 2121

Stroke
The Chest, Heart and Stroke Association,
Tavistock House North, Tavistock Square,
London WC1H 9JE
Tel: (01) 387 3012

Index